Myofascial Release
Healing Ancient Wounds

THE RENEGADE'S WISDOM

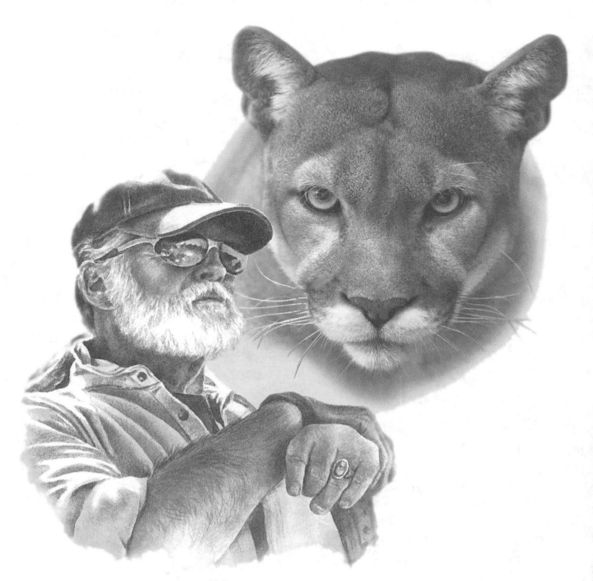

Myofascial Release
Healing Ancient Wounds

THE RENEGADE'S WISDOM

JOHN F. BARNES, PT

REHABILITATION SERVICES, INC., T/A
MFR TREATMENT CENTERS & SEMINARS
MALVERN, PENNSYLVANIA

This edition of *Myofascial Release Healing Ancient Wounds: The Renegade's Wisdom* was printed by Jostens 451 International Blvd, Clarksville, TN 37040. The book was designed by Angela Saxon of Saxon Design, Traverse City, Michigan. It is set in Berling.

©2023 by John F. Barnes, PT
Illustrations by Elaine Verstraete

10 9

Published by Rehabilitation Services, Inc., T/A
MFR Treatment Centers & Seminars
42 Lloyd Avenue, Malvern, PA 19355

Printed in the United States of America

ISBN 978-0-9981009-0-6

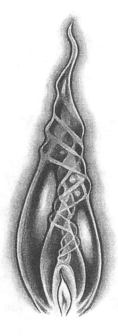

"And the day came when the risk it took to remain tight in a bud was more painful than the risk it took to blossom."

—Anaïs Nin

contents

what is a master?

During my initial education and first few years as a Physical Therapist, I learned how things ought to be by studying books. After beginning to learn the Myofascial Release principles from John F. Barnes, PT and applying them at work, I began to know how things really are by studying mankind, one patient at a time.

So it was during those first seminars that John began to challenge how I viewed things and my purpose. John was patient, waiting for me to walk away from the order and habits that had been limiting me as a therapist/person as I dove into the chaos of personal discovery. I realized I had taken up John's invitation to join him along this path toward Mastery. He has never sugarcoated what would be expected of me or what the outcome may be. He has quietly shown me by example, that every step requires active conscious participation. This journey is less about the steps taken or the event encountered, but is more about activating a perpetual condition of wonder in the face of something that continues to grow one step richer and subtler than my last awareness.

The lessons and gifts that John has generously shared with me are too numerous to list. But the culmination of their efforts has made me not just simply good, but good for something. For this I will always be grateful to my friend, teacher and fellow traveler John F. Barnes, PT the one who has devoted himself to the cause of sharing Myofascial Release with all his focus and strength, with those who want to enjoy the journey. He is a true master.

Rob Maggio, PT, MT, NCTMB
Director, Therapy on the Rocks
Sedona, AZ

While many bodywork modalities may temporarily ease pain, in my experience only the John F. Barnes Myofascial Release Approach® actually allows a physical change in the body that results in permanent pain reduction. As a massage therapist treating people in chronic pain, myofascial release gives me the tools to fundamentally improve my clients' daily lives.

By relaying his own struggle with pain in this book, John shares how he awakened to the real difference that sets myofascial release apart: the link between the brain, body, and spirit that lives in the fascia. Through skillful engagement with the fascia, John teaches how to access the original traumas that became the pain and dysfunction we experience. By healing these "ancient wounds," true wellness is really possible.

It's not hocus-pocus. There is sound science behind what John found in his intuition decades ago. The recent explosion of research on the role of fascia in all bodily systems continues to prove him right: myofascial release is authentic healing.

Treatment of the fascia will continue take a more and more primary place in healthcare. And if healthcare providers want to know the most effective and complete system for healing the true source of physical and emotional pain, they need look no further than this book.

Personally and professionally, my life has been transformed by myofascial release. John has taught me more than a set of skills. Through his example of perseverance and his decades of compassionate action, he has shown me what it means to truly live. Thank you, John.

Jamie Liptan, LMT
Myofascial Release Therapist
Co-founder, The Frida Center for Fibromyalgia
Portland, Oregon

It is not an exaggeration to say that John Barnes saved my medical career. I developed fibromyalgia as a second year medical student. I could find no relief from constant neck and back pain and fatigue. My doctors had nothing to offer me and I was preparing to drop out of school. Then a massage therapist friend recommended the John F. Barnes Myofascial Release Approach,® and after several sessions I could feel things shifting. My pain lessened after each treatment. I felt the release of old traumas and emotions that were "stuck" in my fascia, and with each I felt healthier and happier. I was able to get back to finish my medical training, keeping up with MFR tune-ups over the years.

About six months after my first MFR session, my therapist took an "after" picture of my posture. Compare to my "before" picture, my posture was now in much better alignment, with my head on top of my neck, rather than in front of it. MFR had actually changed my body! But the biggest difference was my smile and light energy, different from my frowning and miserable "before" shot.

I knew I had found something that could help millions of other people suffering from fibromyalgia. My experience with John Barnes MFR completely revolutionized how I look at the human body and pain. Why had I not learned about the role of the fascia in medical school? Unfortunately medicine is slow to change, but the past decade has seen more research into the fascia and myofascial release therapy. John's message over the last 40 years is slowly seeping in. My career mission is to ensure that every patient and health care provider dealing with fibromyalgia, or any chronic pain, learns about MFR. My book, *The FibroManual: A Complete Fibromyalgia Treatment Guide for You...and Your Doctor*, heavily emphasizes myofascial release as a vital component of treatment.

John Barnes has done so much to advance health care, especially the treatment of chronic pain, but mainstream medicine doesn't know it yet. Reading his book, *Healing Ancient Wounds: The Renegade's Wisdom*, will empower you to participate in this health care revolution, along with your own.

Ginevra Liptan, MD
Medical Director
The Frida Center for Fibromyalgia
Portland, Oregon
Author of *The FibroManual: A Complete Fibromyalgia Treatment Guide for You...and Your Doctor*

Being "real" reminds me of the skill of a master, as John teaches us. When we are real, in mastery, we are totally resonating with the now-- open, alert, hearing beyond words, sensing the flow, the balance, the imbalance, and responding with clarity and compassion, as Source would have us do.   For that is our true essence -Source energy, always there, coursing through us as our "chi", working to bring about balance, homeostasis, healing, willing to be "tuned into", and what a joy to live in that space.

Left brained "expertise" appears significantly different from this experience of mastery. Expertise is linear, problem oriented, ego driven, goal oriented. But as John often says, "If you know what you're going to do before you enter the room, you don't know what you're doing". A master enters the room open, alert, in the now, responding not from ego, listening and feeling with compassion for where to respond to this vibrating essence patient or client, staying in that space for the entire treatment, letting go of any expectation or outcome.

As a result - all who are in that energy benefit, even as observers.

Carol M. Davis, DPT, EdD, MS, FAPTA
University of Miami

To me, a master is connected to his instincts. He identifies and trusts his intuition and is able to use his intellect to bring understanding to those who seek the truth.

A master is open to what may seem impossible to others.

He is able to provide the necessary structure to communicate what is not obvious to others... in a way that can be easily understood. And he is really very good at this.

A master humbly leads by example and speaks his truth with confidence.

A master runs the course and persists in the face of adversity, always staying connected with his vision and purpose in life. Strength and vulnerability are integral to his being.

A master encourages the learner/client/patient to feel and be real, to stay connected to their essence and to accept what is...what other choice is there?

To me, Myofascial Release is as important as the air we breathe! I cannot imagine my life without MFR.

John Barnes has lived his life in a way that exemplifies the qualities of a master.

Having first met and learned about the John Barnes Myofascial Release Approach® back in the mid 1980's while in PT school, I feel as though I have "grown up" with MFR. I have witnessed the growth of John's Myofascial Release Approach and the emerging wisdom and insights that he has shared with many thousands over the course of the past, three decades. It has truly been a gift in my own life to be a part of the tremendous transformations that have occurred in the lives of our patients through Myofascial Release and to have experienced such growth and healing in my own life through this wonderful approach.

I feel very privileged to be able to work with John and forever grateful for the positive impact that he has had on my life and growth both personally and professionally. My life and the lives of countless patients and MFR therapists have been richer because of this one man, my friend and mentor, John F. Barnes, PT.

With sincere gratitude and respect,

Valerie McGraw, PT
Chief Physical Therapist
Clinic Manager
Myofascial Release Treatment Center
Malvern, Pennsylvania

preface

My first book, *Myofascial Release: The Search for Excellence* was the technical paradigm and "how to" workbook presented in mechanical/structural terminology. *Myofascial Release Healing Ancient Wounds: The Renegade's Wisdom* delves into the intuitive, therapeutic artistry of myofascial release and the intricacies of authentic healing. It is obviously important to be cognizant and skilled an all of the myofascial release principles to become a therapeutic artist. My goal is to help you significantly increase your effectiveness as a myofascial release therapist. This book is also for the patient/client to enhance and speed their treatment response.

I would like to thank Sandy Levengood and my incredible staff who helped turn *Myofascial Release Healing Ancient Wounds: The Renegade's Wisdom* into a reality. I would also like to express my gratitude to the many patients and therapists who sent in their perspectives on myofacial release and to those who helped with the placement of the patient and therapist perspectives throughout the book, adding another dimension to it's depth and clarity.

I would also like to compliment Elaine Verstraete, whose artistry adorns the front cover and illustrations within. She has a great talent and has captured the essence of myofascial release. Blessings to all of you who have contributed to my life and this book. I hope that our efforts will enhance the quality of the lives of others.

The purpose of this book, *Myofascial Release Healing Ancient Wounds: The Renegade's Wisdom* is to provide you, the therapist, and your patients/clients with a conceptual framework of theories and philosophies that constitute a paradigm or model of the reality of healing utilizing the Myofascial Release Approach. The traditional model of reality that we were taught, while logical, is unfortunately incomplete, yielding limited results in healing and life. Over the years, I have seen many therapists trying to fit the Myofascial Release Approach into the traditional model of reality. This is the equivalent of trying to ram a "square peg into a round hole." It just doesn't work.

It has been my experience that patients/clients can maximize their results when they have been educated about how the old traditional "fix me; treat my symptoms" model of reality can block their healing. Therefore, this book is also for your patients and clients. Although a book could never capture the excitement of a seminar experience, educating your patients and clients on the principles of myofascial release healing and awareness can greatly benefit your efforts, in helping them help themselves. I have purposely written this book in a casual, conversational style that I hope will be easy and enjoyable to understand. It will include commonly asked questions from the Myofascial Release Seminars and treatment sessions. We will zigzag through various topics, with true stories (names changed to protect confidentiality) to illustrate lessons. Many principles and concepts will be revisited from different perspectives to deepen our understanding.

One first learns myofascial release on the mechanical/structural level, and then most realize that there is considerably more depth to this approach than previously perceived. As you hone your skills and sharpen your senses, you begin to treat your patients on a multi-dimensional level, including the physical, emotional, mental, and energetic levels. In time, as the therapist matures in their healing work, she or he connects with their patient as an integrated totality, becoming an evolved therapeutic artist. Myofascial release is the ultimate therapeutic art!

I will be touching on some controversial concepts. Take from my experiences what is of value to you. There are many levels and dimensions of myofascial release. Function on the level that suits you and you will be effective. Consider, however, always being open to new experiences, for there is always the possibility of the new. Remember that we never grow in our comfort zone! Stretch! Come from the perspective of

"What is in my patient's/client's best interest?" and be willing to tap into your fears to become all that you can be.

I suggest that this book be read differently than other books. Allow yourself to experience it visually and with a felt sense. Be there in the moment! Consider stopping at each title, concept, or picture, slowing your breathing, softening your body, and quieting your mind. Think of the concept, and then quietly, without analysis, visualize whatever picture arises and feel whatever emotion emerges. Then ask that picture and emotion to teach you. What does the visual/felt sense mean or symbolize to you? Allow this book to be a profound journey that will take you to a new depth of understanding, wisdom, and therapeutic effectiveness.

The inner journey is not just the most important journey; it is the *only* journey! Let us now travel together as I weave this tapestry, allowing us to connect with our "essence," that state of "being" that brings quality and healing into our lives.

—John F. Barnes, PT

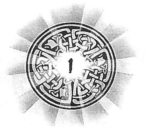

the lightning bolt

A lightning bolt of pain ripped through my body! I lay there stunned. It seemed as if I had slipped into another level of consciousness...a very deep level. It felt like a time warp...a timeless, space-less dimension ...floating and soaring, and then a sense of flow. I felt like I was out of my body. Gradually I became aware of my body, but only the upper half, as if there were no lower half. Then I seemed to slip into another deeper dimension of consciousness, or did it slip into me?

A voice with great authority and wisdom came thundering through me.

You must bring your awareness back into your body now!

"Why" I asked?

You will need all of your awareness, willpower, and courage to handle the responsibilities that lie before you.

"What responsibilities?" I asked.

They will unfold.

"I can't feel my legs."

Move them!

"I can't."

You must focus! This trauma that has just happened to you was initiated eons ago and is now being manifested in your life.

"My legs feel numb."

Good, that means that your awareness is returning. This trauma will significantly change your life forever.

"Who are you? Your voice sounds and feels so familiar."

I am called The Ancient Warrior...I am your guide...I have been with you all of your life...you have thought of me as your intuition, until you allowed your schooling to teach you that intuition was not logical. Now, move your legs!

"It's really starting to hurt."

The pain will be intense; feel it. The intensity will awaken you.

"I am awake."

Barely. It is time for you to be fully aware and move into your power! Your suffering will be the catalyst that awakens you to a deeper reality and will initiate a chain reaction that will affect the lives of millions of people. Move your legs!

Gradually I began to focus. I started to move my legs and slowly, very slowly, got up. What had just happened to me? This whole experience had such a dreamlike quality to it that I was confused. I began to wonder whether it was real. My mind seemed cloudy and as the fog began to lift, I remembered that I had come to the gym to work out with weights. I was preparing for an upcoming competition. No one else was in the gym; even so, I decided to do squats unassisted with over 300 pounds. As I tried to complete the fifteenth repetition, I realized I could not get up. I had been a gymnast when I was younger so I mistakenly decided to roll back, not realizing that when you have a bar with 300 pounds on it, resting on the back of your shoulders, there's no way to release your grip on the bar. I landed on my sacrum and lower back with tremendous force. I was later to learn that I had crushed the disc at L5 and had ripped the ligaments in my lumbar area. That night, after I had injured myself, I was in terrible pain. I was afraid to tell my mother, for I didn't want her to worry. In an attempt to control the pain, I slowed my breathing and softened into the sensations of pain and fear in my body. I eventually drifted into a still, silent dimension and asked for The Ancient Warrior to help me. He said that he would always be there for me; all I needed to do was ask. He went on to share that it was necessary for me to be silent so that I could hear him, and in this way, I would be guided by my intuition. I felt myself go deeper into the stillness, and the intensity of the pain began to lessen. Then I asked,

"I am curious. How do I differentiate between logic and intuition?"

Intuition does not explain...it points the way.

When you're a seventeen-year-old, accidents and injuries happen all of the time. You eventually get yourself up, accept that you'll be sore for a couple of days, and think that it's no big deal. At seventeen, you think that nothing can stop you. The first time I realized that I was having a serious problem happened a few weeks later. I was dating a beautiful young lady, whom I believed to be the greatest thing in the world. It was about the third time we had been out on a date and I was really looking forward to kissing her. In those days you didn't usually kiss anybody until at least the third date. Back in the 1950s, the typical date consisted of going out to dinner and maybe to a movie, and finally going to park somewhere. When it came time for the first kiss, I turned to put my arm around her and my back locked up on me. I was stuck there for a couple of hours in terrible pain.

The most upsetting thing about this experience was not the back pain, but the fact that it messed up the whole evening. Losing out on something that I had so anticipated gave me my first awareness of problems to come. Being young and naïve, I just kept lifting weights, thinking that strength would overcome the pain.

My involvement with gymnastics, football, track, swimming, weight lifting, and karate led to a keen interest in the mind's influence on the body, and vice versa.

I knew in high school that I wanted to be a physical therapist. Physical therapy seemed to be the ideal blend for my personal and professional interests. I was accepted into the physical therapy curriculum at the University of Pennsylvania and graduated as a physical therapist in 1960.

You can imagine my disappointment when I discovered that the physical therapy profession did not appreciate the mind's influence on the body. The emphasis in physical therapy education and treatment was modalities such as hot packs, ultrasound, massage, and some rudimentary exercises. During my time at the University of Pennsylvania and for years after college I tried every form of physical therapy on myself in an effort to alleviate my pain, to no avail. My pain was significantly worsening over time. I was in agony nearly all of the time. Physical therapy and the medical profession basically let me down. The next five years, from age twenty-five to thirty, I could not sit for more than two or three minutes due to the pain. I could barely catch my breath. I was now a physical therapist and was in worse shape than most of the patients I was treating. At that time I was doing a lot of rehabilitation work with stroke patients and paraplegics, in which we would try to get them up to stand and walk in the parallel bars. I would use one arm to support my back and try to hold the patient with the other arm. This awkward dance went on for a while, until I went skiing one weekend and dislocated my shoulder. Now I had one arm in a sling and I had to choose between supporting my back with the good arm or helping the patient.

It never occurred to me to take time off from work. Each time I lifted a patient I was in agony. At this time I had a radiologist friend who begged me to get help. "You can't put up with this any longer," he said. "I have a friend who's a neurologist. Why don't you go see him?" They found that the disc at L5 was completely crushed, and decided that surgery was my best and only option. They removed the disc and fused the spine in the L5 region. The operation made a world of difference; I still had severe problems, but the fusion had at least lowered the intensity of the pain.

I've always thought that every physician or therapist should experience what it is like to be severely injured, and not just for a week or a month, but for a couple of years! It's a whole different story when you are a prisoner in your own body. I felt broken and I *was* broken. It was a horrible, horrible experience! People who have been through a bad experience often report that this event is a catalyst for the positive in their lives. Looking back, that was the case for me. However, when you're in the midst of pain, you get lost in it. For years I struggled. It felt like I was locked in a straitjacket; areas of my body felt like they were stuck in strong glue. I refused to accept that my once powerful body was so limited.

It was through my frustration over being in pain and trying to help myself over the years that I began to experiment with treating myself. I found over time that if I would place my hand on the skin and apply pressure into painful or hard areas of the soft tissue, my range of motion would begin to improve. I eventually discovered that if I slowed down the process and held the pressure for longer periods of time, my pain began to diminish and my range of motion and strength improved even further. This turned into my daily routine. I noted that gentle, sustained pressure without sliding on the surface of the skin produced the best results. I also became aware that as I provided sustained pressure the sensations produced in my body went far beyond the origin and insertion of a particular muscle. It eventually occurred to me that what I must be influencing was the connective tissue, the fascia. I remembered enough about fascia to know that it consisted of two parts, the elastic portion and the collagen portion. Later, I was to discover that "collagen" is an ancient Greek word for "glue producer." Interestingly, when a myofascial restriction is being released it feels like glue stretching. My recovery was so impressive that I realized I must share this with my patients, as well as other physicians and therapists.

I began to use the myofascial techniques with my patients. It wasn't until years later that I had the confidence to begin teaching myofascial release to others. Those techniques that worked well I would modify and refine until I was satisfied with the consistency of the results. Techniques that did not produce consistent results were discarded. It was a long period of trial and error.

It was during this period of experimentation and the development of my approach to myofascial release in the late 1960s and early 1970s that I began treating my twin sons, Mark and Brian. Whenever they were injured, I would treat them with joint mobilization, massage, and myofascial release. They learned myofascial release through their personal experience of it. Just like learning to ski at an early age, it becomes a natural part of who you are and you flow with it. Both of them were intuitive and instinctual therapists before they even went to school to become therapists. Of course, I am prejudiced, but they are both incredible "beings" and therapists. They have taught me a lot!

Brian now has a very successful practice in San Francisco and teaches the Myofascial Mobilization seminars around the country.

BRIAN'S PERSPECTIVE

At nineteen, I fell asleep at the wheel of my car and woke up to a brick wall. After spinning the car around, cracking a telephone pole in half, my car finally came to a stop upside down, over the ridge of the road twenty feet down in a cornfield in the middle of nowhere. I managed to free myself from the car but could only crawl through the field to the light of a farmhouse for help. I called my father from the farmhouse at three in the morning and he found me and drove me home. My father treated me immediately and needless to say, it was a powerful series of myofascial unwindings. I was now the person in need and the recipient of what I had started to learn.

Experiential learning has been a key to my success in gaining a deeper understanding of myofascial release and myself. We learn from our clients each day, for every treatment offers us an opportunity to be partners with our clients in mutual humanness, setting and reaching our highest goals. Our own physical, emotional, and spiritual injuries can become a profound basis for having a very important reference to the world of pain and dysfunction that our clients express that are unique to them.

Our hands are one of the best ways in which to communicate God's love, and myofascial release for me has provided a beautiful bridge in which to communicate this love. In helping my clients move out of the physical restrictions of the fascial system, which tends to restrict their awareness, creating a perceived detachment from their spirit, we can now awaken their mind and body to the magnificent healing power of their essence.

I have been very blessed to have been provided in my life with such an incredible teacher, who is also my father. I have had the opportunity to watch and learn through my experiences with him what it means to be dedicated to a field in which we have an opportunity to care for and teach others how to return to their true essence. His guidance, love and friendship have helped me to become the man and therapist I am today. Thank you dad.

My son, Mark has a very busy physical therapy and myofascial release practice for humans and horses in Boulder, Colorado. He also teaches the Equine Myofascial Release Seminars around the country.

MARK'S PERSPECTIVE

My father's hands are strong, but extremely gentle. They have a certain power that comes with experience; I remember this sense of them from an early age. Most of the truly profound learning I received from my father came to me while in his hands. They have been experiences which are beyond words, and life enhancing, life changing, not only physically when I was in pain, but also promoting perceptual shifts about who I am and the possibilities of who I may become.

I followed in his footsteps, then got lost along the way; he lovingly reeled me in with his heart and hands, and now we walk side by side. I am older now, slightly wiser, and always grateful for my father's hands.

In my teenage years, I spent many Saturday afternoons at his office watching him treat patients. On occasion, he would also treat my brother and me. We have always been amazed at his rapport with patients.

A number of years ago, my father invited me to travel with him to New Jersey to treat a horse. Having no experience with treating horses but plenty of curiosity, I went along.

It was a typical fall afternoon, gray with a hint of moisture in the air. We arrived early to the barn, so we left to grab lunch at a local diner. I asked him what he planned on doing with the horse. He answered that he did not yet have a plan. I have watched my father "flow with the energy" throughout my life in so many situations that this reply did not faze me in the least.

Back at the barn, the first order of business after exchanging greetings with a small crowd of horse-type people talking horse talk was watching the horse in question go around a track. He who was to be evaluated was a two-year-old standardbred. The young horse could not finish the quarter mile as a trotter without "breaking stride" and coming in dead lame.

The horse was in obvious discomfort, even to my naïve eyes. This was the case in our first part of the evaluation, as we watched the young trotter labor around the track, and heard the disappointed exclamations of the crowd.

The trainer brought the horse back to the aisle of the barn and tied him to the outside of his stall. I thought to myself, "Now what, Dad? All eyes are on us, especially you." Calmly, my father circled the horse, looking at what I didn't know. He gently rocked the horse's body, sinking his hands deep into the tissue next to the spine. He then put his hand on the top of the sacrum and rocked it gently back and forth.

My father has this slow, methodical way of simultaneously quieting his patient, and gaining information through a combination of touch and intuition. Much to the initial disappointment of the group that had come to see John Barnes lay his accomplished hands on a horse, he took his time. I believe they were expecting some high-velocity thrusts.

My dad eventually asked for a bale of hay to stand on. He then viewed the pelvis from above, and stated that the problem was in the tissue next to the sacrum. He sank his elbow deep into the soft tissue next to the sacrum, and held it. He held the release for well over ten minutes, following the tissue through to the point of stepping off the bale of hay to continue the release into the hamstrings. Having completed the sacral release, he then took hold of the tail and pulled on it for another four or five minutes. My dad then went to the horse's neck and felt the soft tissues and bony segments there. After a few minutes, he said that the horse had a rotation of one of its cervical vertebrae. He called me over to apply treatment to the neck. Holding the bridle with one hand, I sank my elbow into the horse's neck. After a few releases, I felt a pop. I held this release, following it through many barriers of tissue tightness.

Unconsciously, I slowly sank into a meditative, dream-like state. I began experiencing a very potent communion with this animal. A great sense of joy fell over me, and I had a dream that I was running next to the horse looking into its eyes. For the first time in my life, I had what could be termed a spiritual experience with an animal! When I finally opened my eyes, I saw my father's face with a huge smile. He asked, "Are you done?" I answered "Yes, I think so." The trainer then hooked the horse to a sulky and drove him around the track. The exclamations of the crowd—and especially of the horse's owner—now expressed happy excitement. The horse had not once broken his stride, and was no longer lame. This young horse was obviously moving with greater comfort and ease following the treatment.

This day marked for me the beginning of a great love and appreciation for horses. It also exemplified the valuable kind of information and results one can gain through palpation of the fascial system and treatment through myofascial release. At that time, my father had little knowledge of horse anatomy, biomechanics, or physiology. By relying, however, on his professional experience in releasing restricted fascial tissue in humans, his incredible palpation skills, and his formidable intuition, he was able to have a great effect on the functioning and performance of this equine athlete. This horse went on to become the winningest horse in trotter history!

Mark and Brian have just returned from Athens, Greece where they were teaching myofascial release. Our relationship has been an incredible journey, full of love. I feel blessed to have them as my friends.

Fortunately, myofascial release is very safe. Even when a technique was unsuccessful, I never injured anyone. My patients were extremely pleased with their results and also appreciative of being allowed to return to a pain-free, active lifestyle. It was as a result of these accomplishments that I remembered The Ancient Warrior's prediction and realized that through the myofascial release techniques I had the ability to affect the lives of many. The therapists I trained over the years were able to go home and immediately begin using their knowledge for the greater good of all.

A PATIENT'S PERSPECTIVE

Dear John,

When I broke the bones in my lower leg last November, I knew I was in big trouble. Normally surgery would have been performed, but my diabetes prevented this. My doctor told me it would take months for my leg to heal. They outfitted me with a cast and an electronic bone stimulator and sent me home. Months of therapy helped me get around easier but the pain in my lower leg was relentless. Every move I made caused the non-healing bones to shift in the cast and the pain medication only "took the edge off." My leg felt like a dead stick!

After six months of this, following another trip to the orthopedic surgeon's office with no good news, my home-care physical therapist suggested we try something different. I had the good fortune to be blessed with a therapist who you trained, John, and he said to me, "you've seen some strange things in your life. Well, I do strange things—let's give this a try." I was a nurse for most of my life and had seen many strange occurrences, but nothing prepared me for what was in store. He placed one hand under my cast and one hand on top of it and simply held it there. The diabetes had greatly diminished the sensation in both of my legs, but a wonderful sense of warmth was beginning where he held his hands. He slowly worked from the knee down to the foot. Both of us were aware when he hit the fracture site, but this too was enveloped in warmth. He followed this with what he called "releases" above and below the cast on my knee and toes. When he was done, he passed his hand over the leg, an inch or so over the cast, moving down toward my foot. Although I know it couldn't be possible, I felt the hairs on my leg stand up as his hand passed over. It was then that I realized that the pain in my leg was gone! I was afraid to move, out of fear of spoiling this dream, but my therapist encouraged me to try. I was able to shift my leg around the bed without pain!

John, it has been a few months since this incident. In that time the pain has remained at a minimum, returning only a bit when I started weight-bearing. My doctor was quite surprised when I returned for a routine checkup. He was sure that the electronic bone stimulator finally started to work. I know differently. Thank you for your influence. What you taught my therapist has allowed me to see the future with hope. I can walk without pain. Thank you!

A THERAPIST'S PERSPECTIVE

Myofascial release. Those two words have been the most influential words for me in the last ten years. When I first began to see advertisements for Myofascial Release Training in *Physical Therapy Forum* and *Physical Therapy Bulletin* I thought to myself, "I'll never go to one of those seminars!" They didn't really look technical enough. My model of wellness was very reductionistic at that time.

My wife, who is a physical therapist as well, was exposed to some of John's techniques through another therapist who had taken John's courses. She shared them with me and as I began implementing them into my practice I noticed a profound change in how quickly patients got better. I also was able to treat injuries that had defied traditional therapeutic techniques including patients who had suffered with these problems for years. And this was with just two or three basic techniques that my wife had shared with me. I took these and modified them for various problems that presented themselves. When I combined them with the various manual techniques I already knew, I found that I could loosen joints and mobilize with a lot less force and much less discomfort for the patient.

I still didn't go to the courses. This was probably fortunate, because all the pieces hadn't fallen into place for me in other areas of my life. I might have bolted when I saw the first unwinding demonstration. As it was, the sight of the young woman unwinding was one of the most intriguing images that I had ever seen.

One of the pieces that needed to fall into place came about like this. In my early thirties I began to experience the surfacing of some very strong emotions of sadness. In fact this was probably the first time I had been able to even acknowledge I had any deep feelings at all. These emotions would often come with strong body movements and sensations at the most inopportune times. I had a great therapist and friend who came into my life at that time. I traded therapy for counseling sessions. This made me aware of a whole other dimension to wellness both for myself and my clients.

So when I saw the unwinding at Myofascial Release I, it made sense to me on one level. On another level it intrigued me. It also planted a seed in me that I needed to complete some of the movements started by my counseling sessions. John's ideas and methods helped me to bring together all these experiences that I had with patients and within myself.

In many ways I still had doubts. I left Myofascial Release I with a whole new set of tools and a new perspective. As I implemented this in my practice I began to have patients who would spontaneously unwind.

The unwinding course taught me a lot and eased my fears about working with clients that go through more active unwinding experiences. I have had many others since and each has provided me with new insights.

But the most profound change has come as a result of my Skill Enhancement Seminar experience with John. To be able to feel the work done and see it done as a complete treatment opened my eyes to new ways of doing the work and confirmed some merging beliefs that I had about my own personal and professional growth.

During the Skill Enhancement Seminar we went out on "Therapy on the Rocks Day" with John. When he asked us what we needed to learn there, the word "courage" came up. Let me share a little of what was going on in my life just before we went to Sedona.

I had owned my own practice for seven years with two other partners. Due to HMO's and capitation taking over our area, there were fears that we could not survive. There were a number of PT clinics in our area that lost most of their clientele in a two-week span due to exclusive capitated contracts being issued by the major physician groups in our area. Many of those clinics simply went out of business. So our clinics were sold to a large corporation that promised us that there would be no changes to how we did physical therapy because we were successful. Well, we were sold two more times in the next year. I stepped down as clinical manager because I wanted to treat patients, not do paperwork and meetings. Well, eventually capitation caused policies to come down that minimized staff and increased my patient load to the point where I didn't have enough time to do MFR properly. In addition, I was under pressure to discharge patients before they were finished with the work that needed to be done. My hours were cut to twenty hours per week so that they would not have to pay me benefits. I began to treat clients on a cash basis at a local massage therapy school on one of my off days.

Things were tight and I was very discouraged that the way I had practiced was being destroyed.

My wife was with me as a patient. We were both facing the loss of our jobs due to restructuring. We were being given the choice of one of us going to full time and the other losing their job. My wife was unwilling to work full time because she has always scheduled to be available for our two boys when they are home from school. I was not willing to work full time in a job that was systematically taking the joy of my work away from me. When I was treating clients at the massage therapy school, the day went by fast and I loved the work. We were going to have to make some hard choices. So the word "courage" emerged during that time out during the "Therapy on the Rocks Day Experience."

After we got back we had to make the decision in regard to our work. I told my wife, "I know what the right decision is, but I don't believe that it is the safe decision." We both decided to resign.

Well within three weeks I had a full cash-paying client load. No insurance hassles, no treatment limits, and little paperwork. And lots of time to spend with people. I now have more patients than I can treat. There is sometimes a two-week wait to get in to see me. I have had the opportunity to treat two horses successfully and now I don't have time to develop that branch of the work. I have a tremendous sense of peace about my decision. I know there are no guarantees but there seems to be an order to the path that I have taken.

It is difficult to put into words the gifts that John and

his staff have given to me. To say what they are in words seems to reduce them. I don't know John that well on a personal level, but I do know that the time I have been able to spend with him has provided key influences to my journey. There have not been many people like that in my life.

At one point during our week in Sedona, I was telling John that our patients will sometimes call us miracle workers and John's comment was, "Maybe you are." Maybe we are. Whatever we label it, it sure feels right and it sure feels good.

I would like to end by saying that I am grateful to John and his staff for all their efforts and willingness to share themselves with my wife and with me. You certainly have the ability to help people find meaning in their lives.

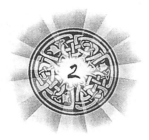

reality is a figment of your imagination

My experience has shown that patients who have an understanding of the Myofascial Release Therapeutic Model of healing usually achieve deeper, quicker, and more lasting results. To those present and future patients, this book is intended to help expand that knowledge. Since the Myofascial Release Therapeutic Model of healing is so different from the traditional model taught to most therapists and physicians, I hope this book will review and deepen your knowledge to help you become a more effective and caring health professional.

The Myofascial Release Seminars that I teach internationally continue to grow rapidly. My schedule is so busy that people always ask if I find it tiring. I explain that since I give every seminar spontaneously, without notes and by responding to each unique audience, teaching stays fresh, new, and exciting. Also, I love what I do, which I believe is the key to a quality life. The therapists I teach are so appreciative that my experience with the seminars is always stimulating and enjoyable for me. My informal seminar teaching style has proven highly effective with the more than 100,000 therapists, physicians, and dentists that I have taught, so I've chosen to continue that format with this book. I'll follow the framework of a typical seminar setting with comments, insights, questions, and answers flowing as they often do. We will zigzag spontaneously from one topic to another and revisit the many principles and concepts from different perspectives, which I hope will benefit all of you, whether you are a patient or a therapist. This may at times provide some chaos for you, but it will actually allow you to have a deeper understanding of the Myofascial Release Approach to healing. Do not let the chaos disturb you; rather, see what you can learn from it.

To many who are taking one of my seminars for the first time, the class is a mixture of curiosity, anticipation, and fear. As the word of myofascial release has spread, therapists take the seminars to deepen their skills. However, many have also heard that the Myofascial Release Approach breaks new ground, challenging them to rethink much of what they have learned. Fear and curiosity are not unwelcome. The seminar room is buzzing with excitement as I scan the room from the stage. A hush develops and I begin the class with an introduction to the work.

The Myofascial Release Approach which I have developed is a whole-body, hands-on approach to the evaluation and treatment of the human structure. Its focus is the fascial system. Fascia is an incredible tough connective tissue that spreads throughout the body in a three-dimensional web. Much like a spider web, it extends from head to foot without interruption.

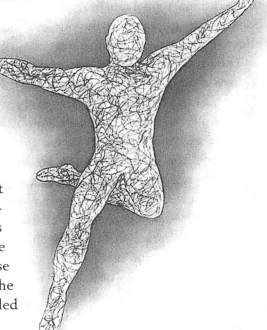

The fascia serves a vital function in that it permits the body to maintain its normal shape and thus keep all of the body's life functions intact. It also allows the body to resist mechanical stresses, both internal and external. Fascia has maintained its general structure and purpose over eons. These functions are evident in the earliest stages of multi-celled organisms, in which two or more cells are able to stay in contact, communicating and resisting the external forces of the environment via the connective tissue.[1]

Fascia supports, protects, envelops, and becomes part of the muscles, bones, nerves, organs, and blood vessels, from the largest structures right down to the cellular level. When all is well, the body functions harmoniously. When injuries occur, however, the fascia has the ability to reorganize along the lines of tension imposed on the body. Physical trauma from direct injury, accident, or unresolved restrictions from the birthing process all can cause the fascia to tighten down in an involuntary attempt to prevent the body from further harm. Inflammation and infectious processes as well as structural imbalances from pelvic injury/ rotation, dental misalignment, leg length changes, and osseous restrictions and/or bony malalignment all can create inappropriate fascial strain patterns. For those interested in a more comprehensive description of how myofascial restrictions and strain patterns can affect the totality of the mind/body complex please refer to my book, *Myofascial Release: The Search for Excellence* (visual standing analysis, pages 37–45).

As an injury remains unresolved, the reorganization of the fascia becomes more pronounced. In its normal state, the fascia is best viewed as the tough, glistening layers in a steak. With prolonged imposition of abnormal stresses, the fascia will tighten, forming new strain patterns. These new patterns add support to the body's misalignment, creating a vicious cycle of dysfunction. This process has the ability to alter tissue and organ function significantly. It has been demonstrated that the transmission of an exposed nerve can be altered by placing human hair upon it; the nerve loses its ability to conduct signals properly. So it doesn't take any great stretch of the imagination to understand how the excessive pressure from myofascial restrictions can produce so much pain and havoc in our bodies. Fascial strains slowly tighten, causing the body to lose its normal ability to act and react to its environment. This tightness, over time, spreads like a pull in a sweater, causing a reorganization of the fibers and twisting their shape. Flexibility and spontaneity of motion are lost, making the body vulnerable to even more trauma, pain, and limitation of movement. These powerful fascial restrictions begin to pull the body out of its normal three-dimensional alignment with gravity, causing biomechanically inefficient and energetically consuming movement and postural patterns.

As J. G. Travell has explained[2], restrictions of the fascia can create pain or malfunction throughout the body, sometimes with bizarre side effects and seemingly unrelated symptoms. Neurological pain is traditionally characterized or diagnosed by observing or measuring the pain, numbness, or impaired sensation along paths, or dermatomes, throughout the body. Fascial restrictions and its subsequent pain seldom follow these dermatomal zones. It is thought that an extremely high percentage of people suffering with pain, loss of motion, or both, may have problems due primarily to fascial restrictions.

It has been estimated that myofascial restrictions can create a tensile strength of up to approximately 2,000 pounds per square inch![3] It is felt that this enormous and excessive pressure of the myofascial restrictions on pain-sensitive structures can produce many of the pains, headaches, and other undesirable symptoms that many people suffer. Most of these conditions go undiagnosed, however, as all of the standard tests, such as radiographs (X-rays), myelograms, computerized tomographic scans (CAT scans), and electromyograms (EMG) do not show fascial restrictions.[4] Many conventional medical, dental, and therapeutic techniques frequently target the symptom, resulting in poor or temporary results. Addressing the cause—the unresolved myofascial restriction—is what is needed to truly solve the problem.

The patient is usually told that there is nothing wrong with them, that time will improve the pain, that it must be arthritis, or that the pain is psychosomatic—it's all in their head! If someone had only taken the time to touch the patient, maybe they could have discovered the problem. Touching patients with skilled hands can be one of the most potent ways of locating fascial restrictions and effecting positive change. Touching patients through mobilization, massage, and various forms of exercise and movement therapy, coupled with the gentle, refined touch of myofascial release and the sophisticated movement therapy called myofascial un-winding, creates a sensorimotor interplay. This experience of contact and movement is the very experience we need to reprogram our bio-computer, the mind-body. Those practicing myofascial release use the skin and fascia as a handle or lever to create new options for enhanced function and movement of every structure within the body. Myofascial release helps remove the straitjacket of pressure caused by restricted fascia, eliminating symptoms such as stiffness, pain, headaches, spasm, and fibromyalgia, as well as restoring range of motion. Through its influence on the neuromuscular and skeletal systems, myofascial release creates the opportunity for patients to "learn" new enhanced movement patterns. Manipulation and myofascial release both are highly effective treatments when they are accomplished with skilled hands and mind. They are designed to be used together to enhance the total effect. Joint manipulation is specific, attempting to improve the motion and function of a particular joint. Myofascial release, however, is a whole-body approach designed to discover and rectify the fascial restrictions that may have caused the effect or symptom.

A THERAPIST'S PERSPECTIVE

I was in my front yard when I noticed a prickly plant growing within my bed of plants. Due to the thorns on the plant I decided to put on gardening gloves. As I was attempting to uproot this plant, I realized it was a vine. I applied a gentle pull similar to an arm or leg pull as I learned in Myofascial Release I to reach into the roots. Once the root came loose an enormous length of vine began to unravel. The vine's attachments were deeply intertwined with a variety of different shrubs and other plants. Each uprooted portion of this prickly vine was about six feet long. To the naked eye it appeared two feet at most.

I instantly thought of the fascial system, likened to this uninvited prickly vine weed. It was firmly rooted and attached to the ground. It had twisted and turned and in growing attached itself to anything and everything along its path, indiscriminate in its surroundings, unaware of its impact on the whole.

I could not help myself from making this comparison. Once it was uprooted on the sidewalk it was larger than the entire plant bed. It seemed almost impossible that so much of its growth and attachments to other plants had virtually gone unnoticed—just like the fascial system.

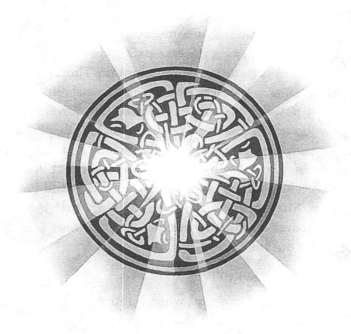

Let's now talk about paradigms, our model of reality. A paradigm is a set of shared assumptions that go unquestioned over time. Each of us is born into a culture, a group of people with a shared belief system, a consensus about how things are and how they should be, a model of reality. The prevailing traditional paradigm that you and I were taught is the Cartesian/Newtonian model of reality that is over three hundred years old.

Have we really moved out of the Dark Ages? For centuries many of the churches of the time maintained an iron grip on the minds and bodies of the populace, demanding total control. Some churches taught of a loving God, guiding and helping us through life, while other churches used the image of a vengeful God, to scare people into yielding to their way and to generate enormous wealth. Descartes and Newton and other scientists of that time were in a fight with the church. Frustrated with their struggle for control, they agreed to parcel out different aspects of the human experience. The church took the spirit, physicians took the biochemistry, psychiatrists took the mind, and therapists got the flesh. Nobody wanted the emotions!

The universe as perceived by Newton and Descartes is a giant machine that functions precisely, logically, sequentially, and correctly. This model of classic physics, which is the basis of our current paradigm, is characterized by arrogance because it allows for only one correct solution. In the field of medical science, this paradigm has reduced human illness to the "biochemistry of disease," completely losing sight of the fact that disease or dysfunction is part of a whole person.

René Descartes, the philosopher and founding father of modern medicine, was forced to make a deal with his church to obtain the human bodies he needed for dissection. Descartes agreed he wouldn't have anything to do with the soul, mind, or emotions; that would be the realm of the church, and he and other scientists could only claim the physical realm. The value of the divisions created by Newton, Descartes, and others is that they eliminated total control by one organization and allowed for diverse ways of expanding knowledge. But now the pendulum has swung too far, in that it has lost sight of the whole being and we erroneously believe that the human being can actually be fragmented and treated as such. We have swung from one extreme imbalance to another extreme imbalance.

Since the Cartesian era, Western traditional medicine has been dominated by reductionist methodology, which tries to explain life by examining the tiniest pieces of it. In other words, the reductionist argues that if you understand everything about the ingredients, you understand everything about the whole. The debatable reasoning of the staunch reductionist is chilling and impersonal: He has eliminated from his model of reality the effect of the mind, emotions, and meaning in life. Essentially, the reductionists are saying that brain function, and feelings of fear, sorrow, and joy, etc., are nothing more than chemical reactions. *That this model has reached its limits and has crossed into absurdity is obvious.* The attempt to fragment humans and their health has been disastrous.

Over fifty years ago, Albert Einstein and Max Planck proved that the current model of reality—the body as a mindless machine that can be mechanically or chemically fixed—was erroneous! Yet this incomplete, inaccurate, and obsolete paradigm is still being taught in nearly all medical, dental, and therapeutic educational programs today. Planck, one of the world's greatest scientists and the father of quantum physics, said, "Science advances one funeral at a time!" We can't wait until these old and dangerous ideas die.

The newly emerging views on holistic health care complement rather than refute the reductionist view, expanding it rather than replacing it. I believe that our new paradigm, the Myofascial Release Approach, has to do with wholeness and connectedness and beautifully complements the wholly modern views of quantum physics. It allows for multiple possibilities and multiple responses. It allows the person to have a role in their destiny and life.

Quantum physics is the awareness and facilitation of interwoven, nonlinear systems in which the whole makes sense of the parts, unlike reductionism, where the parts make sense of the whole. This requires a change of perspective and represents a "breakthrough in science. It connects living biological systems to physics and shows nature to be much more than just mechanical. The whole universe is alive and participating."[5]

Traditionally, medical education taught that emotions are totally separate from structure, that the body is essentially a machine, and when a part breaks down it is to be medicated, surgically altered, or have some form of therapy directed at its symptoms to "fix" it. For years this Cartesian viewpoint or model was accepted and patients were treated accordingly. Certainly this was true in my early practice. My intuition, which I refer to as The Ancient Warrior, has told me many times, "Do not accept the concept that something cannot happen because the scientific literature says it can't. Trust your instincts!"

As time went on, this fragmented, incomplete myth of who we are as humans and how we heal was accepted as truth. This fragmentation led to the overemphasis of our intellectual side in our educational system. Psychologists have been telling us for years that we only utilize about *10%* of our brain. I believe this 10% is our linear, logical, intellectual side. The other 90% of who we are, *our essence*, the creative, intuitive, feeling, and wise aspect, has been ignored and even ridiculed in our education.

Myofascial release is a logical expansion of the very roots of the health professions. It does not necessitate the dismantling of their framework, but rather represents a powerfully effective addition of a series of concepts and techniques that enhance and mesh with our medical, dental, and therapeutic training. We can no longer tolerate paying monstrous healthcare bills for worthless procedures!

Our linear side is a narrow focus. Most of us are stuck in this narrow focus most of our life. We consider this limited focus to be our way of thinking, and it has formed who we have become. We confuse this form of thinking as intelligence. Being stuck in our linear side is like viewing life through a telescope that eliminates billions of bits of information each moment, allowing us to view or access only a small piece of what is available to us. Now consider that at the end of the telescope is a prism that distorts incoming information. This prism represents our conditioning and prejudices. Our intellectual linear side only has the ability to process past information. We have been taught a mode of thinking that only processes limited, distorted, and past information.

We have become "word worshippers," only trusting the written or spoken words of others, or some printout on a machine. Our creative, intuitive, and wise side was stifled early on and we were given dysfunctional messages—no other form of consciousness is valid, don't trust your feelings, ignore and shove down your emotions—while in fact, our emotions are our teachers! Essentially our education was mass hypnosis. We were not educated; we were entranced. Our normal consciousness (linear, intellectual thought) can be called "consensus trance," which creates a loss of our essential vitality. Consensus trance is a state of profound abstraction, a substantial disassociation from immediate sensory/instinctual reality.

What we have considered consciousness is the sleep of daily life. It is as though we are going through the motions of life in a stupor, in a daze. We are on automatic functioning through our habitual patterns that cripple us and keep us from healing and functioning at our maximum level. Basically, we have been mesmerized into viewing ourselves as "thinking brains" whose job it is to figure our way through life. In fact, we are "feeling minds" that perceive sensory information from our environment, processing this sensory information through the microtubules of the myofascial system into our "computer," the brain. The brain converts this information into symbols (words and thoughts), and then sends information (energy) through the nervous system, converting these symbols into action.

Our intellectual side is an important but tiny part of our mind-body awareness and wisdom. Neuroscientists estimate that your mind-body wisdom's database outperforms the intellectual, linear side on an order exceeding *ten million to one!* Science, traditional therapy, and medicine have focused on the smallest part of who we are. The Myofascial Release Approach to healing includes all aspects of our mind-body's powerfully creative, healing potential. It is time we discover who we are! It is time we utilize all aspects of our power and wisdom for our healing! It is time we lead a fulfilling and meaningful life!

I was an only child, and my father died when I was three. My mother was a petite, beautiful woman. She was intelligent and strong willed. She was very wise and told me that she recognized, early on, that I was fiercely independent and very capable of taking care of myself. She loved me enough to guide me, but allowed me to make my own decisions. I have always enjoyed challenge and responsibility.

I remember as a young boy of six or seven being present at adult parties, sitting there being very bored with the adult's conversation. Barely paying attention, all of a sudden I would answer their questions or make a comment. Everyone would stop talking and look at me in astonishment, as if to say, "Where did he learn that?" Prior to my statements, I had never thought or known of what the topic had been. I just heard myself saying it and as I said it; I just knew it was correct. It was as if the answer came through me. My guide had always spoken through me. I have always trusted my inner voice, my guidance, and I thought that everyone had a guide. I now know that we all have guidance from within, but unfortunately our past education and programming has blocked many individuals' intuition and inner guidance.

I believe that, since my father died when I was young and I didn't have any siblings, I had very few role models to mimic. I believe that most children are programmed early on in life through copying their mother's and father's mannerisms, beliefs, and attitudes. My mother, in her wisdom, recognized that I would rebel if she tried to force me into a particular mold. She instead created a strong, positive image of my father. She created a vision, a symbol of masculinity for me to grow and mature into in my own unique way. She would have stopped me immediately if I was in danger or if I took a "wrong road," but she allowed me to forge my own path. In other words, while not neglectful, her loving gentle guidance allowed me to chart my own unique course.

A Therapist's Perspective

I believe it was in the Fascial Pelvis/Myofascial Release course, walking back to the cars after being out on the rocks, that I found myself separated from the group by a chasm. Half to myself I said, "I took the wrong path." John, walking with the group, honed into this across the chasm, and said, "follow your own path." I did. I followed my chosen path back to the cars even though my doubting, fearful voice was saying, "what if you can't get back to the cars this way and you're doing it wrong, wrong, wrong, danger, danger, danger." Beyond all those familiar old voices I felt as if I had just, for the first time in my life, been given permission to simply BE.

I have always been very comfortable with my masculinity. However, I have always viewed true masculinity as a balance between gentle strength, courage, sensitivity, and beauty. I have always cherished my feminine side, my creativity, sensitivity, and intuition, while fully enjoying my masculine side, my strength, courage, analysis, and action. I have witnessed many therapists and patients blossom as myofascial release brings out the latent and underdeveloped talents of their imprisoned masculine and feminine sides, allowing them to become part of their total being.

A Therapist's Perspective

Impressions of John: John Barnes strikes me as a person like Copernicus or Leonardo DaVinci. He is a man with ideas that buck the establishment. He sees a new way of explaining the phenomena he encounters and is not afraid to talk about it. This type of person tends to create a following.

Certainly there is a spiritual aspect to this treatment (the concept of wholeness: we are body, mind, and spirit, that cannot be separated). Oftentimes, when people can't explain things, they credit it to spirituality. But John said in the seminar I attended, this is not a religion, this is something everyone can learn to do.

A THERAPIST'S PERSPECTIVE

Before being introduced to myofascial release I was the epitome of the left-brained, highly disciplined, linear-thinking physical therapist, well trained in breaking the body down into component parts and viewing the "human machine" as a system of pulleys and levers. I entered my first job feeling well equipped to help everybody. Unfortunately, even years after graduation, I still was not seeing the results that I had anticipated (especially patients with TMJ, cervical, and low back pain) and I was becoming extremely discouraged. I felt let down with my profession, as I had been unable to make significant and permanent changes in many of the people coming to me in pain. I was very confused and unsettled, and I was searching. In my personal life, I had never been willing to open up my feelings...even to myself. I was tense all the time, unable to apply the meaning of "relax and have fun." I was experiencing a constant deep, dull ache just behind my breastbone.

It was during this searching phase that I took my first courses (Myofascial Release I, Myofascial Unwinding, and Myofascial Release II) in Detroit, November 1998. During this introduction, I worked with wonderful therapists and instructors. During these ten days, not only were beneficial changes made to my actual physical structure, but by releasing the fascial restrictions I was finally able to let go of enormous amounts of pain, fear, and grief.

Since taking the Myofascial Release Seminars I have had a quantum shift in my way of thinking, and everything else in my life has followed. I am more creative and have opened up my mind to different ideas and, most important, my feelings. I am more settled. In fact, I moved halfway across the country from my hometown in Pennsylvania to Illinois, where I now work in a clinic with a wonderful myofascial release practitioner who has beautiful energy and helps me to grow daily. I am now achieving a level of success with my patients that was unknown to me previously, and with each course I find myself becoming more focused, quiet, and powerful.

I have many goals right now, most importantly to open up my heart. You see the only male in the history of my family to live beyond fifty-one years has had open-heart surgery with four bypasses. I am taking precautionary measures in prevention via normal and alternative health channels and I am working toward releasing the tension throughout my mind-body complex through myofascial release and myofascial unwinding. I am determined to break this terrible family pattern, and to continue in the process of journeying up and down that scary and thrilling trail of healing (aren't we all?).

It is with great joy that I anticipate growing and learning in myofascial release.

✦

[1] Scott, J. Molecules that keep you in shape. New Scientist, 1986: 111:49-53.

[2] Travell JG, Simmons, DG. Myofascial pain and dysfunction—the trigger point manual. Baltimore: Williams & Wilkins, 1983:260.

[3] Katake, K. The strength for tension and bursting of human fasciae, J. Kyoto Pref. Med. Univ., 1969: 484–488, 1961.

[4] Barnes, JF. *Myofascial Release: The Search for Excellence.* Philadelphia: Rehabilitation Services, Inc. 1990.

[5] Ibid.

authentic healing

Myofascial release and myofascial unwinding is, to me, the most profound and deepest form of healing that you will ever experience yourself or be able to provide for others. It's so natural, and you will never injure anyone; it's a skill we were born with and can redevelop.

"I am going to demonstrate a temporomandibular technique now. Would anyone like to come up on the stage to help?"

A young woman with dark hair stepped up to the stage and laid down on the treatment table to be a model for the technique. I evaluated her jaw and found her mandibular motion to be restricted. I placed my hands lightly on her head and centered myself. Her head, neck and jaw began to release and move or unwind. I could feel the energy between the two of us building as her body arched and she began to let out some noise. The condyles of her temporomandibular joint clicked back into place and she released and softened. As I helped her to sit up, I asked the audience if they had any questions or comments.

Question: Could you relate your experience on the table? What did you feel?

I have attended several of John's courses, and never allowed myself the opportunity to be a treatment demonstration. This time, I decided I really needed to experience his touch, and asked him to treat my TMJ. I am grateful. I tend to be rather introverted; not shy, but I don't normally put myself in front of large groups. As soon as I laid down on the treatment table and John entered my energy field, I felt a sense of calm. All anxiety I felt about being in front of a large group while being treated was gone. I believe the technique was to evaluate the lateral deviation in my temporomandibular joint (TMJ) and determine which side needed to be moved back to proper alignment. Sounds very straightforward and technical. I have a chiropractor who adjusts my jaw periodically. It takes about sixty seconds, is very mechanical and never holds more than twenty-four hours. When John lightly placed his fingers on my jaw, the feeling of safety and calm expanded, and I could feel myself become deeply connected with my spirit. I believe I had two or three freeze and thaw responses, because my body began to shake, and then I would get cold. John never changed the amount of pressure. I then began to sense my consciousness, as if I were reaching deep into my history, and simultaneously recalled numerous experiences that have contributed to my jaw problem—not just the auto accident, but other fears and traumas as well. And more important, I began to notice my inability to express the fears around the traumas, and my inability to express feelings that surround emotional insecurities and hurts in general. I had no specific detailed memory of any particular event, just an acute awareness of a lifelong pattern that has accumulated into a tremendous amount of fear, hurt, and pain in my body. I felt completely safe in this experience.

I have understood the theory of expanded consciousness intellectually for years, and have read extensively on the mind-body connection. But this is the first time I have had such a profound "ah ha." While working with me, John maintained light pressure, and gently encouraged me to stay with the moment. My body began to unwind. As I moved on the table, my body found positions that triggered an intense need to express myself. I felt myself begin to expel noise from my gut; no, not my gut, but my core being. As the noise came out, I could feel my spirit shifting, as if that expanded awareness of every event that contributed to this condition began to reconcile. The awareness became more real, more fluid, and the fears began to resolve, again all simultaneously, as if time had no meaning, and cognitive understanding was not present. Just a deep knowing. My jaw went pop, pop, pop, back into place. The tension in my face and head melted away. I felt as if a vise had been removed from my head for the first time in nearly fifteen years.

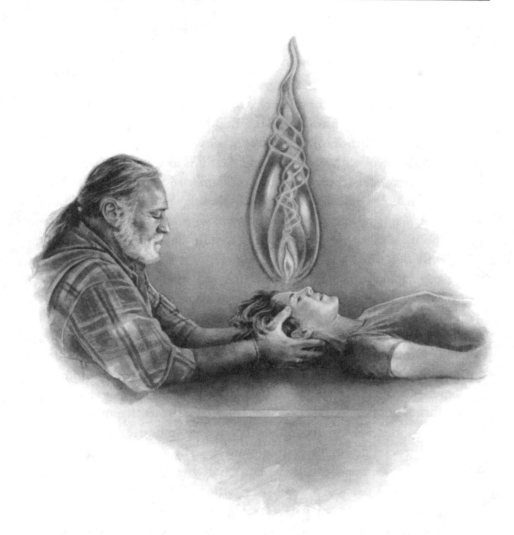

My jaw feels perfect, and my body feels great. It's as if I have rediscovered my voice. Interesting how not voicing my truths have resulted in a messed-up jaw!!

From a therapist's perspective, my understanding has deepened. I now get it! I now know that as I work on myself, I will continue to be able to help others get there, too. With each workshop and treatment, I become more aware and convinced that myofascial release is the right way for me. I have tried everything else, but I really need to stay connected with my truth to be whole again. There really is no other choice.

Question: John, what is the technical explanation of what we just witnessed on the treatment table?

Mind-body awareness and healing are often linked to the concept of "state-dependent" memory, learning, and behavior, also called deja vu.[1] We have all experienced this; for example, when a certain smell or the sound of a particular piece of music creates a flashback phenomenon, producing a visual, sensorimotor replay of a past event or an important episode in our lives with such vividness that it is as if it were happening at that moment. Based on the work of Hameroff and colleagues[2] and my experience, I would like to expand this theory to include position-dependent memory, learning, and behavior, with the structural position being the missing component in Selye's state-dependent theory as it is currently described.[1]

Despite going through years of therapy, many people have not improved much. The problem is that traditional therapy focuses on the symptoms, which are just the tip of the iceberg, a small fraction of the problem. Treating the cause, the myofascial system allows the mind to let go of subconscious holding patterns. My experience has shown that during periods of trauma, people form subconscious indelible imprints of the experiences that have high levels of emotional content. The body can hold information below the conscious level, as a protective mechanism, so that memories tend to become dissociated or amnesiac. This is called memory dissociation, or reversible amnesia. The memories are state-dependent (or position-dependent) and can therefore be retrieved when the person is in a particular state (or position). This information is not available in the normal conscious state; the body's protective mechanisms keep us away from the positions that our mind-body awareness construes as painful or traumatic.

It has been demonstrated consistently that when a myofascial release technique takes the tissue to a significant position three-dimensionally in space, the tissue not only changes and improves, but memories, associated emotional states, and belief systems rise to the conscious level. This awareness, through the positional reproduction of a past event or trauma, allows the individual to grasp the previously hidden information that may be creating or maintaining symptoms or behavior that deter improvement. With the repressed and stored information now at the conscious level, the individual is in a position to learn which holding or bracing patterns have been impeding progress, and then release them. The release of the tissue with its stored emotions and hidden information creates an environment for change.

We all try hard to get better. We use our willpower, but without realizing it, the subconscious keeps pulling us back in habitual dysfunctional patterns no matter how hard we try. Selye[1] described this type of resistance as being "stuck in a groove," something we have all experienced. When something familiar happens we react subconsciously in a habitual pattern, before we can consciously be aware of it to control it. For example, if you were injured in a car accident, every time you see a car coming too fast, you tighten and brace against the possible impact. People replay these past incidents and the automatic, habitual bracing patterns associated with them subconsciously, until these hidden memories and learned behaviors are brought to the surface. Myofascial unwinding helps bring this information to a conscious level, allowing patients to reexperience it and let go, if they choose.

Question: How is it that normal bodily movements or daily activities do not reproduce these memories, emotions, and outdated beliefs?

I believe that these positions represent fear, pain, or trauma. In an attempt to protect oneself from further injury, it seems as if the subconscious does not allow the body to move into positions that reenact the microevents and important microcognitions essential for lasting mindbody change. The body then develops further strategies or patterns to protect itself. These subconscious holding patterns eventually form specific muscular tone or tension patterns, and the fascial component then tightens into these habitual positions of strain as a compensation to support the misalignment that results. Therefore, the repeated postural and traumatic insults of a lifetime, combined with tensions of emotional and psychological origin, seem to result in tense, contracted and fatigued fibrous tissue. This acts to protect us. It protects us from these memories, emotions, and outdated beliefs.

Question: How could we ever know what past events or traumas created the individual's present-day problems?

Good question! We don't know. You and they don't have to know. Myofascial therapists read the body globally, center themselves, and through their touch elicit the piezoelectric effect which charges the patient's system. The wisdom of the patient's mind-body takes them through the past events that it needs to release. The Myofascial Release Approach begins with the present moment, and then working in reverse, myofascial release and myofascial unwinding release the fascial tissue restrictions, thereby altering the habitual muscular response and allowing the positional, reversible amnesia to surface, producing emotions and beliefs that are the cause of the holding patterns and ultimate symptoms.

In order to allow this spontaneous motion to proceed without interference, it is important for the therapist to quiet his or her mind and feel the subtle inherent motions in the patient. Quietly following the tissue (myofascial release) or body part (myofascial unwinding) three-dimensionally along the direction of ease, the therapist guides the patient's movement into the significant restrictions or positions. With myofascial unwinding, the therapist eliminates gravity from the system, unloading the structure to allow the body's gravity-oriented, righting reflexes and protective responses to temporarily suspend their influence. The body is then free to move into positions that allow repressed state or position-dependent physiologic or flashback phenomena to recur. As this happens within the safe environment of a treatment session, the patient can facilitate the body's own inherent self-correcting mechanism to obtain improvement. Myofascial release connects us and our patients with our true essence to allow for authentic healing and a fulfilling and meaningful life.

Question: What do you say to people before they unwind?

Actually I usually say nothing. The least amount that is said the better, because then you don't set up expectations, which often lead to limitations. I don't go into a session to unwind people. I usually start with structural myofascial release work and the unwinding will just naturally happen as a spontaneous part of many treatment sessions, if the patient trusts you and is willing to let go.

In our treatment centers, there are a lot of people who have never heard of myofascial release or of me. We will treat them and they will unwind as part of their treatment experience. They will make progress and reach their treatment goals and we discharge them. A couple of years later they might have another accident. For whatever reason, they might be sent to another therapy facility. Invariably these people come back within two or three visits, saying, "You won't believe what these other therapists were doing. They were putting hot packs and ultrasound on me. They didn't unwind me. What were they doing?" The unwinding was a natural process of healing for them. They didn't question it. They needed little to no explanation.

Question: What can we do initially for an individual? Can myofascial unwinding be used for acute problems?

Myofascial release and myofascial unwinding are the very best things you can do for anybody with acute injuries such as whiplash situations or for any very hypersensitive area. It doesn't have to be a full-body unwinding. Treating a person soon after the injury, and gently letting their body spontaneously move and unwind, the spasms will begin to lessen, their pain will diminish and the range of motion will return. Providing this type of care promptly, as soon as it is determined that they have no contraindications, is the most humane form of treatment which you can give.

We had a chiropractor come to our Myofascial Release Treatment Center in Paoli, Pennsylvania. He was coming down from the New York City area and had a variety of chronic pain problems. After undergoing treatment he was doing quite well and was on his way to us for his last visit, his discharge appointment, and was involved in a five-car accident. Fortunately, he wasn't severely injured, but he was thrown all around the inside of the car. By the time he arrived at our facility, he was really in a state of agitation. Every symptom he'd ever had in his life was flared up. I sat him on the table and unwound him. He spontaneously went through all the motions that had occurred in the car, and within about an hour he was doing very well again and we could still discharge him to go home. We have all experienced or treated patients whose symptoms after a whiplash accident far exceed what could reasonably be explained by the velocity of the accident. Full-blown symptoms have been frequently seen at automobile speeds below ten or fifteen miles per hour. Most victims of even relatively minor motor vehicle accidents usually describe a sense of detachment and shock. The major symptoms of the whiplash may not appear for forty-eight hours and then may progressively worsen for many days, weeks, or even months despite extensive care.[3] In both the forward and backward motions which are involved in the whiplash, the front of the brain (which has the consistency of well-set gelatin) slides forward and impacts the rough and jagged edges of the eye orbits. The orbito-frontal areas of the brain are particularly susceptible to hematomas, contusions, and intercerebral hemorrhages. If the head is turned to either side at the time of impact, a phenomenon called shearing may occur, which can create tearing or bleeding of the contents of the cranial vault.

Psychoneuroimmunology research implies that "every cell in the body can communicate with every other cell." The reason that myofascial release and myofascial unwinding have been so effective with whiplash victims and other posttraumatic injuries may be explained by the fight/flight/freeze response developed by Dr. Peter Levine. He postulates that the fight/flight/freeze response is seen in animals in response to life-threatening experiences. In other words, the preyed-upon animal will flee or attempt to fight, but if run to the ground it will enter a freeze response in which it assumes a state of immobility while physiologically still manifesting high levels of activity of both the parasympathetic and sympathetic nervous systems.[4] Doctor Levine goes on to say that if the animal survives the attack, it will go through a dramatic period of discharge of this high-level autonomic arousal throughout the motor system. This discharge involves trembling, profuse sweating, and deep breathing. This type of discharge is frequently seen after deep myofascial releases, followed by substantial improvement.

In the case of a motor vehicle accident, a holding pattern develops to protect the body against impact. As a result of the freeze response, this subconscious holding pattern is maintained indefinitely, manifesting sustained muscular contraction with resultant myofascial restriction, leading to chronic myofascial pain and tightness.[4]

A PATIENT'S PERSPECTIVE

John, I'd like to share my experience of myofascial release vs. traditional therapy after my car accident. I was in Sedona, Arizona for one week in order to study for the bar exam. This was the culmination of four years of attending law school at night, working days, raising two young daughters, and caring for my mom and grandmother. I was truly uptight at having only one week to cram. I frequently needed to adjust my study position to ease the shooting pain deep in my neck which radiated down my numb right arm. I had been in a car accident a year before which resulted in fractured collarbones and brachial plexus nerve damage. After months of physical therapy, ultrasound treatments, a TENS unit, and drugs, I was finally able to function and resume most of my normal activities, but not without a constant headache and a deep ache in my neck with numbness down my arm. I was too busy to acknowledge the pain except for Advil breaks throughout the day. My sights were fixed intensely on my goal of passing the bar exam and being able to practice law. I allowed nothing to deter me.

Knowing I needed solitude to focus on my studies, my sister offered me the use of her hotel in Sedona for the week while she took your Myofascial Release courses. I was delighted. Upon our arrival, I spread out my boxes of books and notes on the floor and plowed in with a rigid schedule of alternating between eighteen hours of study one day and twenty the next. I was not particularly happy to have my schedule interrupted by my sister's next present to me—regularly scheduled treatments with you. I viewed it as a waste of valuable time. Nevertheless, my sister's blue eyes met mine with such satisfaction and pride in her choice of a graduation gift that I found myself thanking her weakly as my mind anxiously computed the hours away from the books that this dubious gift would consume. She saw the doubt and assured, "It's going to be OK, you'll study better when you're not in pain all the time." Right! As I sat waiting for John Barnes, I was more scared of failing the bar than happy at the prospect of treatment. After all, what could another physical therapy treatment accomplish—been there, done that, for six months three times a week.

A tap on the door announced the entry of John and four therapists. John met my gaze evenly. His eyes seemed to see into my soul, beyond my busy, no-nonsense outer layer to the inner core where I didn't visit often myself. Could he see my insecurities, doubt, and fear of failure? Could he see the ugly little woman I knew I was when the lights were out and no one was around to put on the show for? I stared into his blue eyes and found no judgement. OK, so at least he was honest and not some quack that would hurt me. I met trust with trust and decided I could do this PT stuff once more, at least once.

John introduced his team of highly trained myofascial release therapists who were working with him that week to assist and deepen their own knowledge and skills of the Barnes Approach to Myofascial Release. John walked to the foot of the table and invited me to lie down face-up. He commented to his therapists regarding my position on the table and the obvious leg length discrepancy.

I remember John's hands taking hold of my ankles and saying something about repositioning the way I was lying on the table, so I would be straight. At that point, it was as if my body had a mind of its own and wanted to take advantage of every nanosecond that these knowing hands were in con-tact with me. I felt a warm melding. I stretched my legs far. I had a split second of decision time within which to halt what wanted to move, or go with it. Was I supposed to move, allowed to move? "OK, she's going right into unwinding," I heard John telling his therapists, and the therapists spread around me on the table to support whatever movement I was doing. So, I supposed this was permitted and gave myself permission to move. And what moving it was. A part of me detached from all the activity on the table and thought, "Goodness, this is so strange to be snaking all over, stretching and pushing, but it feels so right." No pressure, no expectations, only silence, understanding, and love. I continued to remember the car wreck.

After dressing, I walked with my sister to the car. We went for coffee. My notes lay by my side. I wanted that next treatment!

I remember the second treatment because simultaneous arm, leg, and cervical traction resulted in my feeling something rearrange in my neck and my headache went away—just like that! That intense headache that had been my companion for over a year was gone. Amazing!

I stopped moving all of a sudden with my neck pushed over to the side and my opposite knee going the opposite direction. I was frozen...and remembering with vivid recall seeing a yellow fire hydrant looming in front, the slow motion of crashing into it, and the feel of my head smashing against the window and my knee crushing into the gear shift. And then I moved again, and froze again, remembering hands holding up my head, hearing the sounds of the saw cutting through the car door, feeling intense cold, hearing voices, seeing fire truck and ambulance lights; and moving again. Then stillness in a heap and hearing John's voice next to my ear suggesting, "Tell yourself you survived." I did. I told myself, "I survived" and I felt all that raw fear of dying and the question of what were my girls going to do without their mom break loose from their very deep and forgotten moorings. Tears came to my stoic eyes, and my small but strong shoulders began to crumple. It was OK to let go in the safety and support of these caring therapists. Soon wonderful hot packs were gently placed on my shoulders. They felt so good after releasing all of the pain and tension in my shoulders. I lay on the table and felt my sister's hand in mine.

*

This explains why traditional therapy's focus on symptoms is not enough for a complete resolution of the problem. Myofascial release and myofascial unwinding release the muscular tension, contractions, and/or spasms which the myofascial restrictions and holding patterns maintain through the "freeze response." The fight/flight/freeze response answers many questions we therapists encounter with our trauma victims.

Unwinding is basically all about trusting. Trusting enough to take your brakes off and to let go. The instant you take your brakes off, your body starts to unwind. Myofascial release and myofascial unwinding initiate the healing process. It is really about getting in touch with your essence. It is your essence or your mind that moves your structure through the unwinding process. We've completely divorced ourselves from the most important part of our being through our training in school and our society, and it's time we open up to all the talents we truly have.

It's really hard for us all to face our fear. We run from it. We were taught to run from it. We were taught not to feel anything. When our fears start to surface, it's a little scary. But I'll tell you, what's really scary is not getting in touch with it! This is what distorts your life and your behavior, and it's what creates disease. Myofascial unwinding is never injurious. You will go through various aspects of tissue memory, and what you will hear from your patients all the time is, "Gee, I'd thought I already dealt with that." Well, they probably had, at least on the intellectual level. We're all good at that, but it's not enough. A complete resolution will only occur once you feel the emotions that were associated with that person or event, and release all of those stored memories. Time doesn't take care of emotional wounds; it covers them up with fascial adaptive layer upon fascial adaptive layer. This is why over time we all solidify and all these physical symptoms manifest themselves.

Question: On what level of consciousness does this occur?

You experience many different levels of consciousness all at once. The fact of the matter is that we're always in all of these different levels of consciousness. We just aren't aware of it, so we remain focused and locked into a narrow, rigid, and linear focus. Unwinding allows you to move beyond that very limited focus and catapults you into your essence, the healing part of you that allows you to go through whatever your body needs to go through. Our limited focus is like an energy program that seems to be stuck; a frozen moment in time. It's an incomplete experience on the subconscious level that has not been resolved. When these various traumas of our lives have not been resolved, it appears that the subconscious is there to protect you. This is what has shut you down into these bracing and holding patterns that you have no conscious control over. You have no awareness of it. Willpower has nothing to do with it. You're out of control of it, which is magnified by having been taught not to feel, not to trust your feelings or your intuition. As you open up to the memories and emotions being stored in your body, your body is now allowed to complete this experience in a very safe manner. I believe that nature wants us to learn from our experiences. The learning may not be on a conscious level, but there will be a learning. And as you receive this learning, your mind lets go, releases, and the body's tissue and structure can then let go. This allows true healing to begin.

Here is a typical scenario. Out of the blue you have an accident. It's as if nature has tapped you a little bit, but you don't pay any attention. It taps you again, smacking you harder each time until you get it. So the sooner you get it the better. It's not going to get any easier. You can't ignore it. It wants your attention and won't quit until it gets it, so you might as well deal with it. The way in which nature works with us is fascinating! The way in which unwinding allows us to open to the learning is also fascinating! Through these unwinding experiences you can expand because now you have access to other levels of consciousness. This is also true of your intuition. Once you get the feel of your intuition's guidance, you have access to it all the time. But you "don't know what you don't know, until you know what you don't know." Unwinding brings you into that space that you don't know. It unlocks the smaller world of the false ego and allows us to expand and identify with the vaster part of who we are.

Unfortunately a lot of meditative practices out there will tell you, "Don't move. Control yourself. Be disciplined." They mean well; they just don't know any better. While being still has value, there is also tremendous value in letting your body spontaneously move. We need both stillness and movement together. We need both! Stillness is important, it's where the answers come through to us, but we need movement to allow us to dispel frozen and scattered energy so that we can move further into stillness! Most of us are always moving to avoid stillness because of pain and fear. Unwinding ultimately allows you to move into deep stillness, and from that silent, still space a sacred and healing motion begins to occur and take you away. Myofascial unwinding is a unique and very special experience. Meditation opens up a doorway, but the unwinding kicks you right through it!

Question: What is a filter from the past?

Unresolved events and traumas from the past become trapped in the tissues. These past experiences become stuck because you haven't learned from them. They create a filter in your life; a rigid, restricted, habitual reaction on a subconscious level from which you now view life. When you face a current situation you react habitually, as if it was the same situation from the past. You are pulled back into that past filter of perception. Unwinding brings an awareness of these subconscious hold- ing patterns, these filters, up to the conscious level so that you can complete them. As you complete the experience, you are now in a position to respond.

John, could I expand on that concept from my own experience?

I told my story earlier of reliving my car accident during an unwinding which occurred during my treatment at "Therapy on the Rocks." The car accident headache never returned after that second treatment. I also went back to "Therapy on the Rocks" for additional intensive treatments following that bar exam study week, and the numbness in my arm receded and is now completely gone. I did visit the site of the accident to see if there was a yellow fire hydrant as I remembered in that first treatment. You guessed it! Here it was across the street just as I had remembered. The unwinding had tapped into my past memory and facilitated a release.

Myofascial release has transformed my way of thinking and being which I bring to living and the practice of law. I am now general counsel for a hospital where at least once a week someone comes by for some of that myowhatchacallit stuff. John has been given a rare and wonderful gift by the Universe, which we are so privileged to share in.

Since her accident, she has been bracing on the subconscious level, fearing she was about to hit the yellow fire hydrant and be killed. I know you've all been through this. Every time you are in a situation or with a type of person similar to one that hurt you, you "re-act" exactly the same way and you have no control over it whatsoever. How many times have you sworn that you will never do that again and two minutes later, you're doing it? And you get so ticked at yourself and the harder you try, the worse it gets. You have this very myopic option available to you and you keep "re-acting," "re-acting," "re-acting." But after you go through the unwinding, you have the ability to respond, which is very different than re-act. Now you have 360 degrees of options available to you. You are no longer living within that narrow perspective which forces you to re-act. You're open now to all sorts of possibilities, because you have released the attachment, the filter from the past. Now you can be back in the present moment. Otherwise you're functioning in past time. It's like you're living life looking through the rearview mirror, which doesn't work very well. This way you can be in the present moment and respond in the present moment. Unwinding may have to take us back in the past into some unpleasant memories and feelings, but that is very healing. Memories never injure. Feelings never injure. No one has ever been injured crying. It is not enough to just stop at neutral, because the potential is enormous. My feeling is that we should always help people go beyond neutral into areas of growth, enlightenment, joy, and ecstasy.

Talking about it will never get you there. Intellectualization will never get you there. It's the experience of it, the feel of it, and that is truly magnificent. This is why we teach all of our patients to unwind themselves. I would really like you to make a goal that you will unwind yourself daily. It doesn't have to take a long period of time. It is your own form of therapy, of stretching, of tranquilization, your own way of growing and enjoying life to its utmost. Myofascial unwinding is the healthiest gift that you could ever bestow upon yourself or another!

You can only take your patients as far as you are willing to go yourself! So it's really our responsibility. You know, I hear all the time, that when you first look into something, it's scary. That's natural. Don't try to stifle those feelings whatsoever, because you can take that fear and convert it into excitement! The thing that everyone says after unwinding, even when they've been dealing with an issue for ten or twenty years and they've been shoving it down for that long is, "That's it? I was so worried about that? I feel so much better now." It's so exhilarating!

[1] Selye, H. *The Stress of life*. New York: McGraw-Hill, 1976.

[2] Hameroff, Stuart R. Quantum coherence in microtubules: a neural basis for emergent consciousness? Journal of Consciousness Studies, No. 1, Summer 1994, 91-118.

[3] Scaer, M.D., Observation on traumatic stress, the whiplash model, Bridges Magazine.

[4] Levine, Peter. *Waking the Tiger: Healing Trauma*, North Atlantic Books, Berkley, CA, 1997.

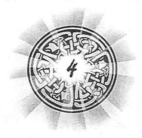

the quantum leap

Stedmans Medical Dictionary, Illustrated 23rd edition, Williams and Wilkins, 1976 states that the word *piezoelectricity* is derived from the Greek word "piezo," to press or squeeze, and "electricity." In other words, electric currents are generated by pressure upon certain crystals. The cells of our body are considered to have crystalline characteristics. Who would have thought that the concept of piezoelectricity could have such profound implications upon our therapeutic effectiveness?

The myofascial system is a piezoelectric tissue. What that means is that when the therapist touches another person, whether it be through traction, compression, twisting, or taking gravity out of the system, the system will begin to spontaneously move, as long as it feels safe. As the system spontaneously moves, it will eventually find a significant position in space that will bring up old memories, emotions, or sensations. These represent past trauma and allow the body then to learn, to shift, to heal.

When you, the therapist, lift a limb or body part with very soft hands, you lift just enough to take gravity out of the system, and then you wait. In most people it might take thirty to forty seconds before you notice some motion. They're making sure that they are safe. If nothing happens after a short time, we then slowly and gently apply traction until we take the slack out of the system. And we'll wait again. The motion that occurs feels like you're floating. It's a very different feel than conscious, voluntary motion. If after one to two minutes motion does not begin, try a little compression, very slowly and gently. If the person doesn't move,

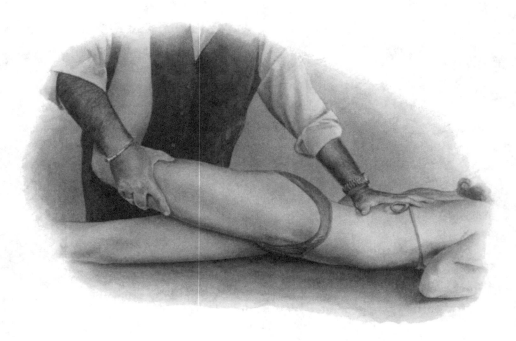

that's fine; that's their choice and prerogative. Develop the habit of moving slowly and gently. If you move too fast, the patient will go into protection. Allow your focus to be very soft. Come from your peripheral vision. The more centered you are, the more powerful you are. You don't force them to do anything. Know that when a person is truly unwinding, they will never injure themselves. Your primary goal is to keep them safe. You'll watch what the body is trying to do and you'll go with it. You stay in the center of the action at all times and that way you can easily handle things. You don't figure anything out. You just go with the action as the therapist. They know what they need, and it'll never be logical.

Myofascial unwinding is the spontaneous movement of the body via the mind. With unwinding, you will achieve tremendous fascial releases three-dimensionally. As with myofascial release, you might get a little sore afterwards or you might feel exhilarated. Everyone will have a different response.

Do not stop while a physical or emotional release is occurring. Not that you will injure the patient, but they will be more agitated than they need to be. You'll be stopping at still points, where the body spontaneously quiets and releases. Still points are very profound. As we take gravity out of the system, the influence of the body's various righting responses and protective responses is temporarily suspended. What's underneath is the unwinding, which has been there all along; but because we're always in gravity, so we're always in a state of protection. This is why we need to take gravity out of the system and create a safe environment. Remember it might take thirty to forty seconds for the patient to take the brakes off enough to start to unwind. Your mind, your memories, your emotions lie within the fascial system, despite what we were taught. When your body finds these significant positions, it will start to release them. Memories will come up which you were not even aware of, memories that you thought you resolved years and years ago, which have been creating so many of your current symptomatic complexes. You don't need to worry, though, because you will not let any skeletons out of the closet that you don't want out.

Question: Can we, the therapists, pick up their negative energy?

It's very important to stay centered so that you don't lose yourself in your patient's problems. We need to be clear in order to help them. As you are learning this work you may pick up some of their stuff, and it's going to be okay because this becomes a mirror for you, highlighting holding patterns within yourself. This then creates an opportunity for you to clear yourself further. But your ultimate goal is to stay centered. For me, the patient's energy flows through me like a mist of information. Remember, energy is simply energy; it is neither positive nor negative. It's our labeling process that calls it positive or negative. We will be getting into the concept of detaching from the outcome later, as it is quite important, and will help you to remain centered.

Question: Do you give patients permission to move?

Yes. They're not used to moving on the table, so they might feel a little strange to do so. It usually happens naturally, but if it doesn't, you simply say, "Slow your breathing, soften your body and if your body feels like moving, just let it go where it feels natural, and I'll guide you." If I'm holding their arm I might say, "If it feels like your arm starts to float, just let it go and I'll guide you." That's all it takes. A nice gentle way of introducing the possibility of motion to them is to have them begin in the sitting position and use the first phrase I suggested.

Question: Do you ever lead them?

There's something I call "testing the waters." I will nudge the person a little bit once in a while, and if they go easily I'll go with them. If they resist me, I will back off. You sort of experiment with the system. You can sense where they want to go, and if you're not sure, just nudge it and if they resist back off. Don't assume you know what they need. You've got to get your ego out of the way, and move beyond "right or wrong."

Question: Do you start a treatment session with unwinding?

I'll start with structural work, but often within the first ten minutes or so they're unwinding. I haven't told them to do it, it just happens naturally. If you're just getting into this, you'll usually work with the structure for a couple of sessions and then all of a sudden, unwinding will just start to happen. You're going to mix it back and forth, because as somebody is unwinding, you're going to be watching for vasomotor response. Vasomotor responses are areas of redness and heat that can be seen or palpated on the patient's body, indicating locations of other fascial restrictions. This form of body language is an accurate way of ascertaining where to treat them next. They'll begin to have certain sensations and you might want to go back to do a cross-hand release or, in some unwindings, they'll be stretching and you'll see exactly where the body is trying to stretch itself. It might need your help, so you might want to get your hands in there and help stretch it or pull that arm a little bit.

Question: Did you say unwinding is always occurring?

We are always trying to correct ourselves. We were just never given the opportunity to complete the process. I think I've mentioned this already, but so many of my patients say to me after they've been unwound, "This is the position I wake up in every morning." The body is correcting itself, but the bed gets in the way and it needs somebody like you or me to help take gravity out of the system or get the bed out of the way so they can do what they have to do.

Question: Is there always a lot of movement?

No, let me bring up another point. Just because someone else is having a vigorous unwinding and yours is very quiet doesn't mean you are doing something wrong. Some of the most profound unwindings will be totally still. You'll be with people and not much is happening and you think to yourself, "Oh man, I didn't do a very good job." They'll come back the next day and say to you, "That was the most profound experience of my life." Whatever happens, happens.

Question: Does the patient resist future unwindings?

No, they really look forward to it. They know they may go through some agitation, but it never injures. It's like letting the pressure out of a steam cooker. You always feel better afterwards.

Questions: Do you need bright lights?

You will learn through the development of your proprioceptive awareness to feel the center of the action. Many times during a lightning storm, the lights have gone out and I can perform Myofascial Release, Myofascial Unwinding, and/or Myofascial Rebounding just as well in pitch blackness. You can feel heat coming out of the body. You can receive as much information from the feel of unwinding as you can from the visual aspect. That's why I want you to soften your focus as much as you can; stop looking for the details and perceive the whole.

Question: What do you do when you are repeating a pattern?

When you have a pattern, it's usually rotary. If a pattern perpetuates itself I'll let it go three or four times, because maybe that's all they need to do. If it continues, then what we need to do is put a little more pressure into the system and just slow them down. You don't stop them; it's like a sea anchor, you just slow it down. Within that pattern, you'll feel a little glitch, and then, all of a sudden, they'll take a new route and you need to get out of the way, and follow their lead again into a new motion.

Question: How long have these techniques been around?

My sense is that various forms of myofascial release, unwinding, and cranial work have probably been around since the beginning of mankind, with many different names. What I see going on is a lot of fragmentation. Somebody does energy work. Someone does muscle energy work. Someone does a little cranial work. Someone does this pressure or that pressure. Too many times it's coming from a left-brain perspective, just focused on treating symptoms so it isn't always from a whole mind-body perspective. I think that you'll find that the Myofascial Release Approach is a synergy. There's a completeness to it, a depth that is very effective.

A lot of courses out there are the "old form" of myofascial release. Unfortunately, they're not waiting long enough, so they only achieve apparent change. They work with the elastic and muscular component and you get results for a couple of days or a week or so, and then everything comes back, because they never released the collagenous aspect! The other big missing piece is the position in space. It's the proper treatment of fascia and allowing the fascia to move via the mind to find its positions in space; this is so significant. So it's that combination of the structural and motion components of myofascial release that gets into the mind/body/emotional/spiritual complex, instead of just the mind or the body or the spirit or the crosslinks as separate entities. When you come from the right-brain perspective it's a whole different situation.

Question: John, I heard you talk about the older forms of myofascial and cranial techniques. Could you expand on this?

As I previously stated, I believe that various attempts at dealing with the fascial system via soft tissue mobilization, connective tissue massage, cranial work, and unwinding have probably been around since the beginning of mankind. But from what I have read and seen, these modalities were applied regionally or symptomatically or too roughly and/or mechanically. In other words, the above were an attempt to force a system that cannot be forced! It was painful to the patient and hard on the therapist, yielding only temporary results. As I gained experience with the myofascial system, I found that it responded quite differently than what I had expected from what I'd learned from the research on fascia. The research, which had focused on the three-dimensional web of fascia in dead people, basically states that you cannot release the three-dimensional web of fascia. I agree; the normal boundaries of the fascial system cannot be altered except surgically or from the enormous force of trauma.

What had been overlooked in the research was the importance of the ground substance and the crosslinks that can develop at the nodal points where the fascia glides upon itself. Restrictions develop from trauma, surgery, inflammatory responses, and poor habitual posture over time. Releases occur within the natural boundaries of the fascial system. Only a portion of the fascial system had been studied, and it was as if the scientific mind did not understand that there is a huge difference between studying a telephone pole and a living tree. My experience was quite different from what I had learned in school and from studying the research on the fascial system. Our model of reality is deepening and expanding with the help of new electron microscopes and sophisticated scientific techniques.

Science is in the middle of a deep-seated revolution. When you look at the evidence that the mind is not confined to the skull, you automatically expand the horizons of research. Many people are now realizing the ways in which we have been limited by these assumptions of science.

My approach to myofascial release is directed at changing the viscosity of the ground substance and releasing the crosslinks that lie within the natural boundaries in the fascial system. My daily experience demonstrated clearly that the myofascial system was moldable within its natural boundaries. It seems full of consciousness, awareness, emotions, memories, and life!

I stopped trying to force this system that could not be forced. I stopped sliding over the restriction. I slowed down and waited for the restrictions to release. I let the inherent motions of the mind-body (unwinding) to occur, and allowed the patients to express their thoughts, insights, emotions, and memories. The results and potential for healing moved into a consistency and a higher dimension that was significant. This deserves your serious attention. I firmly believe that the appreciation of these new, expanded, and refined concepts and principles allows our patients and ourselves to accomplish true, authentic healing.

It seems that the ground substance tends to lose its fluidity when it goes through trauma or an inflammatory response; in other words, it tends to solidify. It is what I equate to pouring glue or cement into the interstistial spaces. It is this dehydration of the tissue, with the accompanying development of crosslinks at the nodal points, that can put enormous and excessive pressure upon pain-sensitive structures and limit the fascial system's ability to glide. This enormous pressure, approximately 2,000 pounds per square inch,[1] can produce the symptoms of pain, headaches, fibromyalgia, and limitations of motion. Remember, myofascial restrictions do not show up in any of the standard tests (X-rays, CAT scans, myelograms, EMGs), so myofascial restrictions are being completely missed and/or misdiagnosed!

Question: What happens if you, the therapist, start to unwind while treating someone?

Sometimes when you are treating people with myofascial release, unwinding them, etc., you may start to spontaneously unwind. You don't have to stop it; it actually makes you more aware and sensitive. Just always keep enough awareness so that your focus is on them and that you are keeping them safe. You don't want to be on the floor blubbering yourself!

When you first start doing this work, a lot of you will still keep trying too hard. You want to do it right. You're worried about what other people think. You'll get past all of that eventually, and as you get better, what you will find is that it just gets easier and easier. We can't force anybody to unwind, nor should we. They will always go into protection if it doesn't feel right.

Give the patient a "control word" like "Halt" or "Stop." Please always respect that instantaneously. If your patient is always saying "Halt," ask them to check themselves out and make it a learning experience. It is their right to stop the process, but have them ask themselves, "Why am I putting my brakes on when I have the possibility to make significant change?" Encourage them to look at their patterns and give themselves permission to stretch beyond their patterns, to give themselves permission to go beyond their comfort zone, where there will be tremendous growth without risk of injury. Let them know they can stop the process at any time. If they start to unwind and get themselves into a position where they may be uncomfortable, they can stop the process again. You can always start the process up again at another time, when they are ready. Give them time to reflect upon this statement: *we never learn in our comfort zone!*

Question: Has an understanding of consciousness eluded brain researchers because they have limited their focus to the brain?

A major international conference was recently held in Cambridge, England, called "Beyond the Brain: New Avenues in Consciousness Research." Speakers included many of the world's most eminent theorists of consciousness experience, including Nobel Laureate physicist Brian Josephson, neurologist Stuart Hameroff, psychiatrist Stanislev Grof, evolutionary scientist Ervin Laszio, and psychologist Charles Tart. The conclusion of the conference is that there is evidence of a shift away from the premise that consciousness is a mere byproduct of brain processes.

Reductionists tend to overlook the fact that neurons are alive. Traditional views of the hierarchial organization of the brain stop at the synapse as the fundamental switch, analogous to bytes in computers. The complexity of neurons and their synapses, however, are closer to entire computers than individual switches. This implies that the mechanism of consciousness may depend on an understanding of the organization of adaptive (cognitive) functions within living cells.

The old way of observing this phenomenon was to try to break everything down into its lowest common denominator: the reductionist model. Until quite recently there have been very few experiments set up to observe the living system. Biology has a long tradition of fixing, pinning, homogenizing, extracting, and fractionating. This unfortunately gave us a very limited and distorted understanding of the interrelationships of the whole living system.

Question: Does this mean that information and consciousness are two words for the same phenomenon?

Yes, I believe that information, consciousness, awareness, your electro-magnetic field, your mind, and love are different labels for your essence.

Question: Are you saying that your mind resides in the myofascial system?

Yes. My experience has been that consciousness infuses our entire being. For years I have taught that fascia, on the microscopic level, is actually a three-dimensional web of tiny, hollow tubules filled with fluid, which carries information. This information, in the form of thermal, electromagnetic, and mechanical energy, is transmitted to all aspects of the mind-body complex via myofascial release for healing on the deepest level.

Question: Is fascia the physical basis for the emergence of consciousness?

Recent discoveries support this suggestion. Two of the leading researchers on consciousness, mathematical physicist Dr. Roger Penrose and Dr. Stuart Hameroff, have stated that past brain/consciousness research had been severely limited by scientists not looking deeper than the synapse of the nervous system. With the help of new, sophisticated electron microscopes capable of incredible magnification, Drs. Penrose and Hameroff have discovered microtubules filled with fluid within the cytoskeleton of the cell.

The famous neuroscientist C.S. Sherrington observed that the cytoskeleton may act as the nervous system of single-cell organisms. Synaptic connections are formed and regulated by cytoskeletal polymers, including microtubules. Drs. Penrose and Hameroff speculated that the cytoskeleton is like a micro-myofascial system within each cell. This micro-myofascial system is made up of a skeleton of tubules filled with fluid, surrounded and interconnected from cell to cell by a viscous ground substance. They go on to suggest that using the quantum field theory, the ordering of the water molecules and the electromagnetic field confined inside the hollow core of the microtubules manifests a specific collective dynamics called "super radiance." Accordingly, each microtubule can transform incoherent, disordered energy (molecular, thermal, or electromagnetic) into coherent photons within its hollow core.

This information supports the continuity of the myofascial system from the inside of the cell to the very periphery of our being and the holographic model of reality in which photons (light) are transmitted as information throughout the mind-body complex. Consciousness (information) is necessary for healing. Consciousness may emerge as a macroscopic quantum state from a critical level of coherence of quantum-level events in and around a specific class of neurobiological microstructures: cytoskeletal microtubules within neurons.

Question: John, how does this relate to treatment of the myofascial system?

This information about how information/consciousness is transmitted through the hollow core of the microtubules to all aspects of the mind-body helps to deepen our understanding of the piezoelectric effect when the myofascial system is treated. The fascia is a piezoelectric tissue; therefore, when a therapist utilizes the gentle, sustained pressure of myofascial release through compression, stretching, or twisting of the myofascial system, it generates a flow of bioenergy (information) throughout the mind-body complex by the piezoelectric phenomenon. This facilitates the extracellular matrix to transform as it undergoes its solid to gel reorganization during myofascial release. Fascia is behaving as an electrically conductive medium that allows this visco-elastic tissue to rehydrate under the sustained pressure of the therapist's hands. This rehydration also allows for an elongation of the myofascial system, relieving the pressure on pain-sensitive structures for alleviation of the symptoms of pain, headaches, and the restoration of motion.

So we are connected—for deep within each cell of our being flows information/consciousness via light energy (photons) throughout all aspects of our mind-body.

The incredible magnification of our new electron microscopes has allowed scientists to see myofascial structures within the cell that expand our knowledge and provide us with a more accurate understanding of our fascial system and its importance to the healthy functioning of our mind-body. There is an avalanche of new information coming out on the deeper structures of the cell, the myofascial system, holography, and the piezoelectric phenomenon. Myofascial release and the other excellent "hands-on" therapies give the therapist powerful healing techniques to effectively, cost efficiently, and comprehensively help their patients realize their full potential.

John, your construct was quite clear. This framework of words will give their intellects something to cling to...a foundation of symbols from which they can soar into experience and knowing. As these young, potential healers grow and mature in this work they will eventually need to let go of theories, words, and symbols. Remember: for those who believe, no words are necessary; for those who don't believe, no words are possible.

Your task, and it is a daunting one, is to lead them out of the darkness and confusion of being "word worshippers" into the light of true experience. Move them beyond trying to compulsively know into "knowing!" No word, phrase or symbol can ever adequately describe any experience. Have these healers use theories as plastic, moldable, ever-changing frameworks from which their intellectual constructs become a springboard allowing them to use their instincts and intuition to flow into true experience.

As The Ancient Warrior was talking to me, I could also hear myself saying to the audience:

"Don't believe a word that I say. Only from your direct experience will you be able to decide upon the value of my words. Experience is the best teacher!"

After class that day, I went to my room and felt the need to continue the conversation about the crippling effect of just relying on words and theories. I slowed my breathing, quieted down and asked, "How do I overcome the resistance to those still interested in the abstract world of words? Those who fearfully cling to the false comfort of words aren't going to like hearing..." I was cut off by The Ancient Warrior as he boomed:

I don't give a damn what they like! My purpose is not to please. My purpose is to guide! That is part of society's self-imposed blindness. Too many spend their lives seeking pleasure, only hearing what they like, desperately staying in their comfort zone! One never grows in their comfort zone! One must leave the false security of their comfort zone to grow. It takes courage to leap into the unknown! Because of their training too many make excuses for their limitations. Where is their curiosity? Where is their courage?

"I agree. Some of the language you use and your intensity amuses me."

I am just speaking your language, so that you will listen and understand. I am mimicking your intensity. Speaking the patient's language lowers their resistance and increases the clarity of communication. Isn't that what you teach your students to do when they dialogue with their patients? Speak their language! No judgement, no criticism, no shoulds; just mirror back their language, especially those words and phrases that have a high emotional tone. Let them look at and feel what they are saying and thinking. Let me mirror back to you. Look at yourself in the mirror of my perception. You have always been very curious. Your awareness comes from a deep stillness. You are like a big cat, a panther. Your courage has been tested many times; your skills have been honed over the years. You sit back and observe in silence. You love nature, beauty, and other beings, but have the prowess and courage to pounce when attacked. So when I speak to you, I offer you guidance, wisdom, and direction in a mode that you will hear. I am usually soft, but can be direct and firm when required.

"I understand and have always appreciated your loving concern and guidance. Even though at times I didn't like what I was hearing, I have always trusted you, my intuition. I appreciate your directness and firmness. I remember the fortune cookie you suggested I pick up one day, years ago...and with your help, I have lived my life in accordance with the message inside that fortune cookie: 'Be as soft as you can be, yet as hard as you have to be.' That to me is balance; each attitude is appropriate depending upon the circumstances, when done with awareness and love."

✧

[1] Katake, K. The strength for tension and bursting of human fasciae. J. Kyoto Pref. Med. Univ., 69: 484-488, 1961.

letting go

One day while treating myself on the floor, something happened with an impact that would change my life forever. While pushing into a tight myofascial restriction, my body started to move spontaneously. It felt right, so I allowed this motion to continue, although I didn't understand what was happening. I then heard my guide, The Ancient Warrior, say something, but it was faint and I didn't understand what he said. As I continued to move spontaneously, I asked, "What did you say?"

Put your hand on your sacrum and push down.

I have learned to trust my intuition, the Ancient One or Ancient Warrior, depending upon his mood, and pushed my sacrum down. It started to hurt intensely and an electrical sensation was fast developing. I was about to take my hand off, for I was concerned that I might injure myself.

Wait until it releases.

I had never heard of the term "release" in that context before. I continued to push my sacrum and all of a sudden my body arched and I heard myself scream. It seemed like I was having an "out of body" experience, as if my consciousness was high above my body watching me on the floor screaming. I then felt like I had gone back in time to when I fell while weight lifting with three hundred pounds. I lay there stunned and confused, but also realized that something significant had just shifted in my mind-body! I recognized that my body had just returned to the position of injury. After the initial soreness wore off, I felt so much better and was moving freely again. All of my treatments worked so much better after that experience. Looking back, I realize that this was my first experience with what we now call myofascial unwinding. Many of the principles that I now teach and utilize in treatment with myofascial release and myofascial unwinding I learned from that initial experience.

After that experience, I was very different as a therapist and as a person. As I treated patients, I could feel a warm, tingling flow of power run through me and into my patients, dramatically improving their results. Many of them now began to spontaneously unwind. They loved it. At times, some of my patients, during unwindings, would express emotion. After they expressed their emotions, they seemed much calmer and more at peace. Initially, I wasn't comfortable with their emotions. When I was a teenager, I was taught that emotions were for the weak, and as a man I was to be strong and tough, so I was tough.

But I noticed that as I was doing myofascial release and as the unwinding began to occur, these warm, tingly sensations would flow through me as the person would release. As they started to become emotional, I started to feel with them. I realized that something much greater was happening than just what I could physically do with somebody. I was learning to get out of my own way. I was learning not to push people so much and to trust that there was a deeper part of them that knew exactly what to do. And a couple of times, when people had become very emotional in the room, that night on the way home in my car, I started to cry. I started sobbing so deeply, I literally had to pull off the road and finish it. I had no choice. I was becoming very concerned, because I thought I was losing it. I've learned that losing it is a good thing, because I started to feel so much better afterwards. I have now come to see how powerful our emotions are and, as they are expressed, our emotions can be our teacher. So, over a long period of time, with many twists and turns, I have been able to synthesize an approach to myofascial release that I can teach to physicians, therapists, and our patients to help them help themselves.

Question: John, after you spontaneously unwound yourself how did you summon up the courage to unwind someone else?

One day I was treating a lady who had been all over the country, seeing many of the leading TMJ specialists and physicians. She had very severe head, neck, and back pain, and a massive TMJ problem for over fifteen years. She was getting so bad that for the last four years she could not open her mouth much further than an inch. I began treating her one night at about eight in the evening. She was my last patient. As I was treating her she started to move. I recognized that she was unwinding. She moved and moved, and all of a sudden she started to move faster than I have ever experienced before. All of a sudden she somehow bounded up in the air. I caught her upside down and held her against my body. She slowly began to writhe down my body and started to scream. I asked, "What's the matter?" She said, "I think I'm being born." Well, I'd never heard of rebirthing back in those days, so I was getting a little concerned. So I asked, "What makes you think that?" She said, "I can taste the vaginal fluid." And I thought, "Oh my God, I've got a real nut on my hands here!" She slid down a little further and really started to scream loudly. I asked, "What's the matter now?" and she said, "It feels like my right shoulder's being dislocated." Eventually she landed on the floor and we both ended up under the table. Her arms and legs were flailing all over the place, banging against the walls.

Now back in those days, my assistants weren't used to noise coming out of the treatment rooms. So there I was, lying under the table, and all of a sudden the door creaked open. One of my assistants peeked in. I just said, "Go home." So the door shut, and the woman kept unwinding for a while. Eventually we ended up sitting on the floor, totally disheveled. We were sweaty and our shirts were all rumpled up and we were looking at each other, stunned. And here's this lady who had not been able to open her mouth for years and her mouth started to open, and open. It opened so much that I was afraid she was going to swallow her own head.

She eventually went home. I didn't get a lot of sleep that night. I was pretty agitated. I was sure the lawyers and the police would be on the front step the next morning. I walked in and my secretary said, "so and so called you," and I said, "I expected she would." I called her and she said, "Oh, John, I just wanted to thank you. I haven't felt so good in fifteen years. I ate breakfast this morning for the first time in years.

My mouth is moving again!" She added, "I never knew anything about my birth before, so I called my mother last night to see if she remembered, and she said 'Oh yes, you had a very difficult birth. In fact, you dislocated your right shoulder'...."

There was something about that experience, as bizarre, wild, and scary as it was to me, that was so profoundly positive; I knew something very special had happened. I think that on some level it gave me permission for myofascial unwinding to happen again. From that day on, so many other people just started to spontaneously unwind. Over the years, I've been able to put together many other pieces and elements to it. It's been a real slow, zigzaggy kind of process, but through it all I've never injured anybody, nor has anyone I've trained.

So you don't have to be concerned. You will never injure anybody. There is an impeccable, amazing part of us that, when we allow ourselves to tap into it, will take care of us. Your mind is your protector and your healer. You don't unwind anybody; you just create the opportunity. If your patients trust you enough, they'll go for it with your guidance. They'll never be injured, and you'll see the most magnificent, lasting changes. Also, it will enhance all of the other structural work that we do.

A question I get a lot is "once you learn to unwind, is that all you do?" No, not at all. We are multi-faceted, multi-dimensional human beings. We all need some "J stroking," an occasional elbow up the back, crossed-hands myofascial releases, cranial work, off-the-body work, some dialoguing, and myofascial unwinding. We need a whole variety of techniques and approaches.

Question: What is the difference between therapeutic pain and injurious pain?

When you, the patient, are unwinding you will experience pain at times, but you will never do anything that injures you. You will many times get into a position in which you will shut down; you will go into protection. We've literally had people come in with bulging discs, pain down the leg, lateral shifts, and as they unwind their body goes into all sorts of positions—flexion, extension, side bending, rotation—and suddenly you hear the disc move back in and the back and leg pain are gone. The body will never do anything that injures itself. It will shut down and go into protection. That's why you never force. The pain that comes up during unwinding is therapeutic pain. The body will protect itself. I've seen this happen over and over again. If they're not doing what you think they should be doing, there may be a very good reason. Just give them permission to do whatever they do. Whatever is in their best interest.

You should not go in with any pre-determined agenda. If you're going to be a master at this, you want to go in each time fresh, as if you've never seen the person before, even if you've seen them many times. Allow every experience, every moment, to be new. Go in with this attitude and you won't get stuck in old patterns. It will be a very powerful therapeutic experience. Trust the patient: if the head doesn't go to the left, we're not going to take it to the left. There's a reason for that.

Question: Does myofascial release affect the acupuncture meridians?

Yes, absolutely. I believe that the acupuncture meridians lie within the physical aspect of the fascial system. It's a well-known fact in physics that if you take a copper wire and crush or twist it, it loses its ability to conduct energy properly. The fascial system is full of melanin, which is our body's superconductor, and the nervous system is full of neuromelanin. When you have fascial restrictions, it is the equivalent of twisting or crushing copper wire. The fascial restrictions are compressing the acupuncture meridians, and as they are being twisted and crushed they lose their ability to conduct the "chi," or bioenergy, properly. So as you unwind or do myofascial release you are opening up the acupuncture channels again, realigning them, and opening up space so that the energy can flow through.

Question: I occasionally find a patient who wants to just curl up during an unwinding. What should I do?

You will find a lot of times that the person will end up in the fetal position. It's good to let them be there as long as they want and as long as it feels right for them. Sometimes, if someone is crying or shaking and it's going on and on and on, encourage them to roll on their side and tuck up into a fetal position. Many times that will complete the process. I will wrap myself around them, put my hand on their head and sacrum and gently tuck them in tighter. They will have the most wonderful experience, one of safety and completeness like they've never had before.

And once they have that sense of safety, then it's theirs. You can talk about it for years, but it will never happen. It's the experience of safety that counts! So it's a wonderful sense of completion and peace.

Question: Why not start unwinding someone on the floor?

That's fine. You can unwind them on the floor or on a low table. But many times people will go through an old fall. Let's say you were a five-year-old child and you were playing on a second-story balcony and you fell off the balcony. On the way down to that cement sidewalk, you're freaking out; there will be still points in the air. You have to be in the air to find that still point to complete the process. Of course when you hit the cement there's a *major* still point! People become lighter when they unwind. Something very interesting happens to your relationship with gravity. But at any time somebody would be too big or moving too violently, you can stop them to go get help, so it is safe.

I was giving a seminar in Los Angeles a number of years ago. It was the first morning of the seminar and at the first break, a lady came up to me and said, "I've never felt this unwinding stuff. Could you just put your hands on me for a second and let me feel it?" She was a tiny little lady, in her mid-forties, probably about 4 foot 9, about 90 pounds. So I put my hands on her and about ten seconds later, she was in a heap on the floor. She just lay there for quite a long time. She eventually looked up at me without moving and said, "I feel like I have thousands of pounds on my body. I can't move." It was time for me to start the seminar again, and she was in the way. She was on a slippery wooden floor, so I figured I'd just push her out of the way, for I knew she'd eventually get up again. So I went to push this woman and she wouldn't budge. By now everybody is watching me, and I'm pushing and pushing and she is not budging. I went over to one of our instructors, a large male, and I said, "I don't know what's going on, but can you help me push this lady out of the way? We have to get on with the seminar." We had these two large males pushing this tiny little lady, and she was not moving. So we eventually gave up and we moved the seminar over.

Well, that was a mistake, because as I started talking to everybody, she started to come around. She was slowly and laboriously working her way up and she eventually got herself to her knees, but then collapsed. She started to push herself up again and collapsed again, like Bambi on ice. So finally she stood all the way up and said, "That was an interesting experience. You know, I'm forty-five years old and all my life I've felt heavy. You know what you reproduced? When I was six years old, I had an anesthesia experience and I've felt heavy physically and emotionally since then. I've never felt this light in all my life." She's come to all our seminars now and done very well.

Another time in Los Angeles—a lot of interesting things happen in Los Angeles—we were doing a group unwinding of four or five people. It's a wonderful experience! It is quite a learning experience, and it's an opportunity to make a massive shift in your life in a very short period of time. A group called me over and as I got close to the group, the lady who was unwinding suddenly bound out of their arms, hit my thigh with her foot, and went up in the air. I caught her by the foot. I swear, if I hadn't caught her, she would have kept on going. Her arms were flailing wildly and stroking the air. Now, I'm not that strong to hold a full-grown adult that easily. It actually felt like she was pulling me up. All of a sudden she became heavy and dropped. I caught her and we guided her to the floor. After she came down, she reported that the unwinding reproduced a drowning accident, where she was desperately trying to get to the top of the water.

During unwinding, people will have these incredible experiences of mind-body memories that have been buried for so long, that have created filters, symptoms, total disorientation in their lives, and it makes such a difference once it all clears out.

Question: Can this help addictive behavior?

As far as addictions go, many times it will get to the core of why they had to anesthetize themselves or developed compulsive or addictive-type behaviors. We are not asking you to be psychiatrists or psychologists. But what we do want you to do, and what we'll help you to do, is to become very effective communicators. This will help you, or the counselor, to speed up the process and deepen it significantly. Most people have all the answers within them. This is why you never lead, and why you'll never injure anybody. What we do is get them to the point where they can get in touch with their own answers, get in touch with the memories that have been blocking their awareness of what's going on. This awareness allows them to heal past wounds.

Question: What do you do when the patient resists letting go?

Give them time. Be gentle. Over time, if this continues to block their progress, let them know that there is only so long that they can hang around the edge of the abyss, trying to decide whether or not to jump. **Dancing around, dancing around, dancing around, enough dancing...LEAP! The therapist creates the safety net so they can take the risk to leap into the unknown. Encourage them to embrace the chaos! Embrace the fear!**

A Therapist's Perspective

John, I've always seen unwinding practitioners symbolically as being like the Mother, supportive, caring, nurturing and cradling. It seems very receptive, loving, and forgiving. In the cradle of a mother's arms or the crescent moon (even reflecting the patient like the moon reflects the sun), I feel are good symbols. Unwinding is feminine (or yin) in nature; myofascial release techniques seem more masculine (or yang) in nature, in a conscious, balanced, and spiritual way. Myofascial release is an active catalyst in the healing process. Often a healing seems to oscillate between these two polarities. That's one way I perceive this powerful healing work.

A Patient's Perspective

I started sobbing as John walked into the room. Without control, I sat up on the table holding my head. I only knew he was "better" than other physical therapists. He was my last hope before they would fuse two cervical vertebrae and deaden all the nerves going into my cervical facet joints.

Even though I knew the surgery wouldn't help, I just wanted the pain, or me, to end. After being bedridden for nearly three and one-half years with severe cervical pain, fibromyalgia, and major depression, I didn't care what the

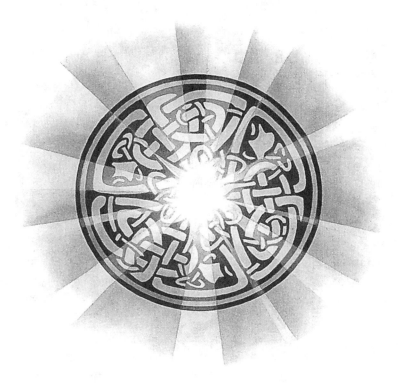

surgeons would do to me. But something told me to listen to my physical therapist, who insisted I go to Sedona, Arizona to see John F. Barnes, PT, at his Myofascial Release Treatment Center "Therapy on the Rocks."

Weeping. Hands spread from cheeks to ears. I couldn't stand the pressure. It was as if someone was blowing up my head from the inside. I couldn't think, I couldn't sleep. I could hardly walk. I just wanted to die. The door opened behind me. A dead silence palled the room. A sweep of air. He appeared at my side. In silence, we met. The depth of his eyes told me he knew and I was safe.

Hardly able to cry out a sentence, I staccatoed, "John, I can't hold up my head anymore. I get so tired, I can't hold my head up." Suddenly, I felt beautiful. As if he could see me as I was. As if he wasn't seeing me, but my soul. It was then I knew, I would survive.

Reality moved in. He asked about how a head injury began this chain reaction of disaster. Then, he moved in like a body mechanic. Checking for imbalances, rotations, restrictions, temperature, and textures, he quickly surmised my situation. Like an artist, he used his hands and his energetic intention to restructure my body. Without ever expecting it, I sat on a chair. He asked me where I was hit on my head. As I took my hand away, he smacked me right on the spot. A second of shock. My body quickly snapped up. I was whirling around in the same motion as my accident. Guided, I dropped gently to the ground. I was re-enacting my experience. The resultant emotions of the injury—regret, sorrow, and anger—spewed out of me. It was spontaneous, unashamed, and seemingly unending. Although I could have stopped it at any time, I knew, as a licensed Ph.D. and psychologist, that this came from the core of my pain. It was necessary for me to heal.

It was a striking beginning and a striking result. After two-weeks of intensive myofascial release treatment by John and his staff of therapists in Sedona, Arizona, the pressure in my head had gone away. It was the first time I felt I could be normal again. Instead of being hopeless, I was extremely hopeful. Instead of shuffling from one point to the other, I was able to hike the beautiful red rocks of Sedona, which is now my wondrous home.

A Patient's Perspective

This week marks exactly one year ago that I attended the Myofascial Release Seminar series. While John told the story of a patient of his, I became riveted to my seat. His patient looked and talked like my sister, who had fallen from a fifty-foot cliff several years earlier and was severely injured. My sister was slowly dying, and I took her to every doctor I could think of. Each of their diagnoses was different. I knew in that moment what was wrong with her and why her body was shutting down. As soon as I returned home from the seminar series, I called "Therapy on the Rocks" to schedule a two-week Intensive Myofascial Release Therapy program for her. The family was angry with me and questioned how I could take her in her weakened condition.

It was an opportunity for me to schedule my Skill Enhancement Seminar at the same time, so the two of us drove from our home in Utah. The drive was long, as we had to stop frequently. She was so weak. The second day after treatment at "Therapy on the Rocks" my sister responded in ways that I can only describe as miraculous. I was holding her legs when I noticed strange shapes come up in my "mind's eye." Shapes like bottle caps, pebbles, brush marks: all of the objects she had laid upon while being rescued from her fall years earlier.

After two weeks of therapy in Sedona, my sister was 100% different. While in Sedona, I learned that my other sister had scheduled surgery to have her coccyx removed. She had broken it thirty years previously, and had been unable to sit or have a normal life for many years. She joined us at "Therapy on the Rocks" and received myofascial release treatments. She is now pain free and just beginning massage school at the age of fifty-five to pursue her dream of helping others through myofascial release.

In one of the classes, John stated that "in this work the extraordinary will become ordinary." I am still in awe of the extraordinary. It occurs every day in my office when I place my hands on the souls of those who come to me for myofascial release. I have been afraid because I am not one of your seasoned therapists who have been practicing this work for a long time. But when I am most afraid I hear the quiet voice of John behind me say, "slow your breathing, quiet your mind, and say to yourself, I am focused, I am clear. Go where the action is. Trust yourself." When I am in this place of silence, I feel the hands and presence of another ancient one. She has taught me wonderful things in the past year.

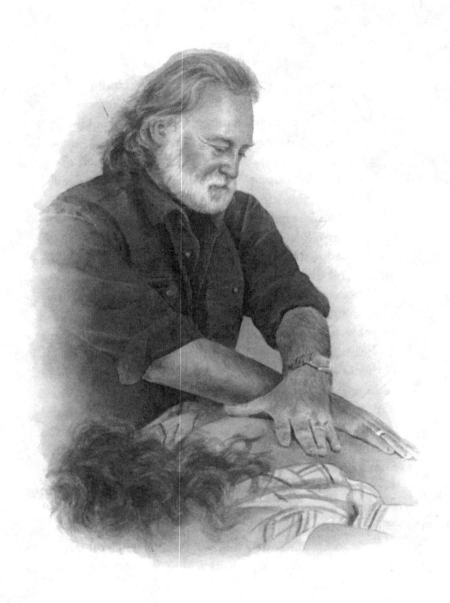

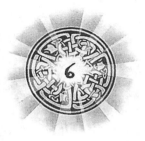

frozen moments in time

For years, I have taught that one of the many benefits of myofascial release and myofascial unwinding is the release of the holding or bracing patterns of the mind-body complex. It seems that during times of trauma the subconscious develops a protective pattern that becomes locked into the mind-body complex like a "frozen moment in time." I believe that it is these "holding patterns" that have frustrated therapists using traditional therapy in their efforts to help their patients have a speedy and complete resolution of their problems.

I want to pull together a number of the concepts and phenomena that we have explored. The Myofascial Release Approach is a very full paradigm with a multitude of principles, ramifications, and possibilities. By revisiting these principles and experiences from different angles, perceptions, and perspectives, it will deepen our understanding. Allow yourself now to absorb this information in a less analytical fashion and engage on an emotional level and a visual/felt sense. In other words, be there with me and the others as they share their experience. Feel their pain, their fear, and their desperation and allow their struggle to touch you. Get in touch with your own personal struggle and let it go. Free yourself! Visualize and feel with your "gut" the upcoming experiences. Flow with it and enjoy. I would like to now weave together this tapestry of concepts, awareness, and experiences to show how they interact, influence, and enhance each other for authentic healing and wellness.

Question: In a release of the freeze response, why do some patients shake during myofascial release?

The tremoring and the shaking that some of you may have already experienced and certainly will experience as time goes on has to do with what is called the "freeze response." A lot of this information came from a book called *Waking the Tiger* by Dr. Peter Levine.[1] You have all heard of the flight or fight response. It turns out there is another response, called the "freeze response." When I read this book I was fascinated because it began to explain, in another way, what my experience with myofascial release and myofascial unwinding had been for so long.

Let's say that you're an animal in the wild and that you're being stalked. When the animal attacks you, you have basically three choices. The first choice for your survival is to flee. If fleeing doesn't work, the second survival tactic would be to fight. If that fails, the third response would be the freeze response. That means you play dead. You've seen that happen with mice and other animals when they are caught. All of a sudden, everything stops and shuts down. Many times, when that happens, the predator will get bored and walk away. So that tactic saves the prey's life. If that does happen—if it's not killed, if the predator goes far enough away and the attacked animal perceives that it is now safe—its system starts to shake and tremble. The freeze response is thawing. It is discharging this tremendous amount of energy that it took to create the immobile state. When that energy is fully discharged, the animal will get up, move into a state of calm alertness, and run off. The animal has just healed itself!

We as human beings have an animalistic, instinctual side, but it's been pretty much denied to us in our society. What happens is that we don't shake off that energy; it becomes stuck in our system. We shut down into fear. We usually immediately are medicated, and this thawing of the freeze response never has the opportunity to occur. To tolerate this, the sympathetic and parasympathetic nervous systems go into a state of hyperarousal and they begin to fight against each other. As I said, it's like you're going through life with one foot on the gas and one foot on the brake. You're exhausting yourselves. This is why so many people are in a state of exhaustion. This encourages us to consider diagnoses like fibromyalgia and chronic fatigue syndrome in a new way. When you finally arrive at a still point, you begin to release. As the energy is discharged, you'll sweat profusely, make noises, and your whole body will tremble or shake. The patient's natural response is to get a little embarrassed and try to shut it down or control it. But the body is rejoicing, exclaiming, "At last, I can let this load go!" and doesn't want to stop. So encourage them to totally let it go. It's the body healing itself. It's the most natural thing in the world.

If for some reason they don't have time to complete the process, you can do the compressive/distractive technique, which is an emergency technique. That will mellow them out in a pretty short period of time. I feel that when you have a massive release like that, it mimics the hypoglycemic effect and epinephrine is poured into the system, so you could give them sugar or orange juice if they need to get right back into a car. But the best thing to do is give them a little time. Let them lie in a room. Give them permission to shake. Put a blanket over them and tell them to go for it and they'll be okay in a short period of time. The shaking from a freeze response is a very healthy experience.

Question: Is the freeze response similar to subconscious holding patterns?

Yes. I believe that the behaviors of fleeing, fighting, and freezing are so primitive that they are thought to pre-date the reptilian brain. These survival tools are found in all species, from spiders and cockroaches to primates and human beings. When neither flight nor fight will ensure the animal's safety, there is another line of defense: immobility (freezing), which is just as universal and basic to survival. No animal, not even the human, has conscious control over whether or not it freezes in response to a threat.[2] When an animal or human is traumatized, it will enter the freeze response as a survival strategy. This state of immobility is beyond conscious control and becomes a vicious cycle, maintaining physiologically high levels of activity of both the parasympathetic and sympathetic nervous systems. This is what I mean by bracing or holding patterns of the subconscious. It exhausts us and thwarts our efforts to help ourselves. We have no conscious control of these primitive responses fighting each other.

Question: Does myofascial release help fibromyalgia?

We treat and help many fibromyalgia patients at our Myofascial Release Treatment Centers. Fibromyalgia is the most recent "buzz word" for fascial restrictions. So, myofascial release and cranial work, and particularly unwinding, can be very helpful for that diagnosis. When you look past the fascial system, it is stuck energy. And what *is* stuck energy but an unresolved emotion. "Emotion" is a Greek word meaning "to move." Emotions are our fuel; they are what moves us! And when emotions are not resolved, they become solidified. This solidifies the ground substance, which tightens the fascial system, and it stays stuck no matter how many times you stretch it. Or, it lets go temporarily, but it pulls back again. This is why it's so important that we release the fascia: we release the mind through the emotions and any belief systems or messages. We are all integrated, so it's not enough just to release the fascia, not enough just to release emotions; we also have to release the belief system, or that will just pull us back into dysfunction. When the message comes up about what that was, whatever that interpretation was, the patient now is in a position to change that if they want to. Sometimes it's just the expression of the emotions that needs to be done at that point, and then all of a sudden, all of the structural work will start to work and will last. Start gently: people with fibromyalgia are very tender.

Question: Why do humans not respond as quickly as animals?

In humans, trauma occurs as a result of the initiation of the instinctual cycle, which is rarely allowed to finish. The duration of the immobility (freeze) response is normally time-limited: animals go into it and they come out of it in a short period of time. When the threat is over, the animal discharges an enormous amount of energy in the form of shaking, profuse sweating, and deep breathing. It then returns to a state of calm alertness. The human freeze response does not easily resolve itself because the supercharged energy locked in the nervous system is imprisoned by the emotions of fear and trauma. The result is that a vicious cycle of fear and immobility takes over, preventing the response from completing naturally. When not allowed to complete, these responses form the symptoms of trauma.[3]

Myofascial release allows for a completion of this instinctive cycle in a safe, natural and effective manner. Working in reverse, myofascial release and myofascial unwinding start with present-day restrictions and compensations. The release of fascial restrictions alters the habitual muscular "holding patterns." With myofascial unwinding, the therapist eliminates gravity from the system. This unloading of the structure allows the body's righting reflexes and protective responses to temporarily suspend their influence. The body, guided by the therapist, can move into positions of past trauma, which allow for a release of the instinctual freeze response in a safe, gentle, and natural manner. As this occurs, myofascial release techniques are utilized to eliminate structural compensations for a resolution of the patient's long-standing symptoms.

Imagine you were injured a couple of years ago. You received ongoing therapy in the form of hot packs, ultrasound, massage, electrical stimulation, exercise and flexibility training, joint mobilization and muscle energy techniques, medication, and psychological counseling, to no avail. All of the standard tests show nothing, and you desperately want to get better. You've been given a multitude of different diagnostic labels and all the experts are telling you there is nothing wrong. You feel imprisoned in a body that won't respond and allow you to play and work again. You feel helpless and out of control. What if something was overlooked? What could it be?

When many of us are injured, we go into a state of disassociation at the moment of trauma in order to survive. Our mind-body experiences an instinctive freeze response, and this positional, physiological memory becomes indelibly imprinted into our mind-body awareness. Because this positional memory becomes disassociated and locked in our subconscious, we have no awareness of it and, without conscious awareness, we have no control of it. This freeze response, over time, creates holding or bracing patterns that eventually produce increased chronic muscular tone, spasm, and myofascial restrictions that eventually become symptoms. Traditionally, therapy focuses on symptoms, explaining why modalities, exercise, joint mobilization and muscle energy techniques, massage and/or medicine can, many times, only produce poor or temporary results. Why didn't good psychological counseling help? Possibly because the majority of psychological therapy is done in consensus consciousness.

In other words, "talk therapy" is on the intellectual, conscious level, while it's our subconscious holding patterns that are perpetuating the symptomatic complex. It's like we want to watch a particular show on television, but we have been tuned into the wrong channel. No result! Myofascial unwinding takes you to the proper channel for healing to occur.

A Therapist's Perspective

I had become frustrated, using traditional therapy, when my patients presented with the same symptoms time after time, never seeming to progress. I was given a book entitled *Bodywork, What Kind to Get and How to Make the Most of It*. I got to the chapter on John F. Barnes' Myofascial Release and instantly knew this held answers for me. I took the Myofascial Release Seminar series in Dallas in '98 and returned home pain-free for the first time in twenty years! I couldn't believe at first that the application of the myofascial release touch could be so profound until I experienced it for myself.

My pain still manages to creep in at times, but I know now that in order to get through the pain, we must first fully experience it and embrace it as our friend...only then can we release it and allow ourselves the chance at beginning to heal. I am more able to guide clients through their own pain now that I've become so in tune with my own. I'm more at peace since having the privilege to share John's miraculous healing energy.

I was *alive*. Alive after experiencing the events of a car accident twenty years ago. I relived those events during a myofascial unwinding in Dallas while John was demonstrating a technique on me. By the time it was over, I had four people with me on the floor. I had cried, screamed, and cried some more, but I was so calm on the inside and pain-free! John said three words to me, "you are alive," during and after that unwinding, and I knew I truly had survived. It was awesome!

It proved the point of tissue memory to me without a doubt. It showed me that it is indeed not only okay, but *necessary* to go into whatever emotion or sensation that is holding us back from opening ourselves to becoming truly "all we can be."...Sorry, but it's true! Only then can we hold the power to help those who are on the same healing journey that we are all on.

I remember seeing John for the first time in Dallas. I had never seen someone with such a powerful and confident air about them, yet so open, loving, and willing to share that power with *me!* He had nothing but encouragement to develop the same qualities that he has, because we all possess the ability to become masters if we just get out of the way and allow it to happen. I was recently in Sedona taking the Skill Enhancement Seminar, and had the gift of working on a wonderful lady who had/was overcoming some monumental adversities, when suddenly John walked through the door, said hi, and sat down and started treating her. Well, the minute he walked in the room, we were all bathed in this wonderfully warm energy, and just knew something was about to happen. She was able to experience a wonderful unwinding and a quantum leap in her healing that I'm sure wouldn't have been possible without him.

Myofascial release frees these powerful, structural restrictions that place enormous pressure upon sensitive structures which produce pain, headaches, and restrictions of motion. Myofascial unwinding guides the patient into significant positions of past traumas. In the safety of the therapeutic environment, the therapist gently holds the patient in these significant positions of past trauma. In these therapeutic positions, the patient's tissue memory releases the instinctual bracing patterns. The freeze response is then deactivated, which allows for continued structural release and elimination of symptoms. The release of tissue memory creates awareness to return the patient to conscious choice and control of his or her destiny. The patient can then progress toward the ultimate goal of healing and health.

A Therapist's Perspective

Well, that week in Sedona brought about some profound changes and experiences. When John began doing some inner oral work on me, there was an extremely sore area on my right palate. I moved into an unwinding experience that would contract my body in a sort of extension position and squash my face to the point that it was difficult to even open my mouth. This would occur in a cycle of contraction, and then relaxation. Afterwards, while alone, I couldn't connect with any event or image that might have caused that position or emotion. As the group was commenting about the treatment afterwards, John suggested that I may have been experiencing a birthing experience. I really connected with that image at a lot of different levels. My mother had twenty hours of labor due to my posterior presentation. It was a preverbal event. I believe that is why I couldn't connect mentally with my unwinding. And it is why I believe that it has been hard for me to make sense out of some fears that seem to be ingrained in my psyche.

In another way that week was also a rebirth for me professionally. I came back with a new confidence in my gifts. My clients noticed the difference right away. I received comments that the treatment seemed deeper, and more profound. There was a willingness by my clients to share more deeply and it was not uncommon for a session to include tears, laughing, sobbing, crying out loud, and/or a whole new sense of release. It brought me tremendous satisfaction and joy that I had never felt before.

This experience is an excellent example of how an unwinding can take us back in time to a significant event. While dialoging has great value, many times the incident will be preverbal and the release will occur not through verbalization or intellectualization but as a felt sense. This is what I would call a physical learning, which is distinctly different from an intellectual learning.

Have you ever noticed that when you become injured, you keep injuring the same place over and over again? I think that when you are injured it hurts, you get scared, and you pull the feeling away from that area to avoid feeling the pain. What's another word for your feeling? Awareness, or your mind. So when you pull your awareness from the area you have no protection. You're out of your body. Since you have no protection, you keep hitting the same damned area, or having more accidents. It's nature's way of saying "get back in there." And with you out of your body, with your mind out there, with no awareness, no protection, the fascia does its job by tightening down to give you some support, some unconscious form of protection. The problem is that if it goes on for too long, you get so tight that it starts to crush everything and you develop physical symptoms.

Question: Why don't we stop at our own still points?

Because our left brain hates still points! To your left brain, still points represent pain, fear, horrible memories. You've lived your life in your left brain, thinking it's all there is to the world. It's doing its job, protecting you from those feelings and memories. The problem is, because we've been deprived of the other 90% of who we are, our essence, our healer, we didn't have this other side available to us to guide us into our still points. Sometimes the patient does need someone else like you or me to take gravity out of the system to help them get up in the air or give them the resistance or traction they might need to complete their process. It's their own mind that takes their own physical structure into positions that are important for healing. When they hit those positions, every physiological event that occurred at that moment will come billowing forth, every sensation, every emotion, every memory, and all the visuals. The body will complete that experience, allowing for an understanding on a very deep level. It does not always include the conscious level. Over time, we can learn to stop at our own still points. One learns that it is what allows us to heal. However, you can't get into some of these positions by yourself, and how would you ever know you needed to be in these positions to heal anyway? People are going to get into positions they haven't been in for ten or twenty years. They will look like a twisted pretzel upside down and they will peek at you through their armpit and say, "This feels great."

Once an unwinding is started, you can touch them just about anywhere. Stay centered, stay balanced. Watch where the action is and just go with the action. Keep your ego out of it. Remember that when the person is unwinding, they will never injure themselves. If you forced somebody into a position, it could irritate or injure them. But when they are unwinding, the person will never injure themself because their mind is their healer, their protector. So we're there just to take the gravity out of the system. We don't unwind anybody. They're unwinding themselves. Soften your focus and you'll see this energy around them. The physical body is moving within this energy, and it is this energy that is moving the physical body. Just watch and feel what the body wants to do and help it out. Stay in the center of the action. Remember that not everybody is going to move slowly. You must be aware at all moments. If all of a sudden they are reproducing getting hit by a car, they're going to go sixty miles an hour across the table. Be there and be alert, ready for anything.

Question: Can you stop the process if they move too fast?

There will be times when it will be very violent. Maybe they were in a high-velocity accident and their body needs to move very fast. If you are not comfortable with it or you are just afraid of it, just say "Stop." You can tell them that this can be done symbolically. Give them a pillow and tell them to hit it, or tell them to go home and beat up their bed. A lot of the time when we have anger or rage come up we are afraid that we are going to hurt someone else. This is why it is important to get it out. If you don't, it may happen. So that is why it is important to hit a bed. It's not enough to just say "I'm angry." You've got to express it fully in physical action. You hear about it all the time: the guy who went to church every Sunday, was a wonderful family man, suddenly took a gun and went up to a church tower and blew off ten people's heads. He exploded. So we have to let the pressure out of the steam cooker, and it can be done safely and symbolically. We have to let the freeze response express itself.

I've never been injured during an unwinding. I've taken a couple of hits, but they were accidents because I wasn't centered. If you are centered, you will never be hurt. There will be times where people start moving all over the place. Just get out of the way. Keep them safe, but get out of the way. You can keep them safe by using pillows to protect them, by moving things out of their way, and by redirecting them as needed. Again, you've got to get the pressure out of the steam cooker. It's like letting air out of a balloon. In these situations, don't even try to find still points. Some people just need to let it out because they're about to explode. When they don't let it out externally, they explode internally.

N

A Therapist's Perspective

I remember in Myofascial Release II, John was demonstrating myofascial release in the mouth. I desperately wanted to disappear into the wall. "I CAN'T DO THAT ONE." Throwing up a prayer, "please God let me get the right person" and opening my eyes to see a sweet gentle face looking down and asking "would you like to be my partner?"

Lying on the table in the dim room saying okay! I trust you and this work, and I will say "NO" if it is too much. Dropping into the willing place, going for the last vestige of that unspeakable night and having it release softly, quietly, gently as silent tears trickled down, dampening my hair. Deep! Deep release! Emotions! Fear, shame, sorrow, and joy mingling with gratitude to the hands whose touch have made this safe and for the sense of safety felt in this group. Thank you!

N

Question: Can this help with paralysis?

Yes. A forty-year-old lady, diagnosed as quadriplegic, was referred to me. She had been in a car accident and her car had turned over. When she woke up she was paralyzed from the neck down. She went for traditional physical, occupational, and speech therapy for about a year and a half, when she plateaued. They gave up on her and she was referred to us. During the first treatment session with me, she went into a spontaneous unwinding and went back to the position she was in during the car accident. She got in touch with the fear of waking up and the horrible feeling of not being able to move and thinking she was dying. She said that after that unwinding, she took the first large breath she had really taken for two years. She felt more at peace. She now is to the point where she can hug me, move her fingers, and she has done seven squats. It's not always going to happen, but imagine how good it feels to them that they are moving again. What happens when we become injured is we leave our bodies, and myofascial release brings our essence back in so we can deal with the situation a lot better.

I would like to share two letters from a couple of very courageous men that I have great admiration for.

A PATIENT'S PERSPECTIVE

In October of 1990, my terrestrial journey suddenly deviated from the norm. Crossing the threshold of tolerance, chaos entered my life in the form of serious injury, challenging me to pursue the meaning behind this event, while redefining my concept of health.

It was over within seconds. Enough time to utter the words, "Oh my God! I can't believe this is happening." In a bizarre moment of sheer terror, my pickup truck rolled, first sideways several times, then managed a hood-over-tailgate roll, landing with an eerie thud upright, with all its tires flattened. A repulsive odor of burnt rubber mixed with gasoline fumes lingered in the air.

I crawled away from the wreckage on my elbows for fear that the vehicle would explode at any moment. Then shock set in. My body shook violently like I was having some wild (Kundalini?) epileptic experience. What felt like a thousand volts of electricity emanated from the base of my spine and assaulted my helpless body. I tried to move my legs and wiggle my toes, but it was hopeless.

A flurry of flashing lights and emergency vehicles soon converged onto the scene. I wondered if this was the way that my script would end? Inside the screaming ambulance, I pleaded for someone to shake me from this petrifying nightmare.

Almost as scary was the cool, steel-gray-looking environment of Intensive Care. The room was a blur of strange faces, blinking lights, and technological sophistication—more than I ever cared to experience—and made for a surreal atmosphere. (Hope seemed to float through opium-loaded syringes.) I craved that morphine hit every four hours. The room spun.

En route to the operating room, fear gripped every cell in my body. They were about to open up my back, exposing the spinal column. They used hardware to repair my broken back—screws, rods and pins. (Three years later I requested that they remove this hardware.) Later, in recovery, the verdict echoed in my mind. According to the specialists, I was a paraplegic and would need catheters to void, drugs to produce erections. Walking was something I would only do in my dreams.

Following this traumatic episode, I endured many months of a "rehabilitation system." Everything was constructed for safe and easy access. I felt totally dependent on others. Doctors, nurses, physical and occupational therapists, dieticians, psychologists, and social workers were a daily reality. My days were a whirlwind of specialization. I struggled through months of rehabilitation just to regain a sense of equilibrium. I would find balance once again, but my lower half, everything below the waist, remained numb, paralyzed. Eventually I mastered wheelchair skills, managed my own self-care and felt well enough to face the real world—a world built for an able-bodied population.

Although my prognosis was grim, I remained optimistic. I resisted tuning out from the world, despite the harsh reality that I was no longer able to work as an interior photographer, enjoy spontaneous sex, ride my knobby-tire bike, or feel like I was participating in our society. I still believed there were avenues to explore.

Paradoxically (ironically?), my journey to heal a broken body, disillusioned mind, and wounded spirit offered an opportunity to open the window to awareness. I imagined an intricate web of nerves jutting out of my spinal column that extended throughout my lower limbs and the rest of my body. I would send my thoughts down those pathways communicating with the rest of my body on a daily basis. (And still do!) Reconnecting my mind to my body required a shift in consciousness and in doing so, my quest slowly revealed insights into this invisible healing energy or Divine presence.

In 1992, guiding my decision to re-enter a therapeutic program, was this will to explore optimum healing. My dedication to striving for optimal recovery was not unlike an Olympic athlete hungry for gold. Our objectives may have been different, but the mindset was comparable. This hunger continued as I selected practitioners who believed in the body's innate capacity to heal and find its own synthetic-free state of balance. My will to heal led me to practitioners who relied on touch as a way of restoring my function.

My physical therapy (at a private clinic in Toronto, Canada) was complemented by massage therapy, shiatsu, therapeutic touch, strain/counterstrain, Reiki, and craniosacral therapy. But the one approach I began to use more often and found extremely beneficial, on many levels, was myofascial release. My commitment developed into a five-year weekly journey into an internal environment.

When therapists first began to address my complex issues, using hands-on approaches, I noticed how my body would resist their efforts. Pain, scars, a fragile sense of self, a broken back, and other interruptions would surface while being touched. Intensives in the U.S. provided the means to calm my system, allowing a natural flow of energy to work through the barriers.

In 1994 and 1995, I attended two-week myofascial release intensive treatment sessions at the Myofascial Release Treatment Center in Sedona, Arizona. The first time I met John Barnes, in addition to treating me with myofascial release, he insisted that we, clients and professionals, all participate in a "grounding" exercise down by a dry riverbed. The trek down was rough terrain, red-rock country. With wheelchair in tow (they carried me down most of the way!), I participated. In Celtic mythology, flowing rivers are one source of Mother Earth's healing powers. But this was a "dry" riverbed?

We found an area for our meditative purposes. Within minutes of our forming a circle, and being still, wildlife peeked out in curiosity. I believe an owl let its presence be known. A gentle breeze took on a spirit-like quality. John coaxed me into the center of the circle, where I proceeded to tightly wrap an imaginary tail around the earth's core. I felt a powerful surge of energy though my legs and out the top of my head. The feeling was transformational—feeling connected to nature's potency was essential for optimum improvements in living.

I began to tune into mindfulness. The calmer, more meditative the state I put myself in, the easier it was for my therapist back home to do her work. Stretching tissue and removing the obstacles that obstructed the flow was an aspect of my therapist's job. My part was to let go of stuff with each exhausted breath. Therapy became this working relationship: the more I worked with her, the quicker this release would be. I felt in complete control of this entire process.

As the years passed, my improvements were phenomenal. By 1994 I had progressed from a wheelchair perspective of the world to walking short distances with elbow crutches and braces. I felt like a toddler discovering the purpose of their feet for the first time! (The feeling is still with me today!) Not only was my ambulating improving, but a year earlier, my efforts at pushing to void were finally being rewarded. I tossed out my catheters. Erections became a Divine gift! I began to date once again and no longer needed drugs to produce ecstasy.

Many therapists helped me push the limits of optimum recovery. These drugless practitioners worked on my body as a whole functioning unit—not as separated parts. Each shared their particular philosophies and techniques for facilitating a healing process. These insightful human beings stressed the virtues of remaining flexible, staying open, and sensing the subtle connection between mind, body, and breath. This insight guided their work, and revealed a higher understanding of the inner mechanisms that make us tick. Therapists using myofascial release not only played a significant role in my understanding of holistic health, but their touch helped me transcend my disability, influencing a healing journey.

Healing is indeed a complex journey, and a collaborative effort is needed. Gentle hands, calm minds and intuition encouraged my mind-body to unwind, relieve pressures, and breathe rhythmically, creating a space that allowed me to melt away myofascial release restrictions. Engaging my mind-body in positive internal dialogue provided a way to tap into nature's healing powers.

Today, feeling the warm spring breeze caress my smiling face while riding my knobby-tire bike is no doubt exhilarating. But recently, I experienced the pleasures of walking (trekking) through the jungles of Costa Rica using a single cane, heightening my sense of accomplishment with every step.

Once harnessed, the power of the human spirit is awesome.

A PATIENT'S PERSPECTIVE

All my life I've been a very active person. I grew up out in the country so there were always chores that needed doing. I raised animals for stock shows, was a competitive skeet and trap shooter, played on city and school baseball and football teams. But for as long as I can remember I have always loved motorcycles. I received my first motorcycle as a Christmas present at the age of eight. I even pushed it into my room and slept with it the first night. When I was in seventh grade I started racing motocross. I started with local events and as the years passed, my love of speed and competitions grew. By high school I was racing all over Texas with good results. By the age of seventeen I was racing expert class and focusing more on motocross than school. During that summer I picked up some good sponsors and decided to make a go at becoming professional. Over the next couple of years I should have received the hint to rethink my decision, considering a few setbacks (knee surgery, broken ribs and a collarbone), but I continued to pursue my goals.

In the summer of 1986 I was nineteen and looking forward to a promising racing season. My motocross bikes were fast and I was in the best shape of my life. My daily routine consisted of weight training, ten-mile bike rides, and hours on practice tracks trying to better my lap times. On June 11, 1986, my life as I knew it changed forever. It was a Wednesday afternoon and I was practicing at a racetrack in a small town outside of San Antonio. I had ridden this track around six p.m. with anticipation of practicing under the lights with many other riders until around ten p.m. On my first lap I was riding about three-quarters speed and went over a double jump that I had passed over hundreds of times, but this time my back wheel caught the top of the second jump and threw me down over the bars. I landed on my head and rolled on my back. I lay on my back knowing something catastrophic had just happened to my body. My legs felt as if they were floating up and away. I was able to move my arms but without feeling or control.

I'm now thirty-three and medically considered a C5-6 complete quadriplegic. In retrospect, the actual accident was painless compared to the ensuing minutes, hours, weeks, months, and years of life-changing events that have occurred.

Rehab was more of an emotional than physical struggle, mainly because I thought the paralysis was temporary and that I didn't need to learn the skills necessary for life in a wheelchair. Within the first year reality set in, and in a big way. I spent a total of ten months in and out of rehab centers throughout the state of Texas. My family was my support and spared no expense finding me the best rehab possible for my quest to renewed independence.

Early on, medical problems consisted mainly of bladder infections, bowel constipation, and leg spasms. I saw one PM&R doc for treatment. He routinely prescribed the medication of the day. Antibiotics for bladder, loads of Baclofen for spasms, and more than I want to remember drugs, laxatives, cleansers, etc., for the bowel problem that would continue to burden me and restrict my life. Without alternatives, I dealt with it. As my life had become more structured with a fifty-plus-hour work week, I was not able to keep my daily exercise program of weight lifting, assisted standing, and lower extremity electrical stimulation in order to keep things moving as best as possible. But even with proper diet, exercise programs, etc., I still had to revolve my life around my damned medication and bowel program, not to mention all the pain. Because of this decreased activity my bowel became more and more of a debilitating problem.

My wife of three years is a physical therapist, and it was a new beginning for us when she took Myofascial Release I. Modern medicine had failed us time and time again. We knew there had to be a better, more natural way to approach these problems. My first experience with myofascial release was an arm pull from my wife on the evening of that first day of the seminar. Afterwards my arms felt two feet longer. Over the next year she continued her discovery of myofascial release and applied it to patients and to me. During Myofascial Release II, John's instructors offered to treat me during break. It took no time at all before I was unwinding off the table. It was an unbelievable experience for me and the others involved. After the initial unwinding my problems improved but I knew my body needed more of this natural healing approach.

Before my two-week Myofascial Release Intensive Treatment, I had dealt with years of bowel constipation and irregularity and had recently been diagnosed with a slipped disc at L5 S1. My slipped disc only increased my initial problems and added many others. Before arriving in Sedona, I seriously thought I would not be able to continue leading my life as I knew it. The pain had risen to an almost unbearable level, and the options given by modern medicine were unacceptable.

My two-week Myofascial Release Intensive with John and his staff was a journey of restoration! Not only did it take care of my bowel problems but also alleviated ringing in my ears and head pain (for which at one time I even had an MRI for diagnosis), TMJ, and blurred vision. Due to MFR my spasticity medicine has been cut in half. I was able to reconnect to my body and see it as whole. My back pain is 110% better, but due to my active lifestyle and long days upright in my chair it comes back every so often. But with the knowledge of MFR we can take care of it with leg-pulls, lumbosacral decompression, etc.

As I write this it's been over a year since my intensive treatment, and things are going great. It's also been over a year since I've seen a doctor for anything at all.

For me myofascial unwinding is the joy of restored movement. Beyond that...I can't put it into words.

Thank you John for restoring life. Mine as well as many others.

*

[1] Levine, Peter. *Waking the Tiger: Healing Trauma*. North Atlantic Books, Berkley. CA 1997.
[2] Ibid.
[3] Ibid.

reclaiming the feminine essence

Fascia has a tensile strength of over 2,000 pounds per square inch! In other words, fascial restrictions have the potential of exerting enormous pressure on pain-sensitive structures, producing pain or malfunction of the delicate pelvic structures. Certainly, not all problems have a fascial origin, but restrictions of the fascia are the cause of many of these problems in a surprisingly high percentage of cases, especially when all the tests turn out negative and medication only helps temporarily, or surgery did not change or even worsened the situation.

I cannot tell you how many times I have heard stories of women being seen by doctor after doctor, taking more and more medication, as months, and then years, pass. Desperation sets in—psychiatrists, therapists, psychologists, surgery, more surgery—nothing helps. In fact, it continues to get worse over time and begins to spread to assorted symptoms throughout the body. The woman begins to wonder if maybe it is "all in the head." Myofascial release is utilized for the treatment of fibromyalgia, menstrual pain and/or painful symptoms of pregnancy and childbirth, recurrent bladder pain and infection, painful intercourse, sexual dysfunction, elimination problems, coccygeal pain, painful episiotomy scars, and the list goes on. These problems can in many cases be substantially alleviated or eliminated by myofascial release, non-traumatically and gently.

Question: My husband and I have been treating patients with fibromyalgia. I have been wondering what might be going on at an emotional level? These patients come to therapy, tell about all of the doctors and psychiatrists they have had to see, and who have put them on one pill or another, but never really seem to come up with a reasonable explanation on a physical and/or emotional level. They are hesitant to dive deep because they have been through the "therapies." What can we do to help them?

What I feel is that the person's body has completely wrapped itself in protection. They are frozen. Protection starts very early, from an emotional crisis or a physical injury. By the time there is pain throughout the entire body, they have blocked out or forgotten what actually started everything. I am treating a girl whose fibromyalgia started as early as high school. I am convinced that this protection, the tissue memory, becomes an armor that eventually leads to completely frozen/solid bodies.

The medical community does such a disservice to these people because by the time they seek alternative therapies they have been on numerous medications and seen psychiatrists because the medications don't work (so it must be in their head). Finally they start to think it *is* in their head, but cling to the name "fibromyalgia" because it is an explanation, a diagnosis. It allows them to feel that they are not alone. The protection starts early on in their lives, but the myofascial restrictions only become thicker and thicker through the "doctoring" process.

Question: John, why do women seem to have more problems in the pelvic area than men?

First, let's examine the pelvic structural and functional differences in men and women. A woman's pelvis is wider than the male pelvis; therefore, the female pelvis is more easily torqueable. My experience has shown that over 90% of women have torsioned pelvises, which can create fascial strain patterns throughout the entire body and head. It appears that most of men's problems in the pelvic area arise from direct trauma; i.e., falls, athletic and performance injuries. A woman's joint surfaces are flatter, and therefore more easily moveable. A woman tends to have less muscle mass than a man does, therefore less support. Every time a woman has her menstrual period or becomes pregnant, relaxin, a hormone that relaxes the ligaments, is poured into her system, making her more prone to trauma. It is also my contention that most women (over 90%) enter the delivery process with unrecognized myofascial restrictions and severely torsioned and twisted pelvises. Under ideal conditions, the myofascial system should be flexible. However, when the baby enters the birth canal, the pre-existing, unrecognized myofascial restrictions within a torsioned pelvis do not allow for adequate flexibility and pliability, and both mother and child are unnecessarily damaged.

We need to consider some of the current diagnostic labels such as fibromyalgia (FMS), chronic fatigue syndrome (CFS), myofascial pain syndrome (MPS), and pelvic/menstrual dysfunction, which really are just the titles given to unrecognized myofascial restrictions.

The following information is paraphrased from an excellent book that I would highly recommend, titled *Fibromyalgia and Chronic Myofascial Pain Syndrome: A Survival Manual*, written by Dr. Devin J. Starlanyl

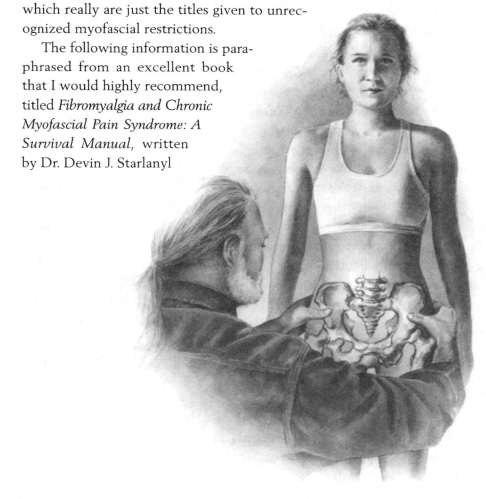

and Mary Ellen Copeland. "With Fibromyalgia, whenever the body enters deep (delta-level) sleep, alpha (waking) waves intrude and wake the sleeper, or jolt him/her into shallow sleep. Neurotransmitter regulation, muscle repair, and many other vital functions take place in delta sleep.... To make the diagnosis more interesting, every person may find different neurotransmitters and hormones and other neutral biochemical modulators affected, to different degrees. Many of the problems are cognitive—what we call "fibrofog" with short-term memory problems and other invisible handicaps. The pain and other symptoms can profoundly disrupt your life."

I would like to add a myofascial perspective to Dr. Starlanyl's insights: when a person with myofascial restrictions lies down to rest or sleep, the tightness of the myofascial restrictions do not allow the muscles to elongate properly. Therefore, this "straitjacket" of myofascial pressure and tightness does not allow the person to rest properly by entering into the deep "Delta State" necessary for rejuvenation. These people never seem to catch up and become chronically fatigued. Lying down with unyielding myofascial restrictions can also compress joint surfaces, the discs that lie in-between the osseous structures, which can then exert excessive pressure on nerves, blood vessels, and muscles. This scenario explains why so many people wake up exhausted with increased pain, headaches, spasm, and stiffness; this becomes a vicious downward cycle, slowly worsening over time.

Then we need to also consider the nutritional, biochemical, and hormonal components. Compound this situation of fascial restrictions and a solidification of the ground substance of the fascial system (the environment of every cell of our body), which are now interfering with people's cellular metabolism, cellular respiration, cellular nutrition, fluid flow, and cellular elimination. Almost all the information disseminated about the myofascial system in school was taken from cadavers. And the focus was on the three-dimensional fibrous web of tissue of dead people. We need to be more aware of another important aspect of the fascial system: the ground substance, which fills the space within the fibrous web and is the immediate environment of every cell of our body! With the advent of new, powerful electron microscopes, we are now able to see the architecture inside of the cell. It is not even *similar* to what we learned in school. It turns out that within every cell is a micro-fascial system, a tensegrity unit capable of both tension and compression, essential to the proper functioning and health of the cell and ultimately the mind-body as a whole.

The matrix or ground substance surrounding the cell is capable of compression, and functions as a two-way highway for the transport of oxygen, neurotransmitters, nutrition, and hormones, and the elimination of toxins.

As I give Myofascial Release Seminars around the country, I meet an enormous number of therapists and physicians. Many of them are on this diet or that, vegetarians, taking vitamins, supplements, or the latest nutritional breakthrough. And yet, despite their good intentions and best efforts, they don't look or feel very healthy or vital, and many still suffer with pain, headaches, fibromyalgia, etc. What have they missed? Consider looking at the myofascial system on the cellular level as a sieve. When we are traumatized, have surgery, or have inflammatory responses to illness, the ground substance of the myofascial system tends to dehydrate. As it loses its fluidity, it tends to become more viscous or solidify. This is equivalent to pouring glue into the sieve. In other words, it doesn't matter how much good food, medication, vitamins, or supplements we put in our mouths; if these substances can't get to and be processed by the cell, of what value are they? What has been ignored in today's health care is the vital role of the ground substance and the microtubules of the fascial system's main function to transmit our bio-energy or life force through the cells to all aspects of our being. Another word for bio-energy is love. Love is our basic and most important nutrition and healing power. Food, vitamins, etc., are just supplements to the important role of love flowing through us. Without love, life is a struggle.

So, as the ground substance becomes more viscous, it impedes the cells' ability to receive bio-energy (love), oxygen, and nutrition and its ability to eliminate toxins. So many people are barely functioning, in a state of exhaustion, poorly nourished, and/or not receiving the benefits of medication or supplements. They are poisoned and living daily in this toxic state with diagnostic labels such as chronic pain, fibromyalgia, chronic fatigue syndrome, headaches, depression, and exhaustion.

Myofascial release can be helpful in relieving pain and headaches, and in restoring cellular health so that we and our patients can again live life fully, healthy, and energetically.

What is fibromyalgia, really? What do fibromyalgia, chronic fatigue syndrome, chronic pain, headaches, pelvic/menstrual pain and dysfunction, and PMS have in common? These are simply different labels of a common denominator, unrecognized myofascial restrictions, which do not show up in any of the standard tests that are now performed, nor have most health professionals been taught how to recognize them. Myofascial release is the missing link in the relief of pain and headaches and the restoration of motion. Fascia surrounds and infuses every organ, duct, nerve, blood vessel, muscle, and bone of the pelvic cavity. Fascia has the propensity to tighten after trauma, inflammatory processes, poor posture, or childbirth. The American way of childbirth is extremely unnatural and can be very traumatic to the woman, especially if she has a pelvic torsion and/or fascial restrictions prior to delivery, and most do!

Myofascial release has helped many women with menstrual and PMS symptoms. Just picture the fascia tightening like a powerful three-dimensional net around the pelvic structures. Then as the woman begins to bloat as her menstrual cycle begins, the combination of fascial tightness and increasing internal pressure begins to exert heavy pressure on nerves, blood vessels, etc. The cramps, the tight back, and all the other unpleasant effects are a reaction to the abnormal internal pressure.

Inflammatory processes, such as endometriosis, can cause the fascial layers to adhere to adjoining tissues, creating pain and symptoms. Many times the fascial tissues will adhere around the bladder and the urethral areas. This creates the environment for infection, since fascial restrictions impede proper elimination of toxins and waste products from the tissues. If the fascia tightens around the bladder it can limit the bladder's potential to enlarge sufficiently, creating frequent or painful urination. When a woman coughs, sneezes, or laughs, urine will tend to seep out since there is no give to the bladder. The label for this is stress incontinence.

A PATIENT'S PERSPECTIVE

My life was in total despair when my husband pulled a brochure for "Therapy on the Rocks" out of a brochure rack on the way to the Grand Canyon on November 1, 1997. He said, "Maybe you ought to try this. You've tried everything else!" I said, "Don't say that unless you mean it, 'cause at this point I'll try anything!" We finished our weekend in Arizona and returned to Illinois, where I soon received the results of my latest MRI. The neurosurgeon said I didn't qualify for a spinal implant to stimulate the nerves to my bladder in order to restore my lost bladder function, but he would like to do another round of testing to determine why I had lost my bladder function after my third cervical disc surgery. I refused to have any more tests and picked up the brochure for "Therapy on the Rocks." I dialed the number and soon was speaking with one of their therapists. Suddenly, peace descended upon me. I felt as though I had come home. Someone understood what I was saying. My prayer to have someone heal my whole body was being answered.

I began treatment the next Monday, and my bladder function returned on Tuesday! The "Therapy on the Rocks" therapists had accomplished in less than forty-eight hours what even the Mayo Clinic had not been able to do in three years! By the end of the week I was off all of the $300-$500 per month medicines I had been taking.

As for John, he was not in Sedona during my first week of treatment; however, his being permeated every minute of my stay in Sedona. The twenty-first of November, less than two weeks after my treatments began, my husband and I met John in St. Louis, an hour and a half from our home. He was presenting the Cervical-Thoracic Seminar. When I walked into the room, John looked up from the stage and time stood still for me. The man who had given me back my life was standing before me in person, and life has never been the same.

Scars from abdominal/pelvic surgery or episiotomy can also create havoc in the pelvic area, as can trauma, causing menstrual dysfunction, pelvic pain, painful intercourse, constipation, diarrhea, and/or hemorrhoids. Recent statistics have shown that hysterectomies are performed, on average, every forty-five seconds in the United States. It has been determined that over half a million of these procedures are deemed unnecessary each year.

Another common problem we encounter is coccygeal disorders from trauma, pelvic torsion, and childbirth. A malaligned coccyx can cause a multitude of problems in the pelvic area, including some of those just mentioned, as well as back and neck pain and/or headaches, due to the influence of the dural tube that connects the pelvis inside the spine to the head. "When the coccyx moves closer to the pubic symphysis, the musculo-aponeurotic fibers from the pubis to the coccyx become so slack that they lose their tonus. If the origin and insertion of a muscle move closer together, a great portion of the muscle's power is lost. Typical symptoms of a sacrococcygeal lesion in a female subject are the inability to sit for long periods of time, declining quality of sexual relationships and cystitis. The coccyx can lead to a general decrease in the motility of the entire body, and it should be checked in people who are devitalized or suffering from general depression."[1]

A Patient's Perspective

Dear John,

The following series of events have been floating in my head since I first heard the word CANCER. Thank you for asking me to write it down. I would never have considered writing these events on paper, but now that I have permission, it is the right thing to do. I have told my husband and close friends what is going on but this does not seem to be enough. My mind continues to bring up possible scenarios (most of them not good) about the "what ifs." The following is the series of events that led me to you for treatment (thanks to my husband).

About a year and a half ago I went for my yearly GYN appointment (for me it's usually two or three years). I was told that I was overweight, that I needed to start taking Tums because I was losing calcium, and that I needed a mammogram. Never once was I asked what types of foods I eat or what kind of exercises I do. (I am presently in better physical condition than before I had my children, thanks to myofascial and craniosacral therapies.) I asked the physician's assistant why I would be losing calcium. Could she see it seeping out of my bones? She stated that it was because I was turning forty, that all women start to lose calcium at this age. I also asked why I needed a mammogram, instantly thinking that she felt a lump. She stated that age again was the factor.

I left the office feeling like I was falling apart. Turning forty was a terrible thing, and I might as well check out nursing homes for the near future. Again I talked to my husband about it, and a few friends. The more I thought about it the angrier I became. It's taken me a long time to feel good about myself and I felt sabotaged (it doesn't take much for me to bruise). After a while people became tired of me going over these events, so I tried to convince myself that the physician's assistant was terribly wrong and that I would not delay my next GYN appointment. I would talk to the gynecologist about the message his office was conveying to women forty and up.

One year later, I went to my appointment. My complaints were very patiently listened to. The remainder of the time I listened to statistical reports from the medical journals about women my age falling apart. I instantly knew where I stood. I mentioned bodywork, exercise, eating right, feeling right, etc.... The gynecologist wants to know where it says all that in the medical journals and where is the statistical report. I knew again where I stood. Results of my exam: I was told that my right ovary is enlarged, I need an ultrasound, I need to receive bloodwork for cholesterol count, I need to invest in Tums, and I need to set up an appointment for a mammogram. What am I supposed to do, get a second opinion and go through the same thing, ignore everything, or hurry to make appointments before I literally fall apart? By this time I am feeling great anger, but I am also feeling scared. What if they are right? I have children I'd like to see get married. My husband and I have great plans for when the kids are on their own. I don't want to have health problems. After feeling mad, scared, and sorry for myself, I decided that maybe I still have some control over my destiny. Forget the Tums, forget the mammogram, go for the simple bloodwork for cholesterol count, and go for the ultrasound. Besides, my ovaries were starting to talk.

The ultrasound was not as easy as I thought it was going to be. It hurts to have a full bladder (stupid thoughts that maybe I hurt because my ovaries are enlarged start going through my head). The technician starts to measure; I begin to start questioning. The more I question the more she is unable to tell me because she is not the radiologist. I hate the lack of control over my own body. The technician has to do the ultrasound vaginally because she is not getting enough information externally. Now my body starts to shake (like the shaking I experienced after having a baby). She tells me to relax. I hate this!!! Now I have to wait a week for the results to come through my doctor's office. I get to receive the information third-person.

The nurse calls to tell me the results of the ultrasound. My ovaries are indeed enlarged, the right more than the left. It could be cancer, it could be endometriosis. Go for a blood test and see the doctor at the end of the month. Great, more tests, another doctor's visit. I could have cancer. I go for the blood test and wait another week. Blood test comes back within normal limits. Yay, I'm safe. I go for the doctor's appointment. He rechecks my ovaries (still enlarged). He talks about my options: laparoscopy to take out my right ovary and/or take out my uterus.

My questions to the Doctor:

> Why take out my uterus when I was not having any problems with it?
>
> Why take out my right ovary when I had the blood test to rule out cancer?
>
> What's going to happen to my left ovary? Is it also enlarged?
>
> Why would you remove everything when I never complained about excessive discomfort?

The Doctor's answers:

> If you have endometriosis, it is a precursor to cancer, and I would even recommend my wife to have her uterus taken out. The blood test is not accurate enough to rule out cancer; it has a lot of false negatives. If we go in for a laporoscopy, the only way we can be 100% sure it's not cancer is if we take the whole ovary out and biopsy it. Not that you have cancer. I think it's endometriosis, but the only way to be sure is to take it out.

I told the doctor that I was going to get bodywork done before he took anything out of me. I told him that I was disgusted with his options.

As soon as I got into the car I started to shake. If I was scared before, I was terrified now. I could not even talk to my husband about the visit because I was crying so hard. I know what bodywork can do but that visit had me doubting my abilities and everyone else's. Why should I believe the doctor when he did not believe in me? *"Because he is the doctor"*.

As a therapist, I started to think about all the things I tell my patients every day, and all the things my teachers have said about bodywork, good/bad energy, etc. I do not want to be a hypocrite. I need to believe in the power of bodywork. I have seen too many wonderful results on our patients not to believe it can be done on me also. My husband and I discussed the options, and I decided to stick with my beliefs. However, the "what ifs" about alternative ways of healing continued to plague me on a daily basis.

This brings me to you. My husband, who is also a therapist, recommends that I see you for myofascial release treatment in the pelvic area. Oh great, I have been avoiding a treatment from you for a long time. What if I start to unwind? Don't get me wrong, I do believe in unwindings, just not for me. Putting my stupidity aside and, I must admit, some of my distrust, I begin to realize how sensible this sounds. "Can we take care of it from the outside?" "No, the damage is done on the inside, the fingers need to feel the tissue, feel the strains, feel the restrictions, hear the story." These thoughts were going through my mind. I agreed to go for the treatment.

I was scared, but you probably knew this. You started the treatment by reading the body. This put me at ease immediately. I am familiar with this. I also realized that you were doing this treatment for me. If I relaxed, I really didn't have to do anything but feel. Take away the thoughts, let my body tell its story even though I was unsure where this would lead. A lot of the treatment did not feel good, but it felt right. The years of strain patterns, thickened tissues were immediately evident. You were doing a release on the left lower quadrant of my uterus and I was feeling the results in the upper ridge of the ilium on the right side. What could create such a strain pattern? Could it have been pregnancies? Most probably! Why would I feel such pressure in my rectum when you are doing releases in the anterior part of my uterus? Every structure in my pelvic bowl relates to the other. Why then, when I asked the gynecologist, *"the doctor,"* whether my enlarged ovaries could have anything to do with my pregnancies and tough deliveries, he said, "impossible"? Could endometriosis develop because of these abnormal tissue strains causing fluid to flow in some areas and not in others, thus causing fascial buildup? I couldn't help but think that my pregnancies and deliveries played a large part in the integrity of my uterus and pelvic strains. I had the exact same discomfort and pain I experienced in childbirth (the rectum discomfort, tissue feeling like it was tearing, etc.) all from internal bodywork. Other types of emotions were also brought to my attention; the lack of control over my own body, the anger over a careless remark from the doctor, etc.

After the treatment sessions I felt relaxed and calm for a few hours. Minor memories would flutter through my mind bringing back childhood embarrassments and also childbearing/delivery memories mentioned above. When I felt anything like a twinge or flutter, my confidence in the treatment sessions lessened a little and doubts settled in. I have mentioned to you, John, that I have a history of constipation. This never really bothered me until I felt all the spasms moving into my rectum during the internal work. A few days after you worked I literally spent the day going to the bathroom. I could not eat (no appetite). Unfortunately my appetite has returned since I have been home.

In conclusion, I know that I have a lot of restrictions in my pelvic area. These restrictions have a history, a history in which I thought I had dealt with. I was wrong, but I am willing to do what it takes to relieve my pelvic area as well as my mind. I feel too many doctors' words and actions are potentially damaging to many womens' psyche. I want to thank you again for your gentleness in dealing with me. If I can feel comfortable with such personal treatments I guess I really don't have to hold on to my fear of physical expression any more.

Question: John, what form of treatment did you give this patient?

I started out treating her by doing a myofascial structural evaluation of her whole body, followed by an energetic assessment. She had a torsioned pelvis with myofascial restrictions throughout the abdominal and pelvic areas.

Imagine that as the pelvis so commonly tightens in these areas, it acts like a tourniquet of pressure wrapped about your intestines, organs, nerves, and blood vessels. It is these powerful myofascial restrictions with a tensile strength of up to approximately 2,000 pounds per square inch that are the cause of so many of the symptoms of digestive problems, constipation and menstrual problems, pelvic pain, reproductive problems, endometriosis, and disease. As I said, myofascial restrictions do not show up in any of the standard tests and therefore create many misdiagnoses.

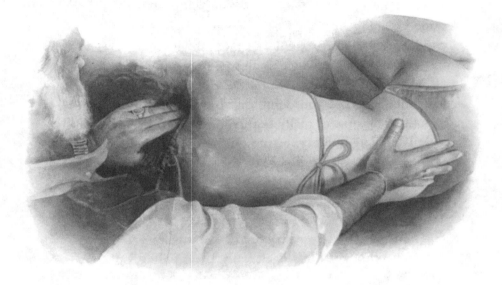

As her treatment progressed I could feel energetic restrictions in her pelvis, spine, and cranium, and the vibrations of unresolved emotion. She had told me that she was angry with her doctor for the way she had been treated and scared. I encouraged her to continue with medical care and followup tests, but to also consider changing her mindset and expect myofascial release to be effective in restoring her to health. I also encouraged her to express whatever emotions might arise. I could sense that she, like many, was in a struggle between the traditional view of health and the myofascial model of healing. I tell my patients stories that symbolically help them gain insights; I never explain the story. It is important for them to develop their own insights and understanding of what that story may mean to them. I told her the following story, *The Grandfather*:

There was a grandfather whose little grandson often came in the evenings to sit at his knee and ask the many questions that children ask. One day the grandson came to his grandfather with a look of anger on his face. Grandfather said, "Come, sit, tell me what has happened today." The child sat and leaned his chin on his grandfather's knee. Looking up into the wrinkled face and the kind dark eyes, the child's anger turned to quiet tears. The boy said, "I went to town today with my father to trade the furs he has collected over the past several months." Here the boy laid his head against his grandfather's knee and became silent. The grandfather softly placed his hand on the boy's raven hair and said, "And then what happened?"

"Some town boys came by and saw me. They got all around me and started saying bad things. They called me dirty and stupid. The largest of these boys pushed me back and I fell over one of the other boys and they all ran away, laughing." Here the boy's anger returned, "I hate them, I hate them all!"

The grandfather, with eyes that have seen too much, lifted his grandson's face so his eyes looked into the boy's. Grandfather said, "Let me tell you a story. I too, at times, have felt a great hate for those that have taken so much, with no sorrow for what they do. But hate wears you down, and does not hurt your enemy. It is like taking poison and wishing your enemy would die. I have struggled with these feelings many times. It is as if there are two wolves inside me. One is white and one is black. The White Wolf is good and does no harm. He lives in harmony with all around him and does not take offense when no offense was intended. He will only fight when it is right to do so, and in the right way. But the Black Wolf is full of anger. The littlest thing will send him into a fit of temper. He fights everyone, all the time, for no reason. He cannot think because his anger and hate are so great. It is helpless anger, for his anger will change nothing. Sometimes it is hard to live with these two wolves inside me, for both of them try to dominate my spirit."

The boy looked intently into his grandfather's eyes and asked, "which one wins, Grandfather?" The grandfather smiled and said, "The one I feed!"

Her second letter:

Dear John,

I would like to give you an ending to my story regarding my ovaries. After my treatment with you, about four months after receiving the advice to take out my right ovary and uterus by the doctor, I went for another ultrasound and blood test to check my status. I had a much better attitude this time around because of the knowledge I had gained after receiving myofascial release bodywork. After playing phone tag with the doctor for two or three weeks to find out the results, I called the office up and said that I was coming in to get the copy of the test results. They immediately thought I was defecting to another doctor and became very short and snippy with me. At this point I really didn't care what they thought; I wanted the results. Despite my doctor's dire predictions and recommendation of radical surgery, the ultrasound report stated that there was no change in the size of my right ovary, and that the left ovary was within normal limits. The doctor finally got ahold of me three weeks after the tests at nine o'clock one evening. He stated that he was satisfied with the ultrasound and the blood test results and that I did not need to come back to the office until my next annual checkup.

I did the next best thing I could think of. I gathered up my anger and reached into the phone, grabbed the doctor by the neck and said: "Four months ago you told me I had to get my ovaries and uterus taken out. Now you say I don't have to come back into the office for a year. What is wrong with this picture?" I just wanted him to be aware that radical medical protocols may not be needed for every woman. How many surgeries are performed unnecessarily? Myofascial release can clear up a multitude of problems, thus eliminating the need to give every woman who walks into his office the same prognosis. I also stressed the need for him and his staff to experience a treatment session to learn more about the techniques. Predictably, he has not responded to my verbal and/or written invitation.

John, I feel that I am one of the lucky ones who did not actually have cancer even though they gave that to me as a possibility. I feel that the enlarged ovary was a warning light that all was not well in my body. If the warning light is taken out, the next time there may not be an option to avoid surgery. I have also found out so much about myself that I never knew existed: I actually have a creative side to me, I am brave, I can take control over my own destiny, I can confront a doctor with my views, and I love and appreciate my ovaries and uterus. Thank you again, John, for treating me, listening to me, and believing in me.

∕

A Patient's Perspective

John, I'd like to share my experience with traditional medicine and my success with myofascial release. My story is a classic example of what you teach us: "Find the pain, look elsewhere for the cause!"

Myofascial release is also helpful in treating vulvadynia and vulvar vestibulitis. Many women and girls suffer from severe vulvar, vaginal, and rectal pain and discomfort. This can greatly impede one's life in many ways. Wearing tight clothing, sexual intimacy, and things as simple as sitting become difficult or nearly impossible.

Vulvodynia is defined by the International Society for the Study of Vulvovaginal Disease as "chronic vulvar discomfort or pain, especially that characterized by complaints of burning, stinging, irritation or rawness of the female genitalia." Vulvar vestibulitis, a common subcategory of vulvodynia, is "pain when pressure is applied to the vestibule, the area surrounding the entrance to the vagina." Vulvodynia is diagnosed when "other causes of vulvar pain such as yeast infection, herpes, skin disorders, and bacterial infections are ruled out."

Here's how it all started for me. In July of 1997, a car accident turned my life upside down. Back pain, leg pain and utter chaos ensued. Two weeks later... pelvic floor pain, unbelievable pain, so severe that I couldn't eat, sleep, feel, or think. I had no idea that my vaginal misery was related to the back and leg pain that was clearly a result of my car accident. I had experienced yeast infections before and assumed that it was just another. But, despite treatment after treatment for yeast, it would not go away. The itching and discomfort became so severe, I could not wear underwear. Nausea and weight loss of nearly thirty pounds ensued over the next few months. My vulva was the color of red construction paper. Missing classes...missing exams...doctor after doctor, medication after medication.... Chiropractors would make me feel great for a day and then the pain would be worse than ever. MRIs, x-rays, gynocologist after gynocologist looking at me like I was crazy, biopsy, trial treatment after treatment, diet after diet, prognoses, diagnoses, labels.

I was in graduate school at the time and went to the university gynocologist. I underwent treatment for everything from yeast and bacteria to foliculitis to scabies.... Yes, I was actually told to put a medication that is used to kill mites on my vulva!!! As if I weren't in enough misery. I was tested for every sexually transmitted disease, with negative results, and finally endured a horrible biopsy of my labia. After injecting several shots of anesthesia into my vulva with a huge needle, this man, with no emotion or support, cut my inner and outer labia using foot-long scissors used to do biopsies of the cervix. It was absolutely unbelievable. When cancer was ruled out after receiving a negative report from the biopsy, he didn't know what else to do with me. So he sent me on my way, mentioning that I might have vulvodynia. It was up to me to find a doctor who might be able to help me. I was so sick at this point, it was all I could do to pick up the phone. The university health center put me on Ativan to calm me down. That was the only relief I got. I would take a pill that would knock me out so I could get some relief from it. I tried every over-the-counter and prescription anti-itch cream; nothing helped even slightly.

After talking to many doctors' offices, going in circles, I visited a doctor in San Francisco who thought I had severe yeast infection. He was going away the next day, so he referred me to a doctor in Palo Alto to get loads of bloodwork and vaginal cultures. I drove about an hour to the clinic in Palo Alto. Before I was even examined, the nurse practitioner said that it sounded like I had vulvodynia and handed me a sheet explaining laser surgery... the new "effective" treatment for vulvodynia, called "noninvasive." I thought I was going to completely lose it. She said that this would be what we would do if antidepressants used to block the nerve endings failed to give me the much-needed relief. Here I was, age twenty-five and being told that they just might have to laser my vagina! I was examined and put on more cream to kill yeast, high dose of oral medication for systemic candida, and put on a yeast-free diet as well as a low oxalate diet, leaving not much to eat. I was more miserable than before. On top of it all, I had to drop out of graduate school because I was too sick to make it to class.

Before long, I flew across the country to stay with my parents because I could no longer care for myself. At that point I had resorted to using lidocaine topically. It barely worked. I began going to an East Coast university medical center and was put on high doses of Elavil, the anti-depressant I had been told about, to block the nerve endings. The only result of this drug was a severely elevated heart rate, to the point where I was sure I was having a heart attack. No decrease in symptoms! So, if I had remained in California, they would have said, "time for surgery!"

Just before Christmas, after six weeks of more doctors, more opinions, acupuncture, chiropractors, herbalists, you name it—worse pain, increasing hopelessness, and spending twenty-four hours a day lying on a mattress on the floor screaming and crying in agony—a gynecologist recommended a physical therapist in Pennsylvania who treats women with vulvadynia as well as back pain. I spoke with the physical therapist, who suggested that I call the Myofascial Release Treatment Center in Paoli, a five-minute walk from the house I grew up in. I thought, "myo what?" I then called and set up an evaluation. I didn't have anything to lose.

The therapists at John's clinic were the first professionals who didn't look at me like I was crazy. They didn't tell me that nothing was wrong with me, and they didn't tell me that I was the worst case they'd ever seen. Not only did they not tell me that I had to live with it, they told me that I did *not* have to live with it... that I had the potential to get better. Finally someone was going to treat the cause... not the symptoms. And the cause was certainly not just where the symptoms were. My fascia was tight... my pelvis was severely rotated, my dural tube was like a rope being pulled taut, my tailbone was tucked under and off to one side, and my pelvic floor was like a spider web all twisted and pulled. No wonder I was in so much misery. My entire body was out of whack.

In May of last year, when John had a cancellation, I was scheduled to be treated by him. I got really nervous. He was to do pelvic work. I thought I was going to flip. But as soon as John walked in the room, a sense of peace came over me. He was so warm and gentle. I knew that I would feel comfortable with him.

I was lucky enough to participate in the Myofascial Healing seminar. I loved it! Again, big time shifts!! I recommend that anyone wanting to enhance their treatments take a seminar or two...or several. John is an incredible teacher. And, it is so much fun!

Two years later, I am significantly better. I attribute all of my improvement to my myofascial release treatments and what myofascial release has taught me. I do home exercises to stretch and release the fascia throughout my body and I continue to receive treatments from wonderful therapists. I work full-time now; I go on hikes, and am able to do most things with a little modification. I now know that I will be pain free 100 percent! There is no reason that I won't be. I have come to recognize an emotional component to my pain and have learned greatly from it. I would have never asked for this, but it actually has changed my life in a positive way.

This is another unfortunate example of the limitations of traditional symptomatic treatment. I emphasize in all of my seminars that you find the pain, look elsewhere for the cause! Rarely is the cause of the problem anywhere close to the symptoms. Symptoms are just the tip of the iceberg. To be effective and comprehensive we must treat the whole person. And as this patient has learned, "I would never have asked for this, but it has changed my life in a positive way." It is important for us to understand that we cannot change the circumstances of our life, but we can change our reaction to it. Embracing our pain, embracing our fear, teaches us on a deep level and has the power to transform us. How has your pain and fear strengthened you?

A THERAPIST'S PERSPECTIVE

I had to face the fact that my sexual desire had disappeared. The urge and the need were gone. This had been going on for about one year and I could no longer blame it on being stressed or busy.

Gradually during that year, I began to develop other problems. I started developing headaches, bloating, fatigue (low energy), very heavy uncomfortable periods, and a lack of enthusiasm for anything. My true self is very playful, creative and sensual. I was no longer inspired by anything, food didn't even taste good. I felt that I was losing myself. My husband began to feel that I was no longer attracted to him and I started to resent him for not understanding.

I visited my gynecologist but did not relate all of the symptoms since I would be labeled "depressed." The pelvic exam was uncomfortable and seemed to reveal fibroids. My physician explained that these fibroids could be the cause of my heavy menstrual flow and discomfort with sex. I would need an ultrasound to confirm them, and if severe enough, the end result could be a hysterectomy. My doctor also explained that I was probably in early stages of menopause. I couldn't believe I was hearing all this at thirty-seven years old. I had no intention of losing my uterus.

Immediately, I contacted a fellow myofascial therapist friend who does a lot of internal myofascial release work in her practice. I knew I would need these treatments. I did follow through with the ultrasound, which showed no evidence of fibroids. My physician had felt fascial restrictions. After this realization I scheduled myself for Therapy for the Therapist, at John's Myofascial Release Treatment Center, "Therapy on the Rocks."

On the trip to Sedona I recognized the anger I had toward my husband. I was ready to move on, to forgive. I was ready to move past all barriers. John and his staff recognized that I was "out of my body," and they gently helped me reconnect with my feminine essence. They lovingly guided me, allowing me to fill my body-mind with the love and light of my true essence. My energy returned, my eyes sparkled again as the color came back into my face. After each myofascial release treatment I felt a little lighter, a little less pain, and my true self was re-emerging.

As I was traveling home I felt full of joy, my mind was racing with new ideas and yes, my sex drive had returned. All of these things happened in a loving, caring environment without surgery or drugs.

A THERAPIST'S PERSPECTIVE

After taking the Myofascial Release I course several years ago, my husband and I would practice the techniques we learned on each other. I received the most benefit from the pelvic floor releases. I could feel vibrations, warmth, and air filtering in as the restrictions melted. There was also an incredible urge to move, which I fought off for as long as I could. When I finally gave myself permission to feel what was going on in my pelvic area to the fullest, I was left shaken and confused. It wasn't until the third or fourth treatment and after my permission to move that I felt a shift in my pelvic area. This area felt lighter (less burdened) and freer.

Little did I know that the benefits to those few releases would come back to me tenfold. I was twenty-seven when I married my husband. I was one of ten in a strong Catholic family. I would not let and/or didn't realize that a sexual relationship with my husband was supposed to be something to be enjoyed. I thought it was just a wifely duty that was somewhat painful. My love for my husband and our desire to have children kept us going. (My husband was a very patient man.) I cannot express enough how those few releases have changed my outlook on making love to my husband. I won't go into detail, but it has been very, very good!!!

Clearing out restrictions, opening up blocked energy paths, and improving circulation throughout the body has benefits more far-reaching than purely at the physical level. Whatever transpired, I am grateful, and will never doubt the power of bodywork. I have received benefits I never dreamed could happen.

The non-traumatic, gentle nature of myofascial release is reassuring in that the patient need not worry, since these effective procedures will not worsen the patient's symptoms or cause harm. Myofascial release can free the structures producing pain and can also relieve the emotional pain associated with past unpleasant events or traumas. The painful memories or emotions from beatings, rapes, molestation, or miscarriages seem to be stored in the body's memory.[2] Many times the woman has dealt with these situations intellectually, but on the subconscious level, the body (the myofascial structures in particular) stores these past painful events. As myofascial release frees the adhered tissue, the trapped emotions and painful memories fade away, leaving the person with a sense of peace. This return to balance is sort of like letting the steam out of a pressure cooker. The comment I hear quite frequently from my patients is "I finally feel like myself again," or "My sense of calm has returned," or "I felt lost and helpless, myofascial release has helped me reclaim my feminine essence!" Myofascial release is not meant to replace the important techniques and approaches that you currently utilize, but acts as a very important added dimension for increasing your effectiveness as well as permanency of results in relieving pain and restoring function and the quantity and quality of motion.

[1] Barral, JP, Mercier, P. Visceral manipulation, Eastland Press, 1988, 261.
[2] Barnes, J, *Myofacial Release: The Search for Excellence.*

if your tears could speak, what would they say?

It's important for people to find their way back to their essence, where they can experience themselves as vast instead of limited. Our shadows block us from our essence. Dr. Carl Jung said, "if you do not confront your shadow, it will come back at you in the form of your fate." The child perceives itself as weak and vulnerable. As they grow up they carry around this entire armor that they put around their heart to protect their vulnerability.

The armor is the shadow. People want to believe that they are strong, but behind that wall of armor lies a very weak, vulnerable child. The shadow creates a lot of our pain and it is absolutely critical to confront our unexpressed pain and emotion in order to heal.

Your role as a guide is to help the patient from being overwhelmed by this tidal wave of fear that emerges. If you want to climb a mountain, but you don't know the way, you ask a guide to show you the best paths; but the guide cannot climb the mountain for you. Each individual must make the journey themselves!

This is the distinction between traditional therapies curing or fixing a physical problem on a physical level. While that is important, it is necessary to take it to another level for authentic healing to occur. Healing is transforming the adversity into whatever experience one needs to learn to free and reclaim one's essence. As the essence emerges from these blockages, healing occurs.

The following is a poem that I read to my patients. It was written by a man who was trained to be a Ninja Warrior as a boy. After years of fighting, he became a Buddhist monk. After receiving myofascial release treatments he wrote this poem about finding your essence behind your armor.

THE SCARED LITTLE BOY AND THE WARRIOR

The sick scared little boy,
Who cringed at night,
He never really grew up.
He just hid inside the armor of the Warrior.
When the day was over and the lights went out,
He would curl up and pray that no one ever found him.
Oh, if they ever found him,
They would surely tease and hurt him again.
So he went deeper and deeper,
Until he found that he could go no further.
He built up walls to keep him safely hid,
And let the Warrior fight to keep people away from them.

The Warrior was strong and smart,
No one could come close to the walls.
But, something happened one day,
And the warrior got hurt.
Although he had been hurt before,
This time he was hurt beyond hope.
As he laid on the ground bleeding,
He cried for the scared little boy,
for he knew he would be found.
He knew they would laugh at him and hurt him again.
He cried so loud that the little boy heard,
and reached out his hand from behind the wall,
he pulled the Warrior behind the wall safe from the world,
then he wiped the blood from his head.
Softly the scared little boy said,

"Sleep now great Warrior, the war is over,
you have done all you can, I will be fine."

The boy frightened and in tears stepped from behind the wall,
not sure of what to do he looked frantically around.
Then he heard the Warrior whisper,
"Be yourself and you'll be fine."
Tears rolled down his face,
as he watched the Warrior die.
But the Warrior smiled as he watched the boy begin to live.

—Vajracrya Daijo Green

The cure for pain...is in the pain!

Let go of judgement to let go of suffering. Our judgements are a weight on the needle of a compass; lift the weight and the needle can point in a true direction, towards truth.

Nature is in absolute order. It's our minds that are in chaos. Our minds create chaos through judgement, doubt, and fear. Once people see that it's not the world that is chaotic, it is their thinking that's chaotic, then they have the power to transform.

Dialogue is one of the many forms of communication that can occur during a treatment session. Academic psychology has emphasized intellectual/talk therapy, which can have value, but unfortunately can also be very limited. Academic psychology has viewed man as a machine, whose goal has been to teach this machine to "cope" with problems. It doesn't recognize the possibility of waking up and going beyond the mechanical. I am not suggesting that you be psychologists or psychiatrists; I am suggesting that we be effective communicators. In recognizing the reality of mind-body awareness, we can allow the essence of the individual to emerge and communicate in its own unique "body language." We never consult, analyze, lead, or tell the person what to think or feel. I believe that we have all the answers within us; through releasing the fascia, allowing someone to move through unwinding into a significant position in space, we gently "open the door," revealing the emotions and/or insights that lie within. This will create an opportunity for the individual to get in touch with their own answers.

Many of the most important aspects of enlightenment are non-verbal in nature. Words cannot capture the essence of this knowledge. Words at times can be useful, as long as we are careful not to confuse the words with the realities. In other words, "don't confuse the territory with the map." Words can never adequately describe experience. Myofascial release enables us to get in touch directly with the experience of our essence, which will express itself in many forms.

Awareness is!

The focus of myofascial release is on tuning into our feelings and emotions, which we believe are our teachers. It is through the felt-sense of our emotions that our mind-body awareness expresses itself. As we release the physical tightness of myofascial restrictions, release unexpressed emotions, and relinquish obsolete belief systems, we clear and reconnect with the power and tranquility of our essence. This is when true, authentic healing occurs.

Let me say something now about the learning process. What I think blocks our healing is our compulsive need to figure everything out. This is important to explain to your patients early, within the first couple of visits. Say something like, "You're very bright, don't you think if you could have figured it out by now you would have?" And they most always say "yeah" and laugh. So you continue, "Look, how about if you give up your need to figure everything out right now. Can you do that?" They'll say, "Okay." The second they give up that need to understand, their progress is going to take off. Because nothing shuts down healing faster than your left brain trying to figure things out. Give them that permission and explain to them, "If you need to know, your mind-body complex will let you know during treatment in the form of an insight, or you may have an "ah ha" experience after a treatment while you're walking home, in a dream, or maybe even a week or two later. You'll say "ah ha," that's what that was all about." You may never know consciously, and you don't have to! Just be open to learning on a level that your wisdom deems necessary for you. Maybe all you needed to do was unwind into a certain position, make a certain noise, express an emotion, or see or remember a scene visually. Get out of your own way and allow that to happen. I'll be here for you to keep you safe. Just keep it simple. Give up the need to know; you'll know if you need to; it's another form of letting go. We don't know what it's like to let go until we truly let go. It's a little scary at times, but as you get into it more and more, you see that it's the most incredible space in the world. It's really a very safe, wonderful, and loving space."

My approach to myofascial release seems to break so many of the rules of traditional therapy. I don't break rules just to break rules. I am interested in what works safely, efficiently, and effectively.

So when someone becomes agitated or begins to cry or expresses some form of emotion, your natural inclination will be to rush in, give them a tissue and say, "It's alright." It is *not* all right! Your act of kindness just blocked them from going into feeling deep enough to allow for a meaningful change.

Instead, encourage them to feel it deeply down to the cellular level. Wait patiently for them to finish. Then when they are done feeling and expressing the emotion, give them some tissue and hold them if they need it. This allows them to go into the depth of feeling necessary for learning, growth, transformation, and healing to occur. Let your patients know that even though they apparently seemed finished, their emotions may come up again in waves. Encourage them not to stifle their emotions, and to feel whatever emotion surfaces deeply, and to express themselves in whatever way they feel is natural, always with an openness to learn. Then for resolution, let it go.

Some sessions will be in total silence; other sessions will be punctuated with questions. The following are some generalized suggestions and questions and/or statements that can be helpful. Stay away from the "why" question. Nothing shuts down healing faster than the question "why?" Why is that? Because the "why" question, the basis of traditional psychotherapy, throws one back into their intellectual, theorizing mode, where they're trying to figure it out.

The inner eye goes blind when it only wants to see why.

Just listen to what they say and simply mirror back to them the same words or phrases that have a high emotional tone. Never lead, just repeat back to them, in question form, their own words. Keep your language in *right-brain* mode, i.e., "what are you feeling?" "what do you see?" "what does that mean to you?" or "what does that represent or symbolize to you?" Also, observe what habitual positions they assume, and gently hold them in those positions. Ask them to go back in time and remember when they were in that position before; what was their feeling or sense and/or emotions associated with that position?

If you notice rapid eye movement, that means that they are processing information. They may be viewing a past scene, feeling an emotion, recalling a memory, or releasing a fascial restriction. This is a potent time to ask them what they are experiencing, seeing, or feeling.

When you ask them a question and they repeatedly say, "I don't know," then ask, "What if you did know?" That question will throw them right into their creative side; you will see their eyes roll back and flutter as they move into an altered state. Remain silent after this or after any question and give them time to access the hidden information.

Another question that can help if they seem flustered is: "What will it look like when you reach your goal?" Most people will look at you, dumbfounded, for they have never thought of that. Never say "if" you reach your goal, always say "when" you reach your goal. Encourage them to visualize it, to feel it; you both should expect it to happen. In fact, their goal is already accomplished; it's just a matter of peeling away the obstacles. So many have been "stung" by others' criticisms and judgements. Other helpful questions are: "Do you deserve to reach your goal?" "Do you deserve to succeed?" "Do you deserve to be loved?" Many people have old messages buried in their subconscious that they may not be consciously aware of. Many people received negative messages early on, such as, "I am bad," "I am stupid," "I am unlovable," or "I don't deserve to be successful and happy."

A PATIENT'S PERSPECTIVE

I felt plagued with tightness in my chest, a heaviness in my heart. I tried meditating upon it, attempting to feel it, to discover what was there, so that I could express it, address it and let it go as I had been learning in my myofascial release treatments. But I seemed unable to access it. I tried all the techniques I knew for self-treatment. I unwound myself, tears would even come to the surface, but I realized it hadn't touched the core of my restriction because the same sensation of heaviness, a burning heaviness, still existed. My physical tissue had not changed. My tears were not originating from this restriction. I even tried making noise from this tight space. Still no change. I was so frustrated.

I received a treatment with John. His confident, loving touch softly connects with my sternum. "I can't seem to reach my own pain. I go in, but can't connect," I tell him. "Try going out to meet it," he suggests, while lifting his hand above my sternum about a foot. Energy begins to stir. I feel reorganization occurring underneath my sternum. He asks me, "What do you need to be able to connect with this?" A wave of hurt stirs within. A flash of judgement enters my awareness. I share with John that I feel judgement is blocking my progress. He then asks me, "What does judgement feel like?" My mother's disapproval comes to mind. I feel my sternum more intensely. Tears flow, I allow myself to feel the disapproval. Fear arises. I feel wrong, like what I'm doing is wrong.

Now I feel anger surfacing. I hear my own thoughts argue, "Why can't I, as an adult, be alright with my own decisions? Why don't I trust myself?" John encourages me to soften in deeper to my body, and feel. I hear myself moan, a deep agonizing moan. It becomes a wail. Deep, deep sadness emerges. I've been unable to trust myself. I've needed approval from others, particularly from those in authority, particularly from my mother. I've wanted her approval, her love. I share what's coming up for me with John. He very calmly and very gently asks, "Are you ready to love yourself? It's time now to mother yourself the way you have always wanted to be loved."

A picture of myself as a little girl comes to mind. She comes to me and asks if she can sit in my lap. I hold her in my arms, tell her I love her and begin to sob. "I love me." John encourages me to say this to myself. "I love me." Then he says, "Now feel the love deep in your heart." The burning heaviness in my chest begins to dissipate.

Afterwards, I feel much lighter. I can take a deep breath of fresh air. Ahhh!

〆

"How has your pain made you stronger?" Stay quiet for a while, with no pressure for an answer. Quiet down, slow your breathing and ask yourself that question. How has your pain made you stronger? Many have interpreted these messages as a truth, set in concrete and therefore unchangeable. These dysfunctional messages have acted as filters through which they have viewed life. Their full potential to live or heal has been limited by these filters or blinders. They expend enormous amounts of energy proving that they are not stupid or bad. They are "re-acting" to and being controlled by the past.

When an old message comes up, ask them to acknowledge it, feel the emotions associated with that message, and if it no longer serves them, to let it go. Then, without leading, ask them to replace it with a more positive healthy message. Use this wording: "What would be a more positive, healthy message for you to believe in and to function from now?" Continue with, "You don't have to answer right now; just plant the seed and allow it to germinate. Give the answer time, and allow your intuition to speak."

〆

There was an interesting experiment that explains why we aren't aware of our filters from the past. Medical students were taught information while drunk. When sober they failed to recall the information; they could only remember when they were drunk again.

This is a form of "state-dependent memory." Myofascial unwinding returns the individual to the "state" or "position" they were in, in the past, and allows these emotions, sensations, memories, and information to surface from a state of dissociation in the subconscious to the conscious level. As this information becomes available to the conscious mind, the individual is returned to a state of awareness. Healing occurs with the clarity of awareness.

Explain to them that there is no such thing as a truth. Shocking, huh? There are interpretations! We all interpret the world in our own unique way; and since that message was not a truth, but an interpretation, we have the power to change that interpretation in any way we choose. All of your early messages and beliefs are interpretations, not truths. We have the ability to change those interpretations in order to provide a healthier message. All of our early teachers and authority figures should be viewed in this light. All of the guilty feelings and fears which they passed down, are interpretations, not truths. Reflect on them and ask yourself if there is a healthier interpretation.

Let's say you're in a car. This happens all the time and it goes back to the freeze response. You're sitting at a stoplight and no other cars are around. You look in the rearview mirror and here comes a truck barreling towards you at fifty miles an hour. The moment before the impact, you create a message. First of all, you think something like, "Oh my god, I'm going to die!" Or, "My neck is going to be broken! My car's going to be ruined; I just put out all this money." All these messages come through simultaneously. At the moment of impact those messages become buried in the subconscious. If you're sitting there at a stoplight, and you don't move, you probably have said to yourself, "I'm a dumb ass! I could have gone through the red light and not have been hit." But because of your programming, you sat there like a damn fool and let a truck hit you at fifty miles an hour. Now you're in pain, and even though the accident was not your fault, subconsciously you are carrying a burden of responsibility, and perhaps guilt, for not taking action. You're walking around feeling like an idiot and you're furious with yourself. Your whole system is stuck in a subconscious holding pattern, and every time you look in the rearview mirror of your car, you freeze up and make the situation even worse. You can't turn your head and it feels like your neck is killing you.

So when those messages come up, say to yourself, "I didn't die; I survived! I'm not a dumb ass. I'm human. Humans make mistakes. It's the way we learn. I forgive myself. I let go." Once you know the message, you can now replace it and create a new, more positive, healthy message, and things will shift.

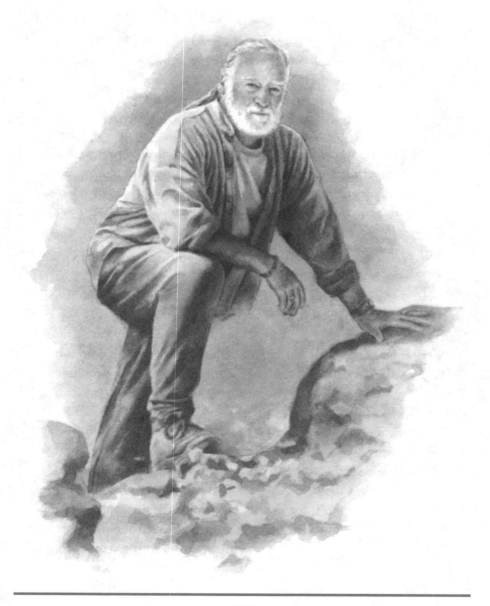

A Therapist's Perspective

Since my first MFR seminar in 1992 I have experienced so many profound moments and have been privileged to view John's wealth not only as an enormously talented therapist but as a deep, loving, patient, compassionate, feeling, and growing human being and friend. Attempting to pick out one example that would encompass all that I feel was too great a task. I began looking for "the pattern" or the "pieces of the puzzle" that would bring my experiences together to help me illustrate my point. When I examined these pieces what I found was myself.

Each and every occasion I have been with John he has guided me one step closer to my true self. My higher self. My whole self, in all of its brightness and darkness. When you are with John you feel his whole presence. In my brightest moments I could feel his pride. His joy for me that I could find my own beauty, sensuality, creativity, and groundedness. Encouraging me to accept and own all that is good in me and not to shrink away from it.

In my dark moments I also felt his total presence, devoid of judgement and criticism. He demonstrated compassion and patience, knowing that the expression of my darkness would bring clarity.

Through it all I have felt totally safe. Loved. Respected. I feel that in that environment anyone can grow to their highest potential, can find their path, can live their journey.

That being said I feel John's greatest contribution has been turning our lightbulbs on. Showing us the path. Kicking the pebble that starts the avalanche. And he has done this to how many thousands of us? I have seen it in myself. In my MFR friends. In all of our patients. It is what totally turns me on to helping out at his seminars. I get a total rush every time I see an MFR I student shift because I know that their life and those of their patients will never be the same.

As we open our hearts and feel, we can begin to face and accept the distortions and perceived weaknesses in our emotional makeup. When we can accept what is, we can transform. Don't worry about understanding the chaos; just accept it for now. Accept it on both the conceptual and tissue level. If chaos is what the patient needs to go through, then encourage them to do it. So, detach from the outcome! Experience the chaos! Lean into the wind! Push your limits! See what you can learn through this. Your patient may be angry with you for allowing them to move into chaos. It is an opportunity that you provide for them. Gently pushing the envelope may be the only way for them to become free.

When you are locked into desiring a particular outcome with a patient, you are biased, which means you have very limited options. When you are centered, you are spontaneous, able to act and respond, totally detaching from the outcome. What you believe to be the cause or reason may not be. Stay in your center, you are then in your power. Do not tilt to one side and try for an outcome. Stay centered! Allow the patients to help themselves.

Question: Do childhood memories also surface?

This is a very important point. A lot of these messages came from a time when you were a teenager, a child, or a baby. You probably are unaware of these messages that drive your life. So when unwinding brings them up to your conscious level, you have the opportunity to create a new message. You as the adult intellectually understands the situation now and thinks it has dealt with it, but this teenager, child, or baby has looked at this situation as an absolute truth and has convinced themself that they are a shameful, a horrible or a bad person. You want to talk to that inner child and say, "It's okay. I'm not bad. I am good; I deserve to be loved. I deserve to heal." It's been said: "Children are great perceivers, but horrible interpreters."

A PATIENT'S PERSPECTIVE

My experience of what I guess I would call tissue memory recall occurred after a three-hour Myofascial Release Session at "Therapy on the Rocks" in Sedona. I will give you some background so that you will understand the full impact of the experience for me.

As a one-and-a-half year old, I was in the car with my entire family, traveling home after Christmas, when we had a head-on collision at seventy-five mph. It was a life-changing moment in my family's life. We all survived, but were all injured in some way. My mother spent a good bit of time in intensive care with punctured lungs, crushed legs, multiple broken bones and lacerations. My father had internal injuries from being forced into the steering wheel. My sister experienced head trauma and a broken arm when she went through the windshield, and my brother lost his spleen when it burst. Asleep in the front seat, I was thrown onto the floorboard and miraculously had only a minor broken leg. Understanding fascia and trauma now in a new way, I can see just how much of an effect this accident had on all of my family.

Thirty-three years later I was in a car with my father, driving home from the airport on my Christmas holiday, when the car behind us pulled out to pass in the fog and ran head-on into a car in the opposite lane. One man was dead when we got to his car, and the other car contained five injured young adults. I felt strangely calm, but was very worried about my father and how seeing this accident would affect him. I really think I "left my body" in order to cope with this situation without panicking. I also thought that this must be destiny—a catalyst for my family to "deal with" our history. I continued to think about the accidents almost daily for several months.

Many months later during the third hour of a Myofascial Release Intensive Treatment, as my therapist was working on my leg, I began to experience intense pain in my shin. My response was to cry. I felt like a little girl who cries when she is hurt, instead of a grown woman. As I was gently encouraged by my therapist to feel whatever came up, I began to see an image in my mind. I saw my family traveling in the car together. I felt my father put on the brakes, and saw the impact with all of us flying forward in the car. I saw my sister go over the seat into the front windshield. I felt myself thrown into the floor, and felt my body close to my mother's legs. At this point I was feeling very afraid and panicked. I wanted to scream "Help my family! Get us out of here!" but had no voice.

I felt myself float out of my body above the car and look down on my family. I saw my brother stunned and looking around him, holding his abdomen. There was a lot of blood everywhere. I felt calm again, but very sad. Then each of my family floated up above the accident too. We all held hands in a circle and watched as they pulled us from the car. I felt everything would be okay then, since we were all together. I had stopped crying now in my treatment. There was a sense of quiet and calm, but of intense sadness.

Later, after this experience, I spoke to my father. I was able to dialogue with him for the first time about the accident and the meaning of it for all of us. This was a powerful experience for me of myofascial release at the emotional level. It changed my life and my relationship with my family. I was able to start seeing how trauma has changed our lives forever. I am thankful to have this deeper "knowing" through myofascial release.

When an experience is scary, there's a part of us that will interpret things as though we were going to die or be seriously hurt. So therefore we walk around with this bracing pattern; afraid to let go because we don't want to reproduce the situation, because on a subconscious level, we think we might die. That's why these experiences are good to reproduce, because now you can let go of that false message and replace it with a positive, life-enhancing one. Towards the end of a traumatic unwinding, ask them to say to themselves mentally, "I survived." This is such a powerful statement!

Some people will cry in every treatment. Allow that to continue for a few sessions, but if it continues they are probably stuck in a pattern. The emotions may be disconnected from a belief. Every thought has an emotion associated with it; every emotion has a thought or belief associated with it. We need to help them connect the recurring emotions with their beliefs. As they are crying, I will say gently, "If your tears could speak, what would they say?" This question has allowed for amazing awareness to surface. Depending on the circumstances you could also ask, "If your fear or pain or inner self could speak, what would it say?" A complete, lasting release occurs when we release the physicality and the emotions and belief system associated with the traumatic event or the person who overwhelmed them, or thrust them into shock and/or a state of disassociation.

Another common scenario I often run into is anesthesia experiences. What does anesthesia do? It knocks out the left brain. Your right brain is recording every moment of what happens to you, whether you're asleep, knocked out, or under anesthesia. There is much documentation about people under anesthesia knowing exactly what the doctor and nurses said, what was on the walls, and what they were wearing. So many times I have heard experiences where the person is being operated on, and the doctor and nurse, thinking the patient is unaware and can't hear, are kidding around with each other. The patient's interpretation was that they were being very cavalier and careless, and became very angry about it. Or they might have heard the doctor say, "I think this person is dying." Your left brain wasn't there to filter this out, to analyze that you weren't dying, so you received that message on the subconscious level. Unwinding then brings up these memories and our interpretations of these memories as embedded messages that we are not even consciously aware of. When the message is brought up to your conscious level, now you can become aware of it, and now you are back into a position of choice. You can keep the message if it works for you, but if it no longer does, then you can change the message. The thing that you have to get across to your patient is that there is no such thing as the truth. We all have interpreted these things as truths, like they are unchangeable and set in concrete. There is no such thing as a truth! I mean that all of your experiences are totally different from one another. You are each making your own interpretations right now, your own truths. So let your patients know that what happened to them in the past was an interpretation, and an interpretation is a message that can be changed.

Let me give another example. Let's say as a five-year-old you did something stupid. We all did stupid things at times, didn't we? But, as a kid, you interpreted that as a life-and-death situation, so from that moment on you have a filter: you always perceive yourself as stupid. Now you are going through your life with this behavioral message, so you're always trying not to look stupid. These are the kinds of messages you want to take a look at because otherwise you limit your experiences in life and respond from a very rigid and narrow framework. Or perhaps you had a bad fall, and you move through life bracing against that fall, because your interpretation right before the fall was that you might die. Over time that created tightness, and eventually neck and back pain. Now you realize you've survived, the bracing's no longer necessary, and you can let it go. The reason for the neck or back pain is gone, and now good therapy is going to start to help you.

Question: Could you explain the scientific rational for these phenomena?

Selye's classic work[1, 2] is concerned with the phenomenon of state-dependent memory, learning, and behavior—the general class of learning that takes place in all complex organisms that have a cerebral cortex and a limbic-hypothalamic system. Pavlovian and Skinnerian conditioning are specific varieties of state-dependent memory and learning.[3]

Memory and learning in all higher organisms takes place by way of two internal responses:

1. A memory trace forms on the molecular-cellular-synaptic level.[4, 5]
2. There is an involvement of the amygdala and hippocampus of the limbic-hypothalamic system in processing and encoding the memory; recall of the specific memory trace may be located elsewhere in the brain.[6, 7]

The limbic-hypothalamic system is the central core to Selye's general adaptation syndrome. The neurobiology of the three stages of the syndrome—the alarm reaction, the stage of resistance, and the stage of exhaustion—help explain the observed outcomes of myofascial release and myofascial unwinding, and illustrate the mind-body integration.

The hormones that are responsible for the retention of memory, epinephrine and norepinephrine, are released during the alarm stage just before the trauma by the activation of the sympathetic branch of the autonomic nervous system. The state or position the person is in at the moment of trauma is encoded into the system as the person progresses into the second stage of resistance. At that point, the system adapts and develops subconscious strategies to protect itself from further trauma, fear, or memories by avoiding those three-dimensional positions that the body is in at the time of the insult. The emotions also communicate this mind-body information by way of the neuropeptides. This creates a vicious cycle of interplay among the endocrine, immune, and autonomic neuromyofascial systems and the neuropeptides.

If this cycle continues for too long, the person enters the third, or exhaustion stage in which the body's defense mechanisms expend enormous amounts of energy, thereby depleting one's reserve and perpetuating or enlarging the symptom complex.

Question: How do you figure out what dreams mean?

Your patients are going to have some very interesting dreams. Myofascial release brings up a lot of dream material. Now, as far as dreams go, don't spend too much time analyzing dreams. That's not what dreams are all about. Just remember your dream and go back into the feeling of it. Ask what those sensations, emotions, feelings, and pictures are all about. Ask how they have meaning for you, and then quiet down and feel for the answers.

You don't have to change your neurosis, just stop identifying with it. Identify with your master self, your essence!

Smoldering under many people's consciousness is a self-defeating message: perfection. Too many are striving for perfection. This early message was thrust upon many by society and families, and they have been desperately trying to be perfect in the eyes of others or themselves. It is an impossible and futile goal!

Remember that it makes absolutely no difference what other people think of you!

We all need to understand that there is no such thing as perfection. Ask yourself and your patients if you and they are willing to reset their mindset and be more realistic. Strive for excellence, that is achievable, and detach from what others think and say about you. If they don't approve of what you do or who you are, let it be *their* problem. Be true to yourself!

Let it be known that whatever the perceived reason or excuse for the pain or dysfunctional behavior, drop the label, visualize their goal and move on. If all they can do is crawl, start crawling!

Tell your patients clearly that what has happened to us is beyond being fair, beyond right or wrong. Life is not fair and this situation will never be made right, but as long as we hold negative emotions toward another person or an event, it is like steel cables connecting us to the past, controlling us. It limits our health and our freedom. Never force anyone. If your patient or client resists say, "Fine. What is the worst thing that could happen if you would cut the cables to the past?" Give them time to answer. Most people say, "Okay, let's do it, I am sick of this." Every once in a while, someone needs to go home and mull it over for a while, but I would say that 95% of the people are willing to go for it right then and there. If they go home, they always come back next time and say, "I have thought about it and I am ready to try this."

Blaming others, or circumstances, is coming from a victim attitude. A person stuck in a victim role is powerless. They are "re-acting," allowing the past to control them. We cannot change the circumstances of our life, but we can change our response to it! This is what it means to reclaim your power. Choose to respond. Accept what has happened. Learn from it and let it go and make the best of it. Quiet yourself, ask your essence for help, and visualize what you want: your goal. This is "responsibility." You now have power to change, grow, release, and heal. When someone is stuck in any kind of struggle, ask them, "What would you need to know, see, or feel to let go of the struggle?"

Question: What if the patient says, "I wish I wasn't born?"

In other words, they are saying, "I am powerless, I don't want to be here." They are stuck in a concept that is inappropriate to leading a full life. They are hiding behind excuses. Have the courage to be here now! We are in and out of our bodies at all times, and it is a matter of awareness. One of the things I say to all patients and therapists is, "The deeper you go, the higher you go." It is about balance. We need to be in both spaces. In other words, you don't want to be just out there. Some therapists are so heavily "in here" and so dense that they have no intuition or creativity whatsoever. And some are so "out there" that they are not here at all; they have limited the use of their abilities. "The deeper you go, the higher you go." You are not going to take away any ability; you are going to enhance their awareness and abilities significantly. You will hear, "I didn't want to be born, I don't want to be here." Well, you *are* here! You might as well do something about it. Life is not a dress rehearsal! Let's make the best of it now!

The hurt we embrace becomes joy.

Question: Can myofascial release be helpful with someone near death?

Yes, it can be very helpful to work in a hospice-type situation. This treatment can help make the transition we call death a much more peaceful, natural process. It helps prepare us. A number of therapists who I know are working in a hospice, and they are doing beautifully with these techniques. Unwinding and gentle myofascial and cranial work can definitely be very helpful.

Question: Are some people scared to come back into their bodies?

Emotional trauma occurs when we are overwhelmed by a perceived threat.

Yes, that is why some are stuck "out there"; it happens a lot. Some people go out of their body and are afraid to come back in and some literally get lost out there. It can be very painful to come back in. We are confronted with our physical sensations, overwhelming emotions, past memories, and our self-judgements. But there is always that connection to bring them back in; there is always the silver cord. The only time that silver cord is severed is when you actually physically die. I will explain more about our luminous essence and the silver cord soon.

Question: Does this relate to past-life experiences?

I don't want anything to block you. It doesn't have to be a past-life experience; what may appear to be a past-life experience may be just your mind's way of representing symbolic lessons in story form. So the only thing that matters, basically, is what is the lesson there? Take the experience from the past life and decide what you can do with it today. And the lesson, whether it is symbolic or real, can change our lives. Those of you who are interested in past-life experiences may want to read *Many Lives, Many Masters*, by Dr. Brian Weiss, M.D.

Question: Are the words "consciousness" and "electromagnetic field" synonymous at all?

Your electromagnetic field is another word for your mind; it's another word for your awareness and another word for consciousness, which is another word for love. When we are hurt or fearful, we pull our feelings/awareness out of the body. What happens then is that the body goes into a survival mode and you go into a fight/flight/freeze response. On a deeper level, you realize that you are not fully protected. Over time, the fascial system, without that flow of energy, starts to lose its fluid content; the ground substance starts to solidify. The problem is that over time, the increasing solidity and tightness limits your motion and starts to produce unpleasant physical sensations, pain, or symptoms. So most people with fascial restrictions are out of their body.

Our mind also can be called our feelings, our emotions, love, consciousness, or awareness. You have a lot of different words that you can use. Use one that your patient or client can relate to so that they don't have to go into resistance. All of those terms are a bunch of words for the same thing. The problem is, in our society, we were taught not to feel. We were, therefore, deprived of the depths of our mind, our wisdom, our creativity, and our genius. So when we are injured, whether it is physical or emotional, what usually happens is we pull our feeling out of the area so that it doesn't hurt so much or is not so scary.

As long as our energy is withdrawn from an area, our energy, or mind, is no longer available to flow though the microtubules of the fascial system, so the ground substance begins to dehydrate. In other words, we begin to solidify in this area. This shortens down the fascial system creating abnormal pressures on nerves, muscles, blood vessels, joints, etc., which in time limits our motion, and produces physical sensations and/or symptoms.

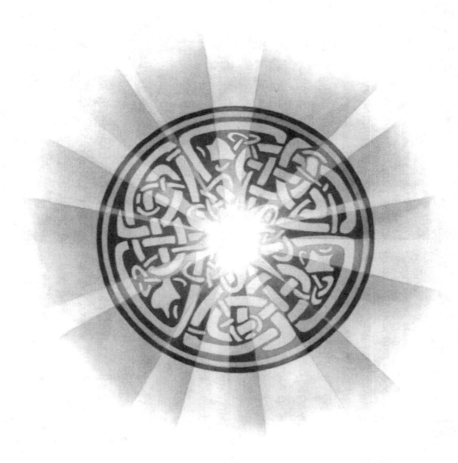

Always explain the "fascial voice" experience to your patients early on in their treatment series. Their full participation in treatment is important to their recovery. Explain that the fascial voice is an important non-verbal form of communication, a body language that can express itself in many forms. As their therapist, you will be constantly scanning the surface of their body for vasomotor responses, areas of redness or heat emanating from the skin. The vasomotor responses guide you to where else this connected web of fascia may also be restricted. Request that they tell you about sensations that may occur during treatment. Tell them to imagine the myofascial system to be like an internal spider web, so when you apply a particular technique, that pressure will be transmitted throughout their fascial restriction, like a spider web.

Wherever that internal spider web is attached it can produce physical sensations, i.e., heat, cold, pulling, pain, numbness. Even memories or emotions can surface, for all is embedded within the myofascial system. This information guides you to "connect the dots" as to where to treat them next. Also, you want to know if they become sore after treatment, or have a flare-up of symptoms. Explain that this is never injurious pain, this is therapeutic pain. Wherever their sensations were "speaking to them" is where to start your treatment session. Remember, find the pain, and look elsewhere for the cause! They are experiencing the "Healing Crisis." In other words, things have to get a little worse before they get better. Healing is a process of two steps forward, then one step back. Over time their periods of relief will become longer and longer.

Healing is not an event—it is a process. Your fears will never kill you—it is the inability to express the body's fears that kills us by creating the environment for Dis-Ease. Remind them that we cannot change the past, but what we can do is change our reaction to it. This has the power to transform their life!

Drink a lot of water! It hydrates the system and flushes out the toxins. Most of us, on a nutritional level, are walking around totally poisoned. We are in a toxic state because the restricted fascial system, on the cellular level, is not allowing us to eliminate all those toxins. The cells are not assimilating food well and are not getting proper oxygenation. This affects us on all levels.

Question: What happens when we hold onto our emotions too long?

You know as a kid, I used to always hear the phrase: so-and-so had a "nervous breakdown," and I never knew what the hell that was. What I've come to realize now is that when we have too much tension built up in our bodies it acts like a pressure cooker, building and building and building until eventually a nervous breakdown occurs. Everything goes haywire. The body is trying to naturally unwind and free itself, but traditionally what has happened in the past is that the person was thrown into a straitjacket, taken to a mental institution, and heavily medicated for years or even a lifetime. What was actually happening was that the mind-body was overloaded, and it started to correct itself through the thawing of the freeze response. Instead of allowing the process to complete itself, which might have taken ten to thirty minutes, this person spent a lifetime on medication or in a mental institution and worried that something was wrong with them because they were emotional and had a "nervous breakdown." Today's straitjacket is Prozac. The breakdown was a healing crisis, a natural response of the body as it attempted to heal itself, and it was thwarted by traditional medicine.

Let your body shake, experience the chaos, go into those significant healing positions, and get in touch with any memories or emotions that may arise. Our whole society is running from pain, masking it, medicating it, never really feeling it. The chapters titled "The Body Remembers" and "Enlightened Movement" in my previous book, *Myofascial Release: The Search For Excellence*, could help to educate your patients further on the healing crisis. "Sometimes, it has to get a little worse before it gets better."

Question: John, I have a couple of clients whom I would like to refer to your treatment centers. How would you suggest I explain the benefits?

Just call, e-mail, or write, and my staff can explain the different treatment programs available. What I have found is that even highly experienced and skilled myofascial release therapists will plateau with some people. Explaining the concept of tissue memory to them and treating them a couple of times a week sometimes just isn't enough to break the powerful hold of the subconscious bracing patterns.

Our experience has shown that being involved in our two- and three-week Myofascial Release Intensive Treatment Programs, where the patient is treated three times a day for an hour each session, does not allow the "bracing" patterns to persist. Our goal is to release the major myofascial restrictions and extinguish the hold of the subconscious "bracing" patterns, so that the person can achieve a deeper and more lasting response. We then send the patient back to you, the referring therapist, with treatment suggestions, for followup care.

What also helps is to have your patients read this book, and my first book, *Myofascial Release: The Search for Excellence* and to view the three Myofascial Release videos that I developed to teach the therapist and/or the patient how to perform myofascial release, myofascial unwinding, and how to follow up with a home exercise and flexibility program.

Question: Is it true that you have designed a healing seminar for patients?

Yes. The Myofascial Release Healing Seminars are for the patient and also for you, the therapist. They are for the human being who wants to heal and live life fully. I believe that by teaching the patient and their loved ones how to take care of each other with myofascial release, we help you, their therapist, to enhance their treatment response, cut their healthcare costs, and provide them with lifetime skills to maintain their health, continue to heal, and reconnect with their essence.

Question: How do you start a treatment session?

In a treatment session, I tend to start with the patient physically. I'll assess and begin treatment with them structurally, letting them talk a little bit and tell their story. They'll tend to ask you questions, tell you what they did, etc. Usually, they'll start to quiet down within a relatively short period of time as you shift your consciousness into an expanded state of open focus. This is when you start to really connect with them on that deeper energetic level, and float with them. As you connect with their essence, that is what really begins to move the structure. The hypnagogic state is a hallucinogenic state. It's that creative state right before sleep or when you first wake up, when you're not quite asleep but you're not quite awake. Letting go is one of the scariest things for us as human beings to do. Initially, you let go of control, and will rebound; in other

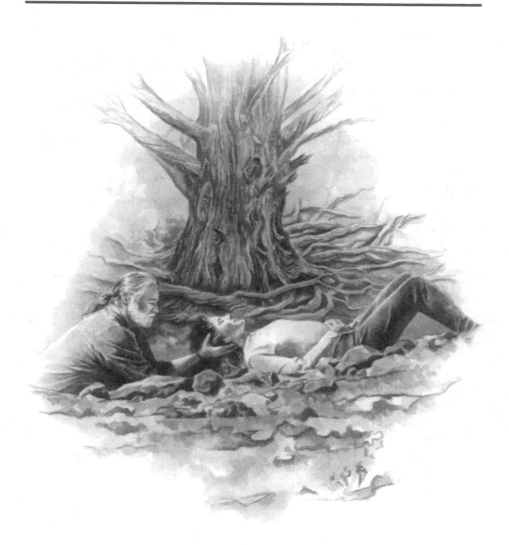

words, you will pop out of that healing state and try to regain control, because fear comes up. You end up right back in your left brain. If you ever
took a rock and threw it along a lake, it kind of skips along the surface.
It hits the lake, rebounds out, and then goes in a speck deeper; rebounds
out again, goes in a speck deeper, until eventually it sinks. So, it's a matter of acclimating to this state until you recognize that it's not really a
fearful place. It was just your fear that kept you from going into this
space, because you eventually will experience the most loving, peaceful,
warm, and creative space that you could possibly ever be in. This is your

center, the same space you go into in a still point. For a moment, now, slow your breathing, quiet your mind, and ask yourself, "Where in my life did I stop being comfortable with the sacred territory of silence?" Close your eyes and quietly wait for an answer.

When you are asking questions, keep your voice soft and low in volume, with a non-threatening tone, and do not insist on an answer. Even if you think that you know the answer, do not push for it. It must come from their awareness and in their own time to be valid and meaningful for them. Too many allow their ego to get in the way. If it isn't working, don't push. Try something else.

Remember: When the horse is dead, dismount!

A Therapist's Perspective

I have found that putting others first is not always the best thing especially when I negate my own needs and feelings to do so. For me this has been a healing journey and a growing journey, one that has taken me through chaos and the emotions from anger to joy. I am now beginning to feel the gentle tugging of my heart leading me at the crossroads of my life. I find security in the knowledge that life's little coincidences are not that at all, but synchronicities that are part of an overall plan and meant to spur me on to learn lessons about myself.

I have begun to awaken to my internal voice. I have been able to slowly get rid of some of the old belief systems that were holding me down, just like excess baggage.

I have slowly started to let go of some of my fear, which has allowed me to act on the feelings of what is right for me. In the past I have identified feelings of discomfort and confusion, but did not realize that these feelings where actually directing me to take charge of my life and make choices that would break me out of stagnation or misery.

I am learning that I have always measured my own success in terms of my own personal comfort and security.

However, the universe measures my success by how much I have learned. I am recognizing that my past intentions of maintaining my life in a comfortable zone have somewhat limited me in my growth.

I try not to look to others for my own happiness now, although it has been hard to convince myself it is really found within. As my own consciousness awakens I feel as though I need to develop my own individual power and authority. I have to sort through my ideas and my belief systems and discard any that no longer serve the process of my spiritual development. I can now recognize that living through rough times presents me with opportunities for spiritual growth. I can (only at times yet) consider difficult situations as being essential to my personal development.

A Patient's Perspective

I am a patient, a former skeptic, and one of many who will tell you some things that you as a patient do not want to hear. On the first day I walked into my PT's office, I was opposed to any hands touching my body. I refused to remove my clothes and put on a gown. I sat, arms folded across my chest, shaking my head at everything he said. Nope. Don't try it. Don't even think of touching me. Don't think I'm taking off my clothes. Don't think I'm cooperating in the least. I'm forced to be here by my orthopedist, and I'm not having any of it. I was terrified, crying inside, and refusing to show him who I really was.

I kept this up, too. Didn't want to "unwind," didn't want to exercise, didn't want his hands here, there, or any-where. I fought, I struggled, I begged and cajoled. Anything remotely spiritual or metaphysical—which I was projecting anyway, and he was mirroring—was dismissed. I was dismissing myself!

That was less than four months ago. How to tell you how much my life has changed? It is not only the personal-ity of my myofascial release therapist, which is loving and

Divinely brought to my life, but it is the techniques he uses, the John F. Barnes Approach, that have brought me to where I am today: a healing, loving, far less self-destructive participant in my own life and in my world—the world I share with you. And I still have so much more work to do, a lifetime of undoing....

What might you not want to hear? You might not want to hear that you have to stop, look, and listen. You might not want to hear that you have to close your mouth in order to hear the world around you, might have to do what someone asks of you, not resist every attempt made to help bring you to peace and health. You might not want to hear that you have to walk directly into the darkness and stand there, feeling it, if you want the light.

You might have to stop fighting, stop thinking, stop manipulating the world around you, in order to be part of it. It is my understanding that according to John Barnes, all therapists must be patients during their studies. They must all feel the hands of others, must all greet their own darknesses, must all close their mouths in order to hear. It is as egalitarian as one could hope: no therapist is held above any patient; all are equal. This, dear friends, is not the way it is "out there."

But in the John F. Barnes Myofascial Release Approach it seems to be so. And by being part of it, we learn to bring it to others, and thus change the world, soul to soul. And if my therapist's techniques, compassion and kindness to me as a patient are any indication, then what John Barnes does and teaches is for me. It may not be for everyone, but it is definitely for me. There is a consistency to their discipline that comforts me—it is an actual method, with proven results. What more could we ask for?

This may not be for you right now. It takes courage to walk into the fires of your fears. Courage to beg your therapist to please help you, please take it away, put out the fires, bring back the light, and have him say, "Only you can take it away, only you can turn on the light..."

[1] Selye H. The stress of life. New York: McGraw-Hill, 1976.

[2] Selye H. History and present status of the stress concept. Goldberger L, Breznitz S, eds. Handbook of stress. New York: MacMillan, 1982:7-20.

[3] Rossi EL. From mind to molecule: a state-dependent memory, learning, and behavior theory of mind-body healing. Advances 1987: 4(2):46-60.

[4] Hawkins R, Kandel E. Steps toward a cell biological alphabet for elementary forms of learning. Lynch G, McGaugh J, Weinberger N, eds. Neurobiology of learning and memory. New York: Guilford Press, 1984: 384-404.

[5] Rosenzweig M, Bennett E. Basic processes and modulatory influences in the stages of memory formation. Lynch G, McGaugh J, Weinberger N, eds. Neurobiology of learning and memory. New York: Guildord Press, 1984: 287-296.

[6] Mishkin M, Petri H. Memories and habits: some implications for the analysis of learning and retention. Squire S, Butters N, eds. Neuropsychology of memory. New York: Guilford Press, 1984: 287-296.

[7] Thompson R, Clark G, Donegan, Lavond D, Lincoln J, Madden IV J, Mamounas L, Mauk M, McCormick D, Thompson J. Neuronal substrates of learning and memory: a "multiple-trace" view. Lynch G, McGaugh J, Weinberger N, eds. Neurobiology of learning and memory. New York: Guilford Press, 1984: 137-164.

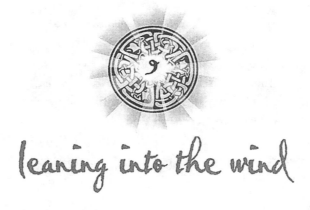

leaning into the wind

In the early 1970s there was a conference in Orlando, Florida. I thought that this would be a good opportunity to take my twin sons, Mark and Brian, to Disney World! I didn't really intend on spending any time at the conferences, since I had found them to be abysmally boring. The only thing that caught my attention as I flipped through the brochure was a dentist that was presenting information on temporomandibular dysfunction.

I woke up the morning of the conference and it was a rainy, dismal day. To my surprise, I felt compelled to get up and go to the TMJ lecture. The dentist was an impressive speaker and the first dentist or physician to ever speak about my strong convictions regarding whole-body relationships and temporomandibular dysfunction. The lecturer went on to say that therapists have much to offer dentists, and dentists have much to teach therapists. He suggested that we work together in helping people with head, face pain, and TMJ dysfunction.

I was so impressed with this man's knowledge and manner that I asked a colleague who he was. My colleague laughed and said, "Why he is the world-renowned, acknowledged expert on TMJ dysfunction!" I followed the lecturer's advice and sent a letter to the local dentists. I explained how biofeedback, neuroprobe (electronic acupuncture), joint mobilization procedures, myofascial release, and therapeutic exercises could be helpful in their efforts to help their TMJ patients. I was not surprised to find that, as with all the other letters that I had sent to physicians and dentists in the past, there was no interest, no reply.

Then a couple of weeks later a local dentist who was writing a book on temporomandibular dysfunction stopped by and was very interested in what I was doing. I invited him and a couple of the other dentists to come over the following week for a short demonstration of biofeedback, neuroprobe, joint mobilization, and myofascial release. After I was finished, the dentist who had originally contacted me said that I was a natural teacher. He said he was giving a TMJ seminar at the osteopathic college, and asked me to be one of the lecturers. I thanked him and agreed to participate.

This created an inner turmoil within me, for the two things that I hated the most were writing and public speaking. I was really afraid to do this, but I felt that it was a tremendous opportunity. As the time for the seminar approached, my tension level was increasing dramatically. On the morning of the seminar, as I drove to the osteopathic college, a sense of panic enveloped me. The fear in me seemed disproportional to the task at hand. I don't remember ever being so afraid! I didn't understand this high level of fear. I had faced fear courageously many times in the past. In football, I enjoyed the ferocious contact of blocking and tackling oftentimes much larger opponents. In karate, I enjoyed the fighting and competition. I was always the strongest in class, and not somebody to be messed with. While I never started a fight, I never backed off and always won the fight easily and resoundingly. I always enjoyed challenge, so what was happening now? My heart was beating fast, I was sweating, and my tie felt like it was choking me. I wanted to turn around and go back home, but I couldn't. I had never backed down before and I wasn't about to now. This fear was different; it felt familiar and very old. *What was happening?*

Go into the fear! Feel it! You are on the precipice of a massive change in your life that will send shock waves throughout the consciousness of millions of your fellow beings. Try to remember your vision so long ago! Your initial purpose was to fight and save your people. Remember your larger vision: to create peace and harmony, and to merge consciousness and love for all beings.

You were criticized and attacked for your thoughts and actions. This is the primal fear that is now emerging in you, for your mission is the same in this lifetime. You are going to merge traditional ways with ancient wisdom. It is time for you to heal your ancient wounds. You must now face this primal fear to fulfill your mission.

As The Ancient Warrior spoke of my vision so long ago, something resonated deep within me. The fear was shaking my whole body. I slowly took off my tie and threw it in the back seat of the car and said, "Yes, I'll just be myself and talk about what I do all day long." I walked into the seminar room and when it was my turn, I gave my lecture and demonstration to about twelve physicians and dentists. Afterwards, I felt good about what I had done. The next day, the dentist called me and said, "You were great. Of all the speakers, you received the highest grade. Would you speak again at my next conference?" I was surprised and agreed to speak again. For the next couple of years I lectured at the osteopathic college and around the United States and also in Canada, Mexico, Bermuda, and Hawaii. I took one of my greatest fears, public speaking, and transformed it into an enjoyable experience.

My skills improved with each seminar. I noticed that within five to ten minutes of lecturing there would be a shift within myself, and everything seemed to flow effortlessly. The Ancient One would start to channel through me and I could feel an instantaneous connection with the audience. Each seminar was a real learning experience for me. At one seminar I felt connected to everyone, except for one man. He just stared at me. He never laughed, no facial expression, no response. I found all of my attention was directed toward trying to get him involved. *Nothing!* After the seminar, the coordinator of the seminar came up to me and congratulated me on my performance. I said, "As hard as I tried I just couldn't get to this one man." He said, "Who are you talking about?" I pointed him out and he laughed and said, "He is from France and doesn't speak any English!" We both laughed hysterically and I got it. Focus on the positive. In every seminar or activity there will always be some that are negative, closed, or skeptical. Focus on those that are open to learn and the others will come along. Be yourself!

Of all the procedures that I taught, myofascial release generated the most interest. In the mid 1970s my private practice was flourishing. However, since I was the only one doing myofascial release, all of the patients only wanted to see me and not my staff of other therapists. I decided to put aside a weekend to teach my therapists some of the myofascial release techniques. I then decided to put a small ad in a physical therapy newspaper to see if other therapists might be interested. My staff thought it was a ridiculous idea. They asked me why would I want to teach others what I was doing? Why give my competition an edge? I didn't see it that way. To me it wasn't about competition. Myofascial release was important and something to be shared. I did agree with one thing that they said: no one knew what myofascial release was, so why would they come? They were right. So I called a physical therapy newspaper and asked if they would be interested in a story about a new approach to myofascial release that I had developed. They sent over a reporter and interviewed me on my approach to myofascial release. They ran the story on me and I placed an ad in their paper the following week. My staff laughed and said it didn't matter; no one would be interested. They said I would be lucky if two or three people responded. They were wrong! The day the ad hit, my phones rang off the hook. Two hundred people registered for my first Myofascial Release Seminar!

I have found that anything I have tried, there was always resistance from others. They may sound well intentioned, but deep down some resent another's success. Listen to what others say, consider it from all angles, but if it is in your heart, and if it feels right, do it! Control your own destiny. Do it and never give up. Never give up! Lean into the wind!

So, we now had over two hundred registrants and the space in the hotel only accommodated one hundred. I created two seminars of over one hundred on each weekend. The next realization I had was that up until that point, I had never spoken to more than fifteen people at a time. Speaking to over one hundred people was a whole different animal.

The first morning of the seminar, I walked into the back of the room and watched my assistant trip and spill my slides all over the floor! I wasn't experienced enough then to have numbered my slides. I was to speak within five minutes. I thought, "If I've ever been calm before, now is the time to be calm." I walked up to the stage, stood behind the podium and began to speak. I had prepared a ten-minute introduction, which I had memorized. A mistake; I do better spontaneously. About three minutes into my prepared speech, I forgot what I was to say. God intervened by having a waiter go through some swinging doors, slamming it against the wall. The noise diverted everyone's attention and I quickly looked at my notes, felt a rush of adrenaline and everything flowed smoothly thereafter. The first day went well, and I spent the entire night reorganizing my slides.

I had received a letter with a special request from a young therapist who wanted to attend my first seminar. She stated that she wore hearing aids in both ears and requested that she sit in the first row so that she could read my lips. We of course granted her request. As the second day of the seminar progressed, we got involved in a cervical technique. After practicing the technique everyone came back to their seats and she was sitting in the front row, right in the middle. I was lecturing and in the process of saying, "These techniques will never injure you..." I noticed that she started to list to one side. Then all of a sudden, she fell to the floor and started to seizure. I ran over and picked her up and carried her over to a table. I saw my whole career flash in front of me and figured this was my last seminar. I centered myself and applied light pressure to the back of her head. Her seizures ceased in about three to four minutes. In a few more minutes she sat up and said that she was fine. She thanked me and asked if she could speak to the audience, which at this point was in a state of shock. They thought that they had just witnessed a "miracle"! I had taken her from a state of total chaos into a peaceful, blissful state in around five minutes.

This very courageous young lady explained to the audience that she was born without cranial sutures. As she grew, without the movement of the cranial plates, her face and head became horribly distorted. She had been featured on a Nova television show documenting the seventeen oral/facial surgeries required to provide her with a normal face and head. She went on to say that she looked so different as a child that many of the neighborhood children would taunt and ridicule her and even be so cruel as to put cigarettes out in her face! She said that she hadn't told us that she had just had hernia surgery a couple of weeks ago. So when her partner lifted her, with so little "give" in her system, the seizure activity was initiated. She said that when I carried her across the room and laid her on the table that she was in a total panic, but that when I touched her head lightly, she immediately felt reassured and her inner voice told her that a major improvement was imminent. She continued, "Sure enough, I felt something release in my head, followed by a calm, peaceful feeling that I have never before experienced." She finished by saying, "This is profound work and I encourage you all to learn this and give your patients the opportunity to experience this work." Afterwards, she scheduled a three-week Myofascial Release Intensive Treatment Program at our Paoli Myofascial Release Treatment Center and has made remarkable improvements. She is truly a courageous and beautiful woman, inside and out.

After the seminar my instructors congratulated me and told me what a remarkable experience it was for everyone. The first two seminars went very well, and when I told people that I was going to schedule another, I was told by the "naysayers" that there was no one else to take the seminars, that was it. I heard The Ancient Warrior laughing in the background: *Disregard those fools. There will be millions upon millions who will benefit from what you are teaching. Never give up! Lean into the wind!*

I scheduled one seminar at a time for the first year, until it became obvious that there was an enormous need and thirst for myofascial release. The Ancient One was right. I have had the opportunity to teach a multitude of therapists and physicians, who are in turn treating millions of people with myofascial release. The seminars are still growing and the Myofascial Release Approach is spreading like wildfire. Despite all of the criticism and attacks, it has been worth it. For years I felt like I was swimming up stream or running the gauntlet. There has been a major shift in awareness and acceptance now. The wave is behind us, lifting us up to greater heights; the demand for myofascial release is enormous and growing exponentially.

A Therapist's Perspective

When I saw the myofascial release ad in my professional journal, I was surprised to see something so progressive advertised so boldly. Myofascial Release I, II, and Unwinding were everything that I expected they would be. John was masterful in weaving his scholarly and rational presentation, exercises developing centeredness and technique training together. (Not to mention some not-so-delicately-worded comments about the existing traditional healthcare system.) I watched him dissolve skepticism and handle know-it-all's.

I was an emotional basket case in intuitive heaven. When I left the seminars I was swinging to the radio. The Kentucky mountains were vibrant with nonearthly colors. I remembered what I had forgotten, where I had been on my path. I was reminded of my spiritual experience that gave me a single commandment: "Grow your character. Read and study all you want, but strive only to grow your character and all else will come to you, when you can handle it."

Later that year, doing "Therapy on the Rocks" in Sedona with John was transformational! My growth in character was apparent, and peace was evident to me and those who knew me.

That first year I took the courses for myself. Now I am retaking them for my clients (and myself—can't be in the presence of a master too often.) I now have a desire and an appreciation for the natural phenomena that arise from being centered and in the flow. Not magic but magical. And it's reproducible!

I am again going for my dreams. It is my joy that my career and service to others demand the same centeredness and detachment as my spiritual path. It makes for an integrated life. I am grateful to John, the visionary who had the courage to teach us to ground, center, and listen as the foundation of every technique and life!

A Therapist's Observations

I was excited to be assisting for the first time at a seminar series. It is difficult to put into words what I got out of the seminar series. I thought it would be great to listen to the lectures and review the material again, but what I did not expect was to find deeper levels of this work. I found that as I laid my hands on the shoulders of the students that were acting as therapists I was starting to feel releases and rhythms that seemed to be happening in the student lying on the table.

When this continued for two days I finally asked John if that could be possible, and was relieved to find out that it was. I did not realize these levels existed. John mentioned to me that there have been many other assistants who had experienced similar awarenesses and have also initially doubted this ability.

As an experiment, during MFR II class one afternoon the assistants viewed John's energy field as a group. Observing John with a neutral screen behind him showed varying levels of pillowy auras as well as more fleeting images. All four assistants saw a white shimmering energy body around his whole body. This white aura widened and brightened as John began a treatment or an unwinding started to occur. Two assistants noted an energy body or guide, off to John's left side, one specifically pointing out that the formation was as tall as the screen.

The instructors saw a very tall, white/gold colored column that extended up above John's head to the ceiling. Two assistants also described streamers in the energy field. There seemed to be a continual shifting of both John's aura as well as his guide as he treated. One could almost predict when a shift was about to happen to the patient, based solely on a shift in John's visual energy field.

Afterward, discussing these observations with John, he assured us that we all possess these fields and they are simply a continuation of our physical bodies. We only need to quiet down to notice.

A THERAPIST'S PERSPECTIVE

Of the many seminars and educators I've experienced, offering a wide range of techniques, the Sedona Myofascial Release Series in '99 was by far the most potent. I found the atmosphere created by John was so affirming and warm. It cradled all of us, facilitating our ability to let go. We were there for *us*, for our own benefit. What we took from that experience to our patients/clients depended upon the extent of our own healing.

When I was treated by John I felt absolute trust of and confidence in his intuition and knowledge of what it was I most needed at each moment. He accessed awareness of obstructions no one there could have known, because I had not revealed those details to anyone.

When I returned from the twelve days of seminars in Sedona several people commented that I looked different, happier, more free.

While repeating Myofascial Release I this summer, a seminar attendee was my therapist. One of the assistant instructors came by and placed her hand on my heart chakra area. Without hesitation I began to cry and let loose. It was as if there was an instantaneous resonance between us.

I am aware, during those seminars, that John and the other instructors are transmitting something to us, in another dimension, to assist our process. And that continues, somehow, even when the seminars are over.

A THERAPIST'S PERSPECTIVE

For me, before myofascial release I was empty. Myofascial release has been an experience of coming into my body, feeling connected. Sort of like seeing the world in color and 3-D instead of black and white and flat. Being around John has been an experience of learning acceptance. I was given permission to be just as I was, never pushed or prodded.

Some things that John has taught me and that made an impact on me are "learning to detach from the outcome" and "letting go of performance anxiety." Of course, those statements were initially meant for treatment, but they transferred into my life. Detaching from the outcome allows me to listen to my higher self and trust to let go of having to be in control. It allows me to be in my center, open to all possibilities.

Performance anxiety extended into my personal life with the "I'm not good enough" feelings. I openly acknowledged that I felt that way while treating, but I didn't realize that I really felt that way about myself.

Sometimes I could describe John's touch as a warm blanket that just seeped into every one of my cells, encouraging those parts of me that were so hidden to come on out. Such a safe feeling. Sometimes it felt like a velvet wrecking ball, flowing through my restrictions, but still so safe and right. I learned to step out of my comfort zone to grow, and heal old wounds. Again, trust and let go of the need to control.

One of the nicest experiences has been to watch the growth and healing of one of my closest friends. She was working in my office so I decided to send her to Myofascial Release I so that she would understand myofascial release on a deeper level. Over the course of that weekend, I saw the life come back into her eyes. It was so beautiful! She is slowly peeling off her layers and taking back her life. I really don't want to think about a life without myofascial release. I have gained a wonderful myofascial release family (who seem to be with me always). I feel that there is a world of growth out there just waiting to be tapped into.

A THERAPIST'S PERSPECTIVE

I heard the sirens and looked in my rearview mirror. Damn! Sure enough the police were right behind me. This scenario was beginning to get a little old. I lived with the anxiety that I was going to be late. I was almost always rushing and I frequently tried to make up time on the road, foolishly praying that somehow time would stand still for me. I knew I had to slow down before I was tragically forced to do so, but once again, I would find myself behind schedule and then off running I would go. I hated being late, and yet I seemed unable to make a shift in my behavior. I also prided myself in having some activity scheduled every night of the week and my weekends were spent flying off somewhere to do something. I loved the adrenaline rush of feeling busy. I was a "rushaholic." I realize now that it was a way for me to feel important and to avoid feelings within that were not so positive or of superhuman quality. But I had no awareness of that truth then. I also prided myself in being unemotional, even-keeled, and not falling prey to some of the usual addictions of youth: drugs, alcohol, and sex. Without realizing it, I had an aversion to letting go of control. I thought it was really weak and stupid. I had interpreted what I learned from my Christian upbringing that it was necessary to maintain control.

I was becoming frustrated in my profession. Only a year out of school and I didn't know what I could really offer my patients that had value. I felt that what I was doing with them I could've learned in less than a month and just as easily trained someone else to do as well. There had to be something I was missing. There had to be more! I was sharing this with one of my professors from my school, whom I had become friendly with and she immediately suggested that I take one of John F. Barnes' Myofascial Release Seminars. Really? I thought to myself. I'd heard some controversial things and wasn't sure it was for me. I feared it might conflict with my belief systems. I might run up against some real weirdoes and feel very uncomfortable. But what the heck, I'd always been adventurous and thought it might be fun to check it out. I had been reading a lot of varying comments in the professional magazines and it had piqued my curiosity. His seminar was coming to my general area in three months and I hadn't planned anything yet for that weekend, so I thought "at least it will give me something to do."

I arose very early the morning of the seminar to drive to the big city. I had treated myself to a room at the classy hotel where the seminar was being given. I was excited! I fell asleep during the relaxation/centering exercise portion the first morning and thought it was just because I had to get up so early that morning. Later I realized that it was really because I had only two reactions to life available to me at that time, conscious and unconscious, and nothing in between existed. I went unconscious to avoid feeling during that centering exercise. I recall sitting in the audience thinking, this is so fascinating! It makes so much common sense that I didn't understand what all the controversy was about, and I wondered why I hadn't figured it out! It seemed so simple and so natural. The concepts did anyway. When it came time for labs I couldn't feel a thing. Wasn't sure what this release sensation was all about, couldn't feel a cranial rhythm (although I did figure this was the controversial part and decided everyone that said they could feel it was just making it up), and couldn't tell where the restrictions were either. I think I did a lot of zoning out while I was the one receiving the work because I didn't feel much then either. Something in me was shifting, however, because I felt a greater sense of ease about myself. Staying at the hotel also did something to raise my self esteem. I had just had a painful breakup with my boyfriend, but here I was feeling like I was going to be okay.

Probably the most powerful thing of the whole weekend though was that John had given me a mini-personal treatment. It literally lasted no more than two or three minutes, but the pain in my knee was gone. I had developed what's called "runner's knee" and was unable to run without experiencing pain and stiffness in my knee, and even was unable to go up and down stairs the "normal" way without pain. I had been concerned because the normally recommended rehabilitation things weren't working for me and all of the more experienced therapists and physicians I had been to couldn't offer me any solutions either. I was much too young to be experiencing pain and limited mobility and I was afraid that I may have to proceed with surgery as recommended by an orthopedist. I knew enough to know that was not an easy route and would've involved a lot of time off work and a painful rehab as well. John had assessed that my pelvis was rotated, placing extra and unnecessary strain on my knee. After two or three minutes he said, "OK, you're balanced," and off he went. Hmmm. A torsion of my pelvis? What from? Everyone else, including myself, had just focused on the knee. After class, I was moving up and down steps easily and upon returning home (well, speeding home—I had a few other things to work on yet), I resumed my running without a problem. Wow! There was something to this stuff! But could I ever do it?

I told all of my patients back at work that there was a way to heal their pain, but they would have to travel to Paoli, Pennsylvania, or Sedona, Arizona…

I started using the techniques as John taught them, not really sure what I was feeling, but it was making a difference in my patients' pain level and their ability to move their stiff joints. I was even utilizing the cranial work, not really believing that it did anything, but I decided I would give it all a try. It reproduced a patient's low back pain just as John said it would happen. I became so excited when the patient reported this that I exclaimed in great surprise and disbelief, "Really?" and then realized I might scare the patient, so I quickly recovered by stating quite coolly, "Oh, of course, that is exactly what was suppose to happen." By golly, this might work, too.

Soon after, I had the opportunity to study manual therapy in the Netherlands for six months, and upon return one of my classmates encouraged me to join her for the unwinding seminar. Whoa! I was doing alright with a few of the techniques from Myofascial Release I, but I knew I had not yet mastered them, and once again, fear of these seminars crept in. Was I good enough to go on? Would there be some new concepts that wouldn't jive with me at this next advanced level? Unwinding was suppose to be kind of weird! I was quite comfortable at the level I was at. Or was I? I was just afraid I wouldn't "get it" and I didn't like the sensation of ineptness or failure. Besides, what if my friend got it, but I didn't? Could I handle that?

Well, my fear of acknowledging that I was afraid overrode my fear of not getting it, so off I went. Besides, this time it was in the same town as my sister lived in and I could write off a visit to her.

I witnessed my first unwinding. It looked pretty weird! John's lecturing about letting go of control. Uh oh, a major roadblock for me here. I heard myself saying, "I'll never be able to do that." But it was so fascinating, I was willing to at least give it a try. I wanted to be able to do it. My performance anxiety was mounting. Just didn't think I could let myself let go. What if something came up that I didn't know about and the illusion that I had a pretty normal upbringing was shattered and I discovered I was a dysfunctional mess? It's my turn. Once again, I find myself trying to act cool. "I'm not afraid." I hadn't realized how much judgement I had toward being afraid. It was not okay for me to be afraid! It was a sign of weakness. Where did that belief come from? And yet, I was so afraid that I was actually running from the truth of this realization. Was this what I was rushing around trying to avoid?

Without knowing what really happened, I felt myself up in the air laughing hysterically and then rolling on the floor. My turn was over. Whew! I had done it! Pure exhilaration! I had no idea what I had just experienced, only that I had done it and had survived. It was actually a lot of fun! What had I been so worried about? I'm okay. No major dysfunctions revealed.

Later, I realized that seminar had been a major turning point in my life. I couldn't explain it. Didn't realize it at the time, but looking back, it was quite influential. I was now ready, partially anyway, to truly begin one of the most fascinating adventures of my life, one that has not ended to this day, one that has dramatically improved my life year after year. Through myofascial release treatments, both giving and receiving, I have embarked on the journey to my soul. I am tasting the essence of my true self. The journey has not always been pleasant, oftentimes full of anger, depression, and a roller coaster of emotions. But it has always been rewarding! Each year becomes easier, more joyful, more full of grace and more understanding of life's many mysteries. Each moment becomes more full of love. Life radiates more beauty!

Today, I admit my fears. I give myself permission to feel them and release them. Today, I unwind easily! It is so natural and second nature to me! I can feel the restrictions, the releases, and the cranial rhythm. Today, I embrace my pain, knowing that it is an opportunity to know myself more deeply. No longer afraid that it will cripple me or limit me, but that it teaches me how to live more in tune with my essence and my purpose. Today, I know that feelings and emotions are God's special gift to humanity. Today, I honor myself, and I have not had a speeding ticket in a long time! No longer a need to rush. And I crave those evenings and weekends where nothing is planned.

My life has meaning, assisting others along this most magical adventure.

I continue, as well, with my own journey, as I believe it has no end. I believe there is no end to the discovery of our potential.

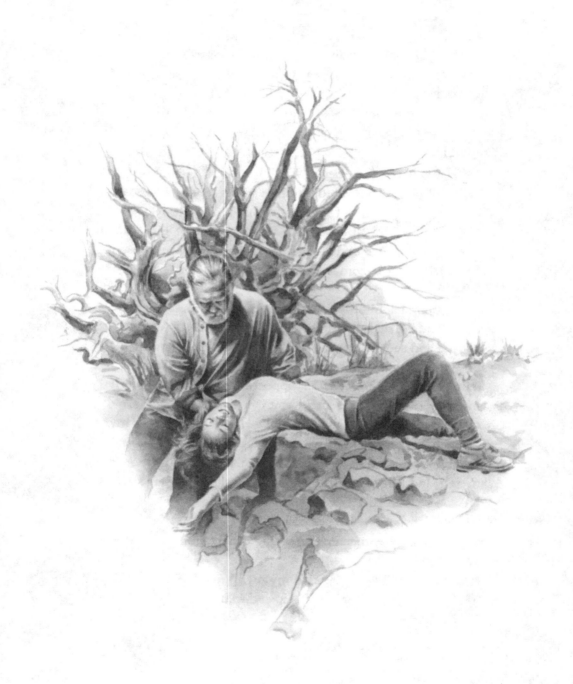

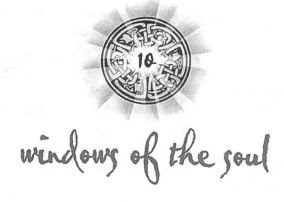

windows of the soul

Still points are the key to successful unwindings. I consider still points and freeze responses to be openings, an aperture into a higher dimension, opportunities for transformation; windows of the soul!

As myofascial release and myofascial unwinding allow a person to move into a significant position in space, a still point or freeze response occurs. The person's energy flows through these openings, or windows of the soul, to a higher dimension. A reorganization occurs; a reversible amnesia becomes conscious. The person moves from a state of disassociation into awareness, and with awareness, transformation becomes possible.

Myofascial unwinding allows the person, with the therapist's gentle guidance, to spontaneously discover the significant positions in space that represent positions of past trauma. These significant positions, still points, are important to recovery.

As these positions of past trauma are found, the person is transported back in time. Every physiological event, every sensation, every emotion and memory important to their healing is experienced. This experience is as vivid as if it is happening at the moment. These replays of mind-body memory, "tissue memory," produce awareness that allows the subconscious bracing patterns to let go of their fearful and powerful hold on the physicality. It releases the tightness, and as the tissue softens, learning occurs. Nature now allows the healing process to commence.

Initially you will miss some still points, but it's really no big deal. You'll just have to come back and find them eventually. No one is going to be injured, and it's the only way that you will learn.

There are a number of ways of feeling the still points. First imagine the head and body being filled with fluid or air. The circumference of the head, body, arms, and legs gets a little bit larger, then smaller, as if it is being pumped. When this pumping motion suddenly stops, this is a still point. Another way of feeling it would be to imagine that the body is moving along as if it has an engine driving it. All of a sudden, somebody flips the switch and the motion stops. Then someone flips the switch again, and the engine starts. When the motion stops, this is a still point.

Another way would be that as their movement stops, the patient gets lighter. You'll actually feel their whole physical structure lighten. And then as the energy comes back in, they seem to become heavier and they start to move again. You'll all have your own way of feeling this phenomenon. I'll just suggest a number of possibilities to you and you'll eventually develop your own feel of it. Initially it might be easier to recognize when they come out of the still point, as they become heavier and begin to move again. This relationship of still points with gravity is fascinating.

Another way to detect a still point is to feel the change in the velocity or quality of the motion. Unwinding tends to feel very floaty and smooth. It may be fast or slow, but there is certain silkiness to it. When you detect a change in the velocity or the quality of the motion, this is the time we step in and influence their motion. We guide them into finding and remaining present with their still points, because this is where significant tissue change occurs. Put a drag on their motion to slow them down and hold them in their still points. Always do this with gentleness. Now again, if they say the key word "Halt" you halt. Back off any pressure you may be applying. Always respect that!

Question: Can you say more about significant positions?

Because the force of past trauma and memory is still embedded in your body and is unexpressed, it has become a frozen moment in time. The tissue solidified; that is the freeze response. The unwinding will take them into positions you didn't think that they were physically capable of doing, that may even look and feel injurious. But as long as the person is truly unwinding, they will never be injured. What is happening is that they are moving into the extreme position that they were traumatized in by that car accident, other past injuries, or painful events, where vectors of force entered their body. They may scream, they may cry, they may struggle as they relive sensations of that past memory or event. They will feel their tissue melt, and those years and years of pain will start to dissipate. With the release of this frozen energy, the physical techniques that we have been utilizing will start to work, and lasting changes will occur in their body.

Myofascial release techniques should be combined with myofascial unwinding. During an unwinding it is often very appropriate to do some type of hands-on technique, maybe a crossed-hands technique or just applying pressure, especially if they are asking for that. They usually know. You can also do an arm- or leg-pull. Just watch what the body is trying to do and go with what it is already trying to do. If it is trying to go this way and you are pushing that way, you are interfering inappropriately.

Question: What happens when the patient shakes?

When the energy starts to flow, they might start to shake. They are having a deep, meaningful release. Still points are windows to the soul! Feel for still points. You need to hold them in the still point until they soften. Remember that when they come out of a still point, they get a little heavier and they start to move again. You might touch key areas once in a while to get them feeling. Remember, this is the key. At the end of most sessions I suggest saying to the patient something like, "What did you get out of that?" "What did you learn?"

You want them to take a look at their belief systems and see what messages come up. Now let them know that they don't need to answer right away; in fact, you prefer they don't answer and don't try to figure the answer out. You may already have talked to them a little bit about this ahead of time, so just say, "I'm going to plant the seed and next time you come in we can talk about this. Remind me." When they discover a dysfunctional message ask, "What would be a more positive, healthy message to believe and live by?"

Question: Why does the patient sometimes start to tremble?

It's a thawing of the freeze response. That's the energy starting to flow. They are deactivating their frozen state and shifting to a more fluid state. It's like wind blowing through a flag. You give them permission to shake or tremble as much as needed.

Question: When should you lift them?

Remember that you're not lifting them! You are just neutralizing the effects of gravity on their system and they will become lighter and float up. If you are lifting them, then back off because that will be your signal that you are not doing the right thing. You are working too hard and thereby forcing the system. There's no reason to do that. You don't have to hurt yourself. You just eliminate the effects of gravity, and they will go up.

I believe that they leave their body during a still point. What I mean by that is that I believe the mind, the energy body, has density and mass, and that's what you feel leave the body. That's why the body gets lighter. It goes out to another dimension and reorganizes. It then comes back through the silver cord, and the body gets heavier again; the energy comes back in. Then, they may go up again. Some really go airborne and do all sorts of flip-flops and unbelievable things. Their energy body is out there in the ozone and their physical body is trying to follow along. A still point could last seconds to minutes. The effects of gravity will eventually bring them back to the table or on down to the ground. We're not lifting or carrying them to the ground; we are simply guiding them down, being sure to keep them safe. We do this by following the movements and energy of the body.

Question: Does the patient always come back in after a still point?

Yes, they'll always come back.

Question: How do we know where to begin?

It doesn't matter where you start the unwinding. You may not really know what is going on; in fact, even the patient may not know what is going on. They come in with symptom complexes, but that's rarely the "core" problem. So they tell you their problem is their shoulder, and it's fine to begin treatment with the shoulder, or wherever their symptom complex exists.

There are a lot of wonderful physicians, dentists, and therapists out there who are very well intentioned, very highly skilled; obviously, medicine, surgery, technology and electronics have done wonderful things for mankind. But there are many conditions where medicine, surgery, or psychotherapy have not been successful. This is where myofascial release and other good manual therapy techniques can be important in the resolution of complex problems.

The medical profession is very good at diagnosing something, putting a label on it, and prescribing medication so you don't feel it. And people go on finding label after label, until they begin to identify with the label. People come in almost exhilarated! "The doctor told me I have such and such diagnosis." Well, what did he do about it? Nothing. But they've got a label now, so they can identify with that label. It makes it real for them. And now they feel something can be done about it. But what is a diagnosis? Nothing but a myopic description of a symptom! And a symptom is just the tip of the iceberg of the entire problem. That label can actually inhibit the patient's progress. They need to understand that they are not "the label." Too many identify with that label and become the condition. So you've got to get them to let go of that label. We need to encourage them to move beyond the label and create a vision of wellness for themselves.

You never guarantee anything to anybody. Follow the same list of contraindications for applying unwinding as for applying the myofascial release techniques. The worst thing that can happen is nothing. If it doesn't help, then it doesn't help, but at least you tried. No further injury occurred. At times, it might be helpful to have them reduce their medication. One always needs to consult with their physician first. The medication can get in the way because it anesthetizes them and keeps them from any depth of feeling. This inhibits them from any real learning that needs to occur to allow for tissue release and any kind of lasting change.

I'll give you a funny example of the type of attitude that you may run up against when this type of thing is suggested. It's very frustrating, and I know many of you have struggled with it.

A man was referred to us at "Therapy on the Rocks" in Sedona. He was a successful businessman and consultant, about thirty-five years old, who had been in a car accident about three years before coming to see us. He was now suffering with a lot of head, neck, and back pain and tightness, but what was most frustrating for him was that he was also struggling with a very severe, short-term memory deficit which had destroyed his career. The poor guy had driven down to see us and it took him eons, because he kept getting lost and forgetting where he was going, who he was supposed to see, what hotel he was going to, etc. Finally he stumbled into our place feeling very frustrated. He'd forgotten where he had a reservation to stay that night. We found out where it was and gave him directions. He called back about five minutes later, and by the time we'd told him where he was staying, he'd forgotten again. This is how bad he was! He was not only frustrated, he was also embarrassed.

He had come down for the Myofascial Release Intensive Treatment Program for three weeks. So the first day we treated him three times. On the second day, during his second treatment, he began to unwind. His head began unwinding, he went into a still point, and he became very quiet and still. While I was holding his head we both heard and felt a whooshing sound. I felt a deep release and he said, "You just got it." His memory came back instantaneously. Obviously he was very grateful. My sense was that his straight sinus had been blocked, creating an internal pressure on his brain, which had created his short-term memory deficit.

The funny part of this story—and the sad part—is that the first day when his memory was still really poor, he had said to me, "If you can help my memory, can I go off my medication?" And I said, "Talk to your doctor first to make sure you have her permission." Now remember, he was foggy and had difficulty remembering things. He returned to his doctor feeling great and told her he quit taking his medication; he no longer needed it. The doctor became furious because he went on to tell her that I gave him permission to go off of his medication. She was not one bit pleased that her patient was doing better, nor was she interested in how he got better. She was furious, thinking that I had overstepped my boundaries by advising him to go off his medication. I hadn't said that. He was mentally foggy. He only told her bits and pieces of the conversation. He forgot to mention I told him to check with her first. The point is that she seemed to care more about protecting her turf than she did about the good of her patient. You can't try to please those types of people. They're beyond that. Don't even worry about it. Don't concern yourself about it. Your job is to please the patient by doing what's right for the patient!

Interestingly, this man recently stopped by "Therapy on the Rocks" to say hello and let us know how well he is doing. In fact, he is doing so well that he just ran and completed the Pikes Peak race, where the athletes run to the top of Pikes Peak and back down! And he is about to run across the United States! That certainly says something about how myofascial release can improve function.

Question: What is helpful for cervical pain and headache from whiplash injury?

Myofascial release, myofascial/osseous release and cervical unwinding are great for headaches and neck pain. This can be done with the patient sitting or in a chair or on a stool. Normally I'll stand to their side and touch them lightly; I'll touch the thorax or shoulder very lightly with one hand and the other hand very lightly touches the top of the head over the parietals. You just wait and relax. Shortly you'll begin to feel this silky, floaty motion. It feels like water running down a hill and follows the path of least resistance. You just go with it. You don't lead, you don't force. You ride along with it. When they stop, you stop with them. Just wait there in the still point until they release and soften and move to another position. Simply ask them to feel. Some still points are very close together. Some are far apart.

Still points and freeze responses are important! One millimeter away nothing's happening; they're smiling. Next minute they're in the depths of something unbelievable. It's that quick and it's that important! So you're going to miss still points occasionally. Nobody is going to be injured. Be aware of them and you'll get better and better as time goes on. If the patient shakes or trembles, that's the freeze response beginning to release. If they express sound, tell them to "bring it up from your belly.

Feel it even deeper!" When you are touching their throat and you notice their lip is quivering or they're trying to make a little sound, simply give them permission to make sound. If that's not enough, usually touching them on the throat or the masseters is enough to trigger them. And when they do make sound, if it comes from the throat, tell them to bring it up from their gut. You may need to touch them there. I act as a surrogate. You listen to their sound. You mimic their sound. Then they make the sound and all of a sudden it gets a little louder and they go for it; and that stuck vibration (sound) is released. If their mouth is open and it looks like a silent scream, or if their throat is getting red, or their mandible or lips are quivering, the first thing to do is just give them permission to make noise. Just say, "Would you like to make noise?" And if nothing happens then, maybe just touch them lightly on the throat or belly. You want it to come from their gut. It has to be guttural. It only has transformative power when emotion is driving the sound.

Question: Do you ever push against the patient?

Sometimes we test the water and move them gently. If they move easily, you go with it. If they resist, you back off. You watch the body language. Some people will need resistance. If they are pushing, try to match it. At some point, if somebody is going through a tremendous struggle, let them really work at it, but at some point, let them win! Sometimes, we need to win. As a child you may have been held down and felt defeated, and now you need to win to complete that experience so that you can let go.

Question: What if the person is having difficulty letting go?

They must feel safe to let go. It's all about trust. Just encourage them to let go, to feel, to soften. Just let your patients know that you are there for them. When somebody is really letting go, they really need to know that somebody is going to be there for them. What I hear all the time from my patients is, "John don't leave me." Say to them, "Just let go." "Do whatever you want." "It's perfectly fine." "Whatever you do or say with me is between us, it's never going to leave this room." "Your expression of emotion is not going to be put on your chart." A lot of people are desperately afraid that if they express emotion or do something weird (and it's not really weird, but from their perspective it is), you will put it in their chart and they might lose their insurance or you'd ridicule them. So just let them know it's okay without pushing them, keep encouraging them to feel and to let go. That's usually what most people need.

Question: Are you saying that positions of the body may bring up therapeutic memories or sensations that psychotherapy hasn't?

Yes, it has been demonstrated consistently that when a myofascial release technique takes the tissue to a significant position, or when myofascial unwinding allows a body part to assume a significant position three-dimensionally in space, the tissue not only changes and improves, but memories, associated emotional states, and belief systems rise to the conscious level. This awareness, through the positional reproduction of a past event or trauma, allows the individual to grasp the previously hidden information that may be creating or maintaining symptoms or behaviors that deter improvement. With the repressed and stored information now at the conscious level, the individual is in a position to learn which holding or bracing patterns have been impeding progress, and why. The release of the tissue with its stored emotions and hidden information creates an environment for change.

A THERAPIST'S PERSPECTIVE

I remember John talking about his treatment room filling with the smell of horse manure while working with a woman who had been abused in a horse barn. I must admit that my reaction to the story was well...horse manure! But one of my friends at work came to me because of a locked shoulder post-endoscopy. We didn't make much progress in the session until she "unwound" and relived her father abusing her; the position I had her in triggered the memory. After the unwinding, which went on for some time and was quite draining for both of us, I thought I would end up with just a little relaxing hand massage. As I started to work on one of her hands, my office smelled of vinegar. I asked her if vinegar meant anything to her, she said "no", but I suggested that if she "found out differently, let me know." A second later she gasped and said, "That is where I went to escape. One place I was safe from my father was in the kitchen when my mother was canning!" She then raised her head from the face cradle, sniffed and said, "Do you smell pickles?"

Question: John, how would you define the myofascial/osseous release technique that you teach?

Visualize how fascial restrictions in random strain patterns can shorten, creating abnormal tensions upon individual or groups of fascicles and the neural, vascular, and osseous structures to which they attach, and which they powerfully influence. These abnormal compressive forces can exert pressure upon the neural structures, creating entrapment syndromes. Fascial compression of the vascular structures can produce ischemic conditions, and the shortening of the muscular component of the fascicle can limit its functional optimal length, reducing its strength and contractile potential and deceleration capacities.

These fascial restrictions can also create abnormal strain patterns that can pull the osseous structures too close together or out of proper alignment, resulting in compression of the facet joints or disk, producing pain and/or dysfunction. This scenario explains why modalities, exercise and flexibility programs, manipulation, massage, muscle energy techniques, neuromuscular techniques and mobilization procedures do not always produce lasting results. I have utilized manipulative procedures for close to forty years and have found all of the above-mentioned techniques to be very helpful. The frustration we have all encountered with poor or temporary results can now be understood by realizing that these procedures affect only the osseous structures or the muscular or elastic components of the myofascial complex. Only myofascial release affects the total myofascial complex—the muscular component and the elastic component of the fascia, the crosslinks that form in the collagenous part, and the viscosity of the fascia's ground substance.

The most effective and comprehensive approach for the reduction of pain and the restoration of the quantity and quality of motion for optimum function is the combination of myofascial release procedures with manipulation procedures, mobilization, muscle energy techniques, and soft tissue mobilization. Then the addition of appropriate modalities as well as exercise, flexibility, and neuromuscular facilitation techniques maximizes and maintains results.

Over the years, as I developed this approach to myofascial release, I have found that release of the fascial system also tends to balance and provide more space between the joint structures of the skeletal system. Trial and error led me to see that some manipulative techniques were too high in velocity or too short in duration, eliciting the body's protective responses or not affecting the environment of the osseous structures, the myofascial system. So the fascial strain patterns that were not released simply pulled the osseous structures back into positions of dysfunction.

This awareness through my experience led me to develop an expanded method of myofascial release called myofascial/osseous release. To help clarify, myofascial release is one end of the spectrum, where the therapist uses the fascial system as a handle or lever to relieve the pressure on pain-sensitive structures and/or mobilize the osseous structures. At the other end of the spectrum, myofascial/osseous release techniques focus on utilizing the osseous structures as handles or levers to free the skeletal structure and its environment, the surrounding myofascial system.

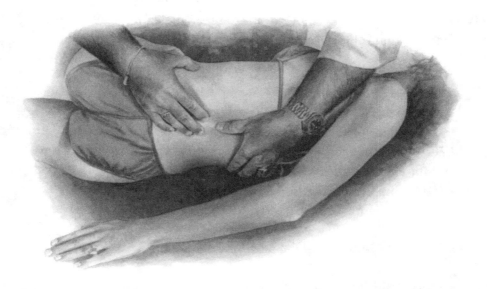

The very important difference from other mobilization, muscle energy, and manipulation procedures is that myofascial/osseous release techniques are performed very slowly following the fascial releases three-dimensionally. The fascial system does not release quickly or all at once. This time factor is essential for lasting results. The feel over time is like a rope unraveling, releasing a strand at a time. This creates a changing of tension that is followed by the sensitive, trained hands of the therapist in a three-dimensional manner, like taffy untwisting and stretching. Myofascial release and/or myofascial/osseous release techniques are safe, easily learned, and highly effective in reducing pain and restoring motion and optimal function on a permanent basis by treating the entire myofascial/osseous complex.

Question: What are the principles of "off the body" energy work?

There are principles to it that are similar to myofascial release. You learn to focus your "light energy" hand, not just your physical hand, to hook into their energy. Your physical hand is there, but your "light energy" hand is actually doing the work, acting like a magnet and starting to draw the energy like a weed. It's the same principles of myofascial release basically, you start to move the energy, you'll feel it get stuck, so instead of ripping it out, because you want to get the roots of the system, you stay there, and eventually you'll feel it give a little more and a little more. Then, as it starts to move, you sweep it a little bit more and then more vigorously. The whole idea is to break the dam, the frozen emotion or belief that is blocking the flow of energy, and start to move it.

Question: Do different areas emit different vibrations?

There is a difference. There are so many differences that I can't give you a quick synopsis of it, but just know that over time, you will learn to get a sense of those differences. For instance, a rib is going to emit a finer vibration than a vertebra. And emotions are going to send off certain energy; when someone is emotional you'll be able to feel the vibration in and off the body. I'm to the point now, when I'm close to somebody, I am totally aware of their emotional state, and when somebody's really in a state of negative emotions, the energy feels like a boiling cauldron, everything feels very agitated.

So, over time, you'll get more of a sense of it. Just know that no matter what the feel of the energy, it's telling you where they need physical intervention; it's telling you that you need to get the energy flowing. There are various forms of energy work that are out there. Only doing energy work is like shoveling fog. The trouble with just energy work is that it is not paying attention to the fascial system, which is creating and/or maintaining the restriction of the energy. We need to combine myofascial release with subtle energy therapy for maximum results.

A Therapist's Perspective

The phrase "Go deeper than the urge to make noise," and "Go deeper than the urge to move" have been most meaningful to me as I have again and again in my life been faced with my old pattern of staying stuck in my chaos. That phrase urges me to really face the energy that is stuck and to face the part of myself that I do not want to see. It urges me to listen and to honor the still point that the chaos of movement and noise prevent me from attaining. So many times in my life have I wanted to not hear or feel, not listen and be numb. "Going below the urge to move or make noise" is a call to me to be alive, to be present, to be in the moment and not in the past or future, to be NOW.

A Therapist's Perspective

Before Myofascial Release I, I was an angry, rageful, quiet and introspective person living in an abusive relationship. Taking Myofascial Release I in 1985 altered my life drastically and swiftly. I was sitting in the center aisle, and as John walked by, sometimes he would put his hand on my shoulder. I couldn't stand it and was shaking constantly and finally asked the person next to me to switch seats with me. At the end of Myofascial Release I, the lights were turned down and John started unwinding someone.... As I looked up, I saw John with a white light field around him. At this moment my childhood came flooding back to me. I had returned home to the energy I knew of and saw as a child. The energy I saw many times around people I had considered to be safe in my life. The energy I had used and played with as a child. The energy I had lost track of and sight of. I had this new clarity around my eyes. I was able to read road signs and return home safely and swiftly from Baltimore with no wrong turns or getting lost (this was not a normal occurrence).

John's presence brought me safety, balance, and stillness. John's touch was firm enough to give me boundaries and gentle enough to ease my child's fears, and find the soft and loving side of life. I felt he could handle my rage and bring up my laughter. John and the therapists he has trained were able to touch my pain. John gave me permission to release my anger, to laugh uncontrollably, to touch my patients and to care about my patients. John's classes have given me new vision, new hope, and a new direction in life.

I'm now in a loving relationship with a wonderful man and we have a beautiful daughter. I surround myself with healthy relationships and treat myself kindly. I love my work and patients love it too. I'm able to shift out of my stuff and stay out of it for extended periods of time, experiencing joy....I have less guilt and more determination. I'm able to make goals, set goals and change my goals if I want. I have permission to be me after all....

Thanks to you, John, and all the very lovely therapists whom have touched my body, emotions, mind and soul....

You are welcome. You mentioned safety, balance, and stillness, which are essential for healing to occur. The concept of windows on the soul can be explained by the engram theory. Fascia is an integral part of the entire body architecture. The fascia of one region becomes contiguous and confluent with the fascia of its adjacent regions. There is virtually no cell in the living organism that lies outside the fascial influence. I believe that during traumatization or development of the structural imbalance, a proprioceptive memory pattern of pain sensation and motion is established within the central nervous system. Beyond the localized pain response from injured nerves, these reflex patterns remain, perpetuating the pain and dysfunctional movement patterns beyond healing of the injured tissue, similar to the experience of phantom limb pain. Myofascial release, myofascial unwinding, and myofascial rebounding reprogram the central nervous system by resetting the proprioceptive sensory mechanism.

The fight/flight/freeze theory, the engram theory, and the proprioceptive memory concept seem to have a common denominator. Our internal alarms are ringing and can't automatically readjust after their initial activation.

This high level of neurological activity shuts down physiological processes. This internal exhaustion and disharmony can eventually cause dis-ease. The triad of myofascial release, myofascial unwinding, and myofascial rebounding deactivates our internal alarms, i.e., our protective mechanisms, and allows the mind-body to return to rest and the balance of homeostasis. When homeostasis is achieved, healing commences.

A THERAPIST'S PERSPECTIVE

John, would you allow me to share my thoughts on the connection between engrams and myofascial unwinding?

As John says, we are gelatinous electromagnetic fascial beings of intelligence. During myofascial unwinding, the body taps into stored memories of specific movements or series of movements, as well as the emotional responses correlating to those movements, called the sensory and emotional engram patterns.

Engrams are located in the sensory side of the cerebral cortex and are the body's means of arranging into meaningful sequences the firings of the primitive reflexes to control motion. The motor system follows the pattern of stimulation it receives. A sensory engram is a sensory record of a particular gesture or series of gestures that is a remembered sequence of sensations from all of the species' past and current experiences. It is an "ancient/now" simultaneous pattern, subject to immediate change, and operating within the confines of the connective tissue. The body adapts to restrictions in the connective tissue network, which are functions of habitual movements. The Sensory engram adapts to any movement restrictions, and at the same time those same restrictions are a product of the sensory engram. Likewise the emotional engram develops its own signature response pattern directly correlated to the cerebral cortex perceptions. Negative fear thoughts can result in the body responding by protecting itself with preparing for flight/fight. Since the brainstem is only responsive to the "now," if the cerebral cortex perceives danger, the body will respond in real time to danger, whether it is imagined or actual.

Unwinding can access the engram and feed new information into the sensorimotor loop. During unwinding, the body moves into a "still point" where the new information is evaluated and integrated, accepting new beliefs or insights and responding accordingly in the musculature to open space and free movement. The pain-spasm-pain cycle is interrupted on a most intimate level, beyond the physical structure. The fascial voice of unwinding seeks balance and homeostasis among the entire being...emotionally, physically, and spiritually.

Another Perspective

John, I agree, and would like to add that we are referring to the memory template that is created within the brain in response to a trauma or experience within the body. This is a technical way of describing the mind-body connection. Our brains are not unlike a sophisticated computer. All information is stored on a disk, and how it is stored is an exact replica of the experience itself.

During the process of unwinding, when your body is moved into a tissue memory of an emotional or physical nature, the still point or freeze response is a window of memory or awareness that opens. And within that window is the doorway to recovery if the body is given an opportunity to let go of or move beyond the physical or emotional connection to our being at that current moment in time.

The healing, as I believe personally, is within the complete acceptance of this occurrence, the surrendering to it and the emotional process of experiencing the trauma or situation fully. Very often that means experiencing something to its fullest, expressing oneself fully and then asking oneself or others for complete forgiveness for our response or being at that time, and then if possible filling that engram template or space within your body with love and light. Within this process of awareness, the body is able to detach from the hold this has on our current being. Sometimes there are messages to our being…we all must remain willing to move through this to view its purpose to ourselves in the present—to let go.

A Therapist's Perspective

John, I recently had an interesting and rather disturbing experience with which I was hoping you could help me.

My neck has bothered me on and off for the past few years. Typically, my wife would work on it and things would resolve, but our lives had been hectic, and a few weeks passed without a treatment. The pain had started in its usual place, on the left side of the neck, but this time was spreading down into the left shoulder and rib cage. I could feel the fascia tightening down, all emanating from one spot in my neck. I was trying to continue with my busy schedule of treating patients, coaching my daughter's gymnastic team, etc., but this neck thing just kept getting worse. After an afternoon with gymnastics, I was attempting to relax when a sensation began to move through my left shoulder, chest and rib cage. As I sat there I could feel the fascia tighten in my chest like I was caught in a vise! Each breath became more painful until I was only able to inhale slightly without extreme pain. My wife was convinced I was having a heart attack. I took three ibuprofens and prayed. After forty-five minutes my breath finally returned but not without pain. John, what could have caused this?

It sounds like the chronic and recurrent neck tightness resulted in myofascial osseous restrictions that slowly tightened and spread throughout the years. Then sometimes the slightest thing can throw people over the edge and send them into an acute situation and/or emergence of new and expanded symptoms. It's the "straw that broke the camel's back!" The fascia around the chest and heart were probably already tight, and maybe a rib or two disarticulated. A rib out of place is excruciating, making it hard to breathe, and it can mimic a heart attack.

What was interesting was that after the chest pain continued for two to three days I began to experience an intense burning sore throat pain on the left side of my throat, followed quickly by intense headaches and flu-like symptoms. My physician ordered a chest x-ray as he thought I had spontaneous pneumothorax, which of course I did not have, but he could not see how the neck pain could be related to the sore throat and headaches. My left-sided chest pain, sore throat, and headache slowly subsided, only to be followed by a fever blister on the left side of my mouth! How can these events possibly relate to my original neck pain?

Let's take our focus down to the cellular level. Fascial restrictions not only put excessive pressure on the heart and blood vessels, nerves, bones, muscles, etc., but the ground substance which is the very environment of the cell begins to solidify. This then can cause inefficiency in the cell's ability to metabolize, breathe, and eliminate waste products. The cellular environment becomes toxic, diminishing the immune system's ability to defend us from invaders. In other words, we become more prone to sickness, chronic fatigue, and disease.

With this in mind, let me expand a little more on how the fascial system, when restricted, can negatively impact upon the functioning of the heart. A fascial sheath called the pericardium surrounds your heart. For years I have been teaching that myofascial restrictions in the chest can create problems in the efficiency and effectiveness of the pumping mechanism of the heart.

The following is paraphrased from a front-page article in the *Wall Street Journal*, November 3, 1999.[1] There is an emerging hypothesis that humans are hobbled by genetic machinery geared to defend them more from prehistoric dangers such as saber-toothed tigers than from chronic ailments. Dr. Karl Weber is an expert in heart-muscle mechanics. He observed that half of the deaths of heart failure patients result from the heart pumps gradually giving out. Half occurred suddenly. An athlete's heart under the microscope looks like filet mignon; in a heart failure patient the heart looks like stewed beef. The difference in failing hearts, Dr. Weber and colleagues found in research done mostly at the University of Chicago, is an extraordinary abundance of fibrous connective tissue in the spaces between the cells. This makes the muscle stiff and like an old bellows, unable to contract effectively.

So what does all this have to do with a saber-toothed tiger? The human circulatory system developed over millions of years, when surviving an attack by a predator presumably required the ability to preserve blood pressure, to make clot-promoting platelets, and to retain salt and water. Once the circulation is stable, the same system stimulated the repair process, which includes laying down the fibrous scaffolding on which new cells are assembled into tissue. Once the repairs are completed, the system retreats and the body returns to normal.

Dr. Weber isn't alone when he argues that congestive heart failure triggers this system. When the heart fails to pump adequate blood to the body, he says, the kidney senses low blood volume. It thinks it's the Sahara Desert, he says. The survival mechanisms kick in. But by helping the body to preserve salt and water that it doesn't actually need, and to lay down fibrous tissue it doesn't need, the defense mechanisms worsen the situation. The result is a chronic and potentially lethal feedback loop that never shuts off. The body, Dr. Weber says, becomes a house divided.

While this *Wall Street Journal* article was focused on the heart, these phenomena can apply to the entire body's fascial framework. This sounds exactly like the fight/flight/freeze response! The myofascial system will become restricted with excess fibrous tissue from trauma, inflammatory processes and unexpressed emotions. Today's saber-toothed tigers are the stresses of modern life, cars coming at you, horns blowing, work, and relationship problems.

Unlike animals that are naturally expressive, with a life full of motion and action, we are taught to "be nice," don't feel or express your emotions. Our mind-body defense mechanisms are triggered and never extinguished. Our inner "alarms" are ringing and we slowly spiral down into a dysfunctional spiral. Our systems become exhausted and eventually "give out." Symptoms appear to spread, and gradually worsen.

Another factor to consider is the excessive use of anti-inflammatory drugs. Traditional allopathic medical approaches to relieving patient complaints have focused primarily on masking symptoms through the use of drugs. *Dorland's Illustrated Medical Directory*, 25th edition, defines inflammation as "a localized protective response elicited by injury or destruction of tissue, which serves to destroy, dilute or wall off...both the injurious agent and injured tissue." In reality, inflammation is a necessary and essential protective response in the healing mechanism. Any attempt to disrupt this inflammatory stage will, in effect, retard the natural healing process. This "walling off" process is then not allowed to dissipate and can cause fibrous buildup on the cellular level. I believe that this thwarting of the complete inflammatory process can cause sickness, fibromyalgia, endometriosis, pain, and tightness that insidiously develop over time.

Emotional trauma can tighten the myofascial system as much as physical trauma and uncompleted inflammatory processes. Remember that we have an elastic component within the elasto-collagenous complex, and the skeletal musculature also lies within the fascial system. Stress in and of itself is not bad; it is our reaction to stress that can create problems. If we don't feel, express, and learn from stress and our emotions, we then habitually brace against life, against feeling submerged emotions, and against future fear of pain and stress. Our training from society programmed us with a set of rules that worked against our health, against expression of our true self, and against living life fully.

We have all had our hearts "broken!" If this perceived pain or loss was not integrated and expressed, these unresolved emotions can turn into myofascial restrictions, and many will eventually end up with physical heart problems as the result.

I'd like to quote from Marianne Williamson's wonderful book *A Return to Love:*

"When we were born, we were programmed perfectly. We had a natural tendency to focus on love. Our imaginations were creative and flourishing, and we knew how to use them. We were connected to a world much richer

than the one we connect to now, a world full of enchantment and a sense of the miraculous.

So what happened? Why is it that we reached a certain age, looked around, and the enchantment was gone?

Because we were taught to focus elsewhere. We were taught to think unnaturally. We were taught a very bad philosophy; a way of looking at the world that contradicts who we are.

We were taught to think thoughts like competition, struggle, sickness, finite resources, limitation, guilt, bad, death, scarcity, and loss. We began to think these things, and so we began to know them. We were taught things like grades, being good enough, money, and doing things the right way, are more important than love. We were taught that we're separate from other people, that we have to compete to get ahead, that we're not quite good enough the way we are....The thinking of the world, which is not based on love, began pounding in our ears the moment we hit shore.

Love is what we were born with. Fear is what we have learned here. The spiritual journey is the relinquishment—or unlearning—of fear and the acceptance of love back into our hearts. Love is the essential existential fact. It is our ultimate reality and our purpose on earth. To be consciously aware of it, to experience love in ourselves and others, is the meaning of life....

We came here to co-create...be extending love. Life spent with any other purpose in mind is meaningless, contrary to our nature, and ultimately painful....

Love isn't material. It's energy....We experience it as kindness, giving, mercy, compassion, peace, joy, acceptance, non-judgement, joining and intimacy.

Fear is our shared lovelessness, our individual and collective hells.... When fear is expressed, we recognize it as anger, abuse, disease, pain, greed, addiction, selfishness, obsession, corruption, violence and war.

Love is within us. It cannot be destroyed, but can only be hidden..."[2]

—From the Introduction of *A Return to Love* by Marianne Williamson

✎

[1] Winslow, R. Heart failure patients get new hope, thanks to a forgotten drug. Ron Winslow, *Wall Street Journal*, 11/3/99.

[2] Williamson, M. *A Return to Love.* Harper Collings, New York, NY. 1992.

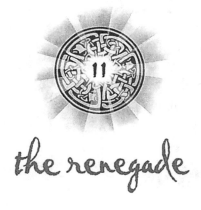

the renegade

As one becomes more experienced on this path, interesting and some-times startling phenomena begin to occur. One is struck that maybe the physical symptoms are just a superficial veneer, that possibly there is another dimension that has to do with our imaginal consciousness, a symbolic world of ancient wounds that, when allowed to be connected to the present physical sensations, creates an opportunity for learning, growth, and resolution of present-day problems.

Possibly many of the patterns we have in this lifetime are symbolic or representative of a similar type of experience from earlier in our lifetime, or perhaps even in another lifetime, that was never totally resolved. So, nature has given us an opportunity to do something about it again. And when you start to see these past life experiences, you start to see patterns in your life that came from those ancient wounds. As you return to those ancient wounds, they allow you to become more aware, so now your present-day, dysfunctional pattern can change. You no longer keep injur-ing your neck; or that old back pain that has been bothering you for so long goes away, because you learned from and transformed what origi-nally caused it. So we must look at all of the experiences that come up for us as a possibility. Also, it can be helpful to look at the symbolic level, the image level of this phenomenon.

Past-life experiences certainly are controversial, and as I said earlier, you don't have to believe a word I say. It is not really important to the treatment process whether you personally believe in past lives or not.

Past-life experiences really may be no more than your mind's way of representing a lesson to you in symbolic form, for that is the way your right brain works, via stories, pictures, colors, feelings, and that type of thing. Regardless of what we believe, it is not up to us to be judgemental and force our belief system on somebody else. We need to support the situation, go with the action, and speak their language. Let's say somebody is unwinding, and all of a sudden they start to express that they are on a battlefield, and there is snow on the ground and they are freezing. They perceive that it is the eighteenth century and they have a spear in their body. You don't say, "that is ridiculous!"

Keep your communication in right-brain language, saying one of the following: "What do you see?" "What do you feel?" "What does that mean to you?" "What does that represent or symbolize to you?" Those phrases are basically right-brain language. You stay away from "why." Nothing shuts people down faster than the question "why," because that throws them into their left brain to try to figure things out. You will feel them shut down if you do ask "why." The "why" question is the very basis of most psychology and psychiatry. Figuring it out gets in the way of healing. If they need to know why, it will come up, and, just like when we are waiting for them to unwind, it takes a little while for the right brain to process through the left brain and turn it into left-brain language, words. So, give them a little time and let them know that when you ask them a question, they never have to answer. There is absolutely no pressure ever to answer, and if they do answer, it may take a little time. Don't keep peppering them with questions. The answers may come up as a word or thought, or it may come up as a feeling, a picture, a symbol or an emotion. All of that is valuable information.

In any event, I have experienced what appears to be my own past life. I have died a number of times in my unwindings, and for me, as I moved into that so-called death space, it was a wonderful place. It took away all of my fear of dying. It has allowed me to live life more fully! The Dalai Lama has said in his book, *The Path to Tranquillity* that, whether one believes in a religion or not, and whether one believes in rebirth or not, there is not anyone who doesn't appreciate kindness and compassion.

Don't have an agenda; just be open to whatever. Allow yourself to find your own mind-body's way; it has its own agenda and wisdom. Many times either in this life or in other lives, the person, when unwinding, may go back to early childhood. Don't talk to them like an adult. You have an adult body lying there, but you have a four-year-old mentality surfacing; so talk to them like a four-year-old. They may also go back into times when they were pre-verbal, so don't expect them to talk. They may just need to gurgle or make noise or cry. They may go back to times where they are not speaking English. Don't expect them to answer your questions. They may not understand. And also, do not call them by their name, because they may have had a nickname when they were younger. It could just throw them into confusion and into their left brain to try to figure out what's happening. Or if there is such a thing as a past life, they may have had a different name or they may have even been the other sex! So Ralph today may have been Alice then. Go with the action, whatever it is. It is always fascinating!

Question: Would you tell us one of your ancient wounds in a past life?

I was in Denver finishing the second day of the Myofascial Release I seminar. As I stepped off the stage students swarmed around me, thanking me, and asking questions. I have always been happy to answer serious questions and feel that there are no stupid questions. In fact, it can be very interesting going to the core of a concept. We tend to take things too much for granted, so we get lost in the labels and lose the essence of what we're actually saying or questioning.

It was getting late and this one therapist kept peppering me with a question that he kept rephrasing in different ways; it was obvious that he had an agenda. He already knew the answer and was more interested in showing the others and me what he knew. Eventually, one of my instructors came up and distracted him and I walked out of the door and into the elevator. This guy had agitated me and I found myself agitated that he had agitated me! As I entered my room, I was asking myself, "what was it about this therapist that I found so annoying?" He symbolized the constant resistance to what I believe in and teach, and the mindless resistance to change exhibited by some. I was about to delve into my feelings deeper when the phone rang. It was one of my instructors, asking if she and the three other instructors could get together; they needed treatment and sensed that I did also. I reluctantly agreed.

I was aware that my usual deep, inner calm was missing. I felt tired and was in deep resistance to being with anyone, let alone to being treated. As I got off the elevator and walked down the corridor to their room, I stopped and turned around to go back to my room. I decided that I would rather be alone. As I swung around, my intuitive voice, The Ancient Warrior, boomed..."GO!" I have trusted my intuition implicitly since my earliest memories.

I entered the instructor's room. The lights were dim and we decided the order in which we would be treated; I would go last. Their treatments went well, but I felt unusually tired. They suggested that I lie on the bed. One therapist cradled the back of my head; the other three touched my torso and legs. I quieted myself and nothing happened for a while. I told myself mentally that even if nothing happened, this felt soothing. Eventually a very subtle, slow, spontaneous motion began in my body. I felt like I was being transported back in time. I went deeper and deeper and I became aware that my motions were speeding up and I could feel a rumble deep in my belly. A charge of energy was quickly building momentum. The rumble in my belly started to feel like a freight train. I exploded and was now airborne fighting powerfully, throwing all four people around like little sticks. I was furious! They leaped on me and held me down in a spread-eagle position with each one pinning my limbs down with all their weight. My fury went beyond anything I had experienced before. The spread-eagle position and the feel of their weight on me catapulted me into another time. I saw mountains in the background, it was dusk and I had just been lassoed and pulled off my horse.

I was caught! I couldn't believe it...I was caught! I was a Native American, glistening with sweat and I could smell the "white man"; I hated the smell of white men! They had me spread-eagle and were beating me. The rumble in my belly escalated into a frightening power that exploded in me. I roared, throwing all four into the air. The sound of lamps crashing and the therapists falling on me brought me back into present time. We were all in shock, stunned at the force that had exploded from deep inside of me, a force that had thrown four full-grown adults high in the air. I was still panting, with a low, rumbling growl coming from my throat. They were shaken and it took me over ten minutes to return fully to the present time.

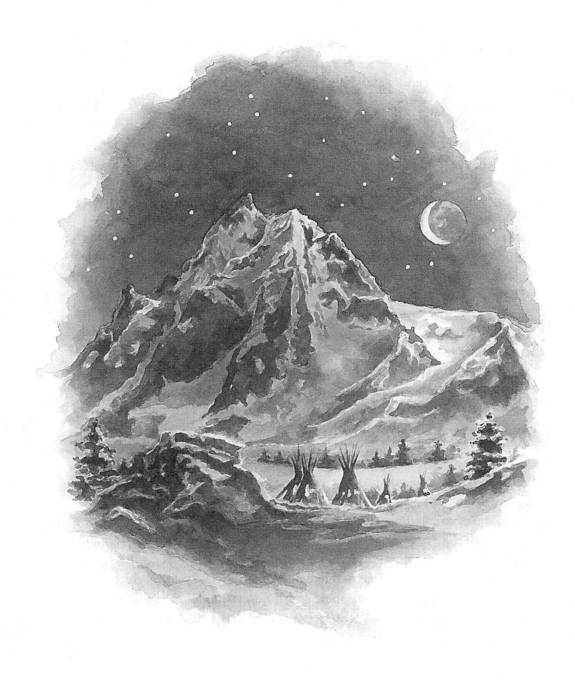

We decided to lie on the floor and quiet ourselves. A vision that was implied by The Ancient Warrior years before began to play in my "mind's eye." I saw hoards of white men, with guns streaming across the prairie. I saw that if we didn't do something my people would be killed. My tribe had already been under attack by the white men, but nothing of the magnitude seen in my vision. I shared my vision with my father, who was the Chief and leader of my tribe. I told him we should put our differences aside with the other tribes and join forces to protect us; there is strength in numbers. He refused. He could not forgive the grievances he held against them.

My ideas were eventually rejected and I was causing too much turmoil. I felt that it was best to leave the tribe with a few trusted friends to see what I could do on my own. I found it impossible to change the minds of those interested in the status quo. I was now called the "Renegade," and the only one who stayed with the tribe but knew of my whereabouts was my wife. I started to loot the white men's storehouses for guns and ammunition. Over time I gained quite a following with many of the braves from different tribes who were willing to fight and defend our tribes. Our successes in stealing guns began to threaten the white men. As the leader, they saw me as a threat and they started to hunt for the "Renegade."

I started to return to normal consciousness and felt devastation at having been caught. We all decided to call it a night and go to bed.

Question: John, did this all seem real to you when it happened?

Yes. When you go into the past with unwinding you don't *think* about it; you actually *relive* it, with all your senses, in vivid detail. This can generate tremendous force. There is the force within the memory that is trapped, like a volcano trying to erupt, which can eventually create dysfunctional behavioral filters and symptomatic complexes. As this force is expelled during myofascial release, the myofascial system releases its hold on the physical, emotional, and intellectual components of our being. Basically, the fight/flight/freeze response is extinguished, releases occur, and healing can commence.

Question: John, you always encourage us to be open to learning from a past situation or pain, to be able to let it go and grow. What did this ancient wound teach you?

This ancient wound symbolized for me my struggle for people to wake up from complacence, the trance of the status quo, the need to respond to change when change is necessary. We need to combine the strengths of the linear, intellectual side with the prodigious power of our creative, wise side. Instead of fighting, let the "East" meet the "West," to synthesize and be whole. This strengthened me, for I saw that I was on the "right track"; however, I was depressed because it appeared that I had lost my fight.

Question: Was this the end of the story?

No, a few weeks later I asked some of my therapists to treat me, and it turned into an unwinding and the story continued... I, The Renegade, was fighting with these men, and one hit me on the head and knocked me out. As I awoke I was tied to the back of a horse being dragged through a stream. They were trying to drown me. Water was filling my lungs and I was gasping for air and choking and then everything went dark! I lay still and the unwinding finished. I was distraught. I interpreted this as the end. I had died! I had lost my fight! I had let my people down!

For months after that experience I was depressed and sad. I was confused. Why put out all this effort, if it was doomed for failure? I felt like I had the rug pulled out from under me! This period of personal chaos was coupled with professional chaos. I was being attacked in the professional newspapers for what I believed in. I was in the national physical therapy headlines weekly. Traditional therapists who had never met me or taken my seminars called me every derogatory name possible. They even called me a "Renegade" for defying the traditional ways!

On January 15, 1991, my organization sent out a nationwide brochure that cost close to one hundred thousand dollars. My years of experience had enabled me to predict the response. On January 16 the Gulf War broke out. Hardly any response. I might as well have burnt the money. With the possibility of war, people were scared to travel and the mentality was why educate myself, if I may have to go to war or die? Attendance at the seminars plummeted. I was lecturing to a miniscule number of people at each seminar and losing tens of thousands of dollars each seminar. This went on for a long period of time. I was confused, but there was a spark deep inside of me that wouldn't die. Everyone told me that I was crazy to continue. We were paying our bills, but barely. It was very bleak. One night as I lay in bed I felt very alone, and emotions welled up deep inside me. I asked The Ancient Warrior what I should do.

Don't stop. You have lost the battle, not the war. Summon your courage and continue.

I feel like I've had my vision taken from me. I don't know where to go.

No one can take your vision from you. Let adversity strengthen you. Go deeper and you will reconnect with your vision. Ask to be unwound again.

The next day my schedule was full, treating patients until nine in the evening. About three that afternoon, I received a call from a friend. He said a mutual friend whom I had trained called him to relay a message to me; she'd had a dream that I was in a desperate struggle, and needed to be unwound. He said that they would be over around nine when I finished treatment that night. I thanked him, but said that I couldn't, that I had to leave right after seeing patients to drive to New York City to give a Myofascial Release Seminar the next morning. He interrupted me to explain that she was from Maine, and was already on a plane flying down. I appreciated her kindness and I remembered The Ancient Warrior's suggestion and reluctantly agreed. After the last patient that night, the three of us went into a treatment room. She explained that she didn't know me that well, but that her dream was so vivid. She said she felt so grateful to me for what I had taught her; myofascial release had changed her life and her patients', and she felt compelled to help. In her dream she "got" that I was too stubborn to ask for help.

The unwinding started and I returned to the darkness as I lie in the creek. I was very still. The two therapists stood over me as I lay on my back. All of a sudden I saw my arm burst out of the water and grab the White Man's neck! I then threw a punch and hit the other, knocking them down. I was alive! I had pretended to be dead! I had fooled them! As they went sprawling, I picked up one of their pistols and shot three of them. Then I leaped on a horse and escaped. There was one left, but I was free!

I was jubilant. I couldn't believe that I had spent months feeling sorry for myself. The two therapists were brushing themselves off and I picked them up and apologized for knocking them around! We all laughed and hugged each other and I thanked them for their help. On the ride up to New York I was so happy and grateful. It was midnight and there wasn't much traffic on the New Jersey Turnpike. I was driving at about sixty miles per hour when all of a sudden I was somewhere else. I saw myself again as the "Renegade." I had white owl feathers in my hair, and wore deerskin boots and a loincloth. I was leaping off a cliff, descending quickly, and then smashing my tomahawk into a man's head. I yelled in victory... I had just killed the fourth man! I had circled back, tracked him and pounced on him from the cliff above. In my vision, I then turned into a powerful panther, which is my power animal.

Just as suddenly, I was back in my car driving through the oil refinery area of the New Jersey Turnpike, as though nothing unusual had happened. I don't know how long that experience took in real time, maybe an instant, for I was still in the same lane driving at the same speed. This was such a powerful lesson to me to NEVER GIVE UP! When adversity strikes, go inward to that deep well of strength that lies within all of us. Maintain your vision and never give up!

Some people would call that crazy. But my experience has been that we all have another dimension where our power, creativity, and wisdom lie, and we can learn to tap into this inner strength at will. And as we learn to do this, we can teach our clients and patients to do this, for this is the dimension where our ability to heal lies. Interestingly, the seminar attendance picked up that next week and grew steadily and we returned to sold-out attendances.

A funny thing happened to me a few months after that. A friend of mine who is a psychiatrist invited me to a workshop. It was being given by a psychic who was affiliated with the Edgar Cayce Foundation and who had decided to come "out of the closet" in this workshop. The problem was that I had been working for two months straight with no days off and the weekend of the workshop was the first weekend that I had to rest. My friend was very excited and I didn't want to let him down, so I went. It was a small group of ten people; except for my friend, I didn't know anyone. I liked the speaker; he was very articulate and seemed solid. But I found myself grumbling to myself that this was very rudimentary and here it was my only weekend off and I am sitting here listening to concepts that I am very familiar with. All of a sudden The Ancient Warrior said,

Stop it! A master always looks at each situation as a fresh moment, ripe with opportunity.

So, I quieted down as I heard the speaker say, "pick someone you don't know, pair up and sit facing each other." A young lady of about twenty-one, whom I had never met before, got up and asked if she could be my partner. I agreed. The instructor asked us to quiet our minds, pull our energy back, and sit there in silence. After about five minutes I felt jolts go through my body, and my partner screamed! The instructor ran over and asked her what happened. She said she didn't know. She said we started to quiet down and relax, and all of a sudden my partner—she pointed at me—"turned into a shimmering Indian, with white owl feathers on his head. He jumped off a cliff and hit and killed a man with a hatchet. And then he transformed into a huge cat, which pounced at me!"

She said she didn't know what she was doing there. She'd been out shopping with her girlfriend, she said, pointing to another lady across the room. She added that she was a hairdresser and was not familiar with this type of thing. Her friend had heard about this workshop from a friend and thought it might be fun. She said, "Wow! What an experience. This sure beats shopping!" I went over to her at break and said, "I didn't mean to scare you." She said, "It's okay. It was worth it. I feel lighter and calmer than I can ever remember feeling. Thank you!"

We spend so much valuable time lost in this incessant internal chatter. We can get lost in the rumination of our linear side for days, weeks, months, or unfortunately for some, a lifetime. A master is always in the present moment, in his or her power. Opportunity abounds in the now! The perspective of the present moment is eternal and gives us the power of clarity and awareness. Healing occurs in the present moment! It is essential that the therapist be in their center. Their patient will feel the experience of the "now." It is in the space of the present moment that authentic healing and growth occurs and transforms us into our full potential.

Question: John, it seems that the more I learn about myofascial release, the more I question. I am perceived as the expert in my area and I find this a bit hard to deal with.

Henry Miller, in *Wisdom of the Heart*, wrote, "I obey only my own instincts and intuition. I know nothing in advance." You are the best at what you do, but you need to remain open at all times. Nothing will limit your power and effectiveness more than to think that you have it all figured out. Always view yourself as a beginner, always discovering, always willing to fail. Be open to what the body is telling you, and be ready to respond to it. The expert already has things figured out, already knows what is wrong, and already knows how to fix it. Nothing could be more limiting. If you know what you are going to do when you walk into the patient's room, you don't know what you are doing! Myofascial release is all about constantly following your intuition. Be like a cat, curious with all of your senses keenly aware, and respond to the moment. View yourself as the beginner, and let others view you as they will.

[1] Reflection on writing. *Wisdom of the Heart*, New Directions Press, Norfolk, Connecticut, 1941. See page 331 in Wu Li Masters for full reference.

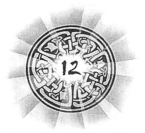

if they walk into the room, they will walk out!

I had an interesting call a couple of years ago. I don't usually respond to phone calls when I'm treating. One of my assistants knocked on my door and asked, "When you are done, is there any way you can get on the phone? We have a person who is very insistent on talking to you and seems very upset." I was just finishing up, so I picked up the phone. He said, "John, you don't know me, but one of my therapists took one of your courses a couple of months ago and it's good stuff, isn't it?" I said, "Yes it is." And he said, "And that unwinding stuff, I like that a lot. He taught me how to do some of it and it's really been helping people." I'm thinking I've got a patient waiting. I can hear all this noise in the phone in the background. And he says, "The reason I'm calling you is, we got this guy unwinding in the clinic right now, and he won't stop unwinding!" And in the background, I could hear all this thrashing and groaning and moaning. And he says, "What do I do?" I gave him a couple of clues. He put the phone down and I hear him walk away. More noise. I hear footsteps back to the phone. "John," he said, "he's still moving around a lot." So I said, "Well, what happened to him?" And he said, "Well, he was run over by a pea picker." Now I don't know what a pea picker is, but he said it's a large machine that picks peas and it has huge tires on it. Then we hear screaming, the phone drops, and the man runs away from the phone.

When he returns he says, "John you're not going to believe this, but I just saw the tractor treads go across his chest! John, he's not moving right now." He said, "John, he died!" And I said, "Well don't worry about it. He'll come back." I told him what to do, and he went away for a little while and came back and said, "You were right. He's breathing now and says he's feeling pretty good now."

What will happen with the unwinding phenomenon, is that you will be taken back to exactly what happened to the patient at the moment of injury. I don't want to tell you anything that scares you, but I want to prepare you for anything. I have treated a number of people who have appeared to die while I was working with them. They become cold and still. They stop breathing, and there is no energy in their body. When this happens to you the first time, it will tend to freak you out a little bit. But if that happens, just pretend that I am kneeling next to you whispering this in your ear: "If they walk into the room, they will walk out!" If they fall over in the waiting room it may be time to call the medics, but if you're unwinding them, remember, "If they walk into the room, they will walk out," and they will have experienced the most amazing changes.

Sometimes you will see physical manifestations occur during or following unwinding. I've treated a lot of abuse patients and cult victims, and you will notice when you are treating them that whip marks appear across their back or rope marks around their neck. You will smell drugs come out of their mouth. I think what happens is—and again, nobody has any proof of this, I'm just trying to put some sense into some of these experiences—is that somehow these energy patterns, these memories, are locked in the energy field. Consider our electromagnetic field as our mind. Our mind is not just in our physical body, but beyond our body. So when the body physically moves through that electromagnetic field, when it hits the still point, it finds these frozen memories, that allow the energy that has been frozen in time to start to flow through the physicality. It flows through the fascial system's microtubules to the brain, our computer, and converts this energy into symbols which in turn, via the neural system, convert the energy into physical action. I've literally treated people whose eyes become black and blue, and I hadn't touched their head. All of a sudden they had a memory from when they were ten years old when they were hit in the eye with a baseball, and they've had eye pain and sinus problems since the incident. Ten minutes later the black and blue mark goes away, and within a day or two the eye pain that's been bugging them for thirty-some years goes away and their sinuses clear up.

I often laugh when the people take my course and they go back to a remote area in Iowa or Nebraska and they say, "Well, I have nobody to talk to about this." And I want to answer, "Do you think I had anybody to talk to when I started?"

I actually began developing this Myofascial Release Approach as a result of my own back injury and the excruciating pain which resulted from it. Maybe I should go back a little bit. My father died when I was three. I was an only child. He'd owned a gentleman's farm, and after he died my mother continued to take me up to the farm for the weekends and summers. We lived on top of a mountain that was surrounded by thousands of acres of forest. I was alone a lot, and to break the boredom, I would go out into the woods by myself and play. I found that I had a good sense of direction, so I used to play a little game with myself. I would go out in the woods and purposefully get lost and try to find my way back home. It didn't always work out, but after a while I became pretty good at getting myself back. It almost seemed like I was out of my body, looking down at myself. From this high vantage point, I could make my way through the woods and find my way back home. In Pennsylvania, the summers, especially August, were very hot and humid. So at midday I would find a big old tree that had a lot of shade, and I found that if I would sit down under the tree and become very quiet, eventually all the birds' sounds would pick up again. The birds and animals would actually come to me.

So, I think early on I learned the value of silence and quieting down. And maybe at the time I was having out-of-body experiences, but I didn't have that label for it. It seemed very natural to me and I didn't think that there was anything unusual about it. The other thing that was interesting to me was that my mother would occasionally go into the local town to shop and I would ride in with her for something to do. I had no interest in shopping, so I found myself, even from an early age, going into this particular bookstore and just sort of browsing around. Eventually I became interested in different philosophies and comparative religion. As I read all of these different philosophies, it seemed to me that they were all saying the same thing; it was just from a lot of different perspectives coming from different cultural contexts. There was an image in a lot of these philosophies that I use today. I'll get more into this later when I talk more about how people tend to leave their body and how we need to all bring ourselves in. A lot of us are out there without even realizing it, and I think some of you are very aware of it but don't know how to come back in. So, anyway, as a child I was very in tune with my intuition. A lot of you were probably very intuitive as a child also, but school pretty much beat it out of you. Intuition had to be shelved in school, for school was about memorization.

You have heard it said that some people are "out to lunch"; for some it's a prolonged lunch. Some people are to the point where the pilot light is on and that is about it. And that is really a way I would describe most people who are stuck in their left brain. Their pilot light is on, they are functioning on automatic, but there is not a hell of a lot of awareness in there. They are just going through the same routine over and over again. It is not our fault; this is the way we were trained. It is not until we wake up that we realize what a daze we were in. All of our energy and awareness has been taken out of our bodies because we weren't allowed to feel; everything has been concentrated in our head. People are out of touch with what is really happening, and when they are stuck in their head they are out of their body. In that state you are very vulnerable and can become injured quite easily. When you are truly aware, you will not be injured. You are totally protected.

I was referred a patient from the West from one of the therapists that I have trained. The patient was a Native American man, a very large man, about six foot five in height and weighing 280 pounds or more. He was solid and very angry. He was the foreman of a logging mill that has huge conveyer belts with tongs that grab massive logs and drag them along the conveyer belt. Evidently something jammed in the machinery and the men couldn't fix it. So they looked him up to see if he could fix the machine. As he got close to the conveyer belt, he slipped on some grease on the floor and triggered the machine. His head got caught in the conveyer belt. He says that his head was forced through a hole the size of his fist. Now this says something about our cranial bones being able to move to protect us.

So, he is caught by his neck, and nobody knows what to do. One of the men suggests that they reverse the machine. He says "No way!" This is an incredible guy. He says, "Give me my wrench" and somehow gets his own head out of this machine with the wrench. As he is freeing himself from the machine, his ear rips off and it is hanging on by a thread. He reaches up, rips it off and throws his ear on the ground, and says, "I don't need this damn thing anyway!" His men are freaking out. They say, "No, no, go see the doctor." "Doctor?" So he goes to see the doctor and the doctor sews his ear back on. Now here is something about this man's work ethic: he shows up for work the next day.

When he finally arrived at my clinic, he said that he felt like he was dying inside; he was in such horrible agony. He had undergone various forms of therapy for years and continued to have horrible head, neck, and back pain, and was just barely getting by. Eventually he was sent to a therapist who has taken a lot of my courses, and this therapist was the first person to ever help him. They eventually came to a point, though, where progress had plateaued and the patient was still struggling with his pain and ability to function in life. The therapist recommended he should come to my clinic and participate in my Myofascial Release Intensive Treatment Program for three weeks. The first day he was very, very angry. A spontaneous unwinding did occur in his treatment with me and as I mentioned, people seem to become lighter when they are unwinding. He started to move off the table and I was holding this 280-pound man just by his sacrum quite easily, so he realized that I could handle him, and that created trust. Anyway, about the third day or so I was working on his head. Now when I treat people and animals, I communicate with them verbally, but I also communicate with them through pictures and feelings.

We have become "word worshippers" in this society. We have been deceived into thinking that the only valuable form of communication is words. Words are actually the weakest form of communication. Words just create the target or the context. It is your creative mind, that functions with pictures and feelings, which creates true communication This is how you can communicate with all animals and infants, and you also can communicate with an adult human being at a very deep level that way. I was holding this patient's head, and a deep level of communication began in this way between us. All of a sudden he whipped around and said. "Do you know what you are doing?" I said "Yes." He asked, "How do you know how to do that?" I said "Well, I've been doing it for a long time. My guide, my intuition, The Ancient Warrior taught me." He said, "Well, I have been able to do this for a long time too, but I never told anybody, because I thought they may think I was crazy. My grandfather was a shaman (the Native American healer). When I was growing up my father was a very bad alcoholic and he used to beat me every day, horribly. The only way that I could survive was to leave my body, as my grandfather had taught me." I have found that many children who were abused and/or molested survived these ordeals by leaving their bodies. The problem is that now their awareness interprets their body as a painful or fearful place and doesn't want to or has forgotten how to come back in. Without our awareness in our body, we cannot heal. We are only existing, not living life as fully as possible.

I am going to tell you this story, then I am going to go back and describe why we need to do each step here. I said to him, "I understand. I recognize that you have been out of your body as a way to survive and I highly respect that skill. I want you to know that I will never take that skill away from you or discourage you from using it. But I would like your permission to allow you to expand that skill. Because as long as you are out there, you have no awareness in your body. You have no healing energy. There is no way in the world that I or anybody else in the world, no matter how good we might be, can help you. You need your awareness to be in your body for it to fully heal. It is really important to acknowledge this skill and to establish your intention to expand upon this skill rather than trying to change it. This is a survival skill that most of us have developed, whether we are consciously aware of it or not. If you try to take it away, you will meet resistance and healing will be impossible."

I continued, "What I am going to ask you to consider doing is learn how to come back in your body again. Would you be willing to do that?" He said "All right." I said, "Well, I want you to also understand that there is a possibility (don't say that this *will* happen; say that it's a possibility) that it may reproduce some pain, fear, or some old memories that are not very pleasant. The old feelings or memories will not injure you. You need to feel them and see them to allow your body to learn so that your mind-body can start its healing process. It doesn't have to be a conscious learning.

"I want you to know that you are very good at being out there, so you can pop out at any moment that it might become too intense. So are you willing to try that?" You have to obtain their permission and let them know clearly that they are in control and give them the steps that are going to occur. Always let them know they have an escape route. Usually, I will ask them, "You know what it feels like out there?" And they say, "Oh yes." "I am going to take you in and out. There is a different feel when you are out there, versus when you are in here. We have to learn through feel, so that you can compare the sensations and that will give you back your control. It is not enough just to think about it."

I use visualization. This goes back to the story I told earlier about when I was young. When my mother would take me to town, she would go shopping and I went to the bookstore, and I started to look into different philosophies and different religions. I started to see over time that many were saying the same thing, but just different words from different cultural contexts. It was interesting to me that in many of the different books I read, they described an image, an "energy body" of ours, that lived within us, that had not been recognized in our culture.

They described it as a luminous essence, a shimmering, beautiful, luminous essence that is in every aspect of our body and beyond, and is capable of traveling. It is connected to our physicality by a silver cord through the umbilicus. I always ask the person if this image resonates with them. I say, "I am going to give you an image and if this feels comfortable we will use it, but if you have another image or access route into your body let me know and we will go with that." All that matters is what works for them. Some people do prefer to come in through their head or through a wound. It may look different; it may be a different color. In any event, I described this luminous essence, this shimmery cloud or mist to him, and he said, "Yes that is exactly what it is to me." I continued, "I am going to ask you to come down this silver cord into your belly button and I am going to ask you to fill your body up like an empty vessel with this luminous essence. I am only going to ask you to stay in for a couple of seconds and whether you even want to stay or not, I want you to leave again. We need to go back and forth a couple of times. There will be different feelings and you need to compare the feelings to gain control."

So, usually I am touching them somewhere. Most of the time I will be touching their head very lightly. I want to be non-invasive so I whisper to them. He quieted down and I talked him down through this silver cord. I could feel the energy coming in. What I have found with most people is that it is very tentative at first. It kind of taps in a little bit and just sort of floats near the surface. And then I asked him to leave. Next I said, "Now I am going to ask you to come in for about ten seconds, and even if you want to stay longer, I'd like you to leave at that point." So, we went back and forth. And then eventually I could feel his energy coming down into his body. Zzzzt…a buzzing energy, that actually feels like a weight coming back into the body. Within two weeks this man's symptoms were completely resolved. He'd gone back and returned to work full time, needing no medication whatsoever.

It is all about feel. This is why I suggest that when you touch somebody as they are unwinding, touch any area that is hot or vibratory. That is showing you there is energy blockage there. Or simply touch them at any of the key areas and ask them to feel. A very simple formula would be to suggest: feel, breathe, and soften into this area, be willing to learn from it and let it go. Just keep encouraging them to feel, getting them out of their heads and out of the intellect. Or, you can quiet them down, do a little cranial work or transverse plane releases, anything gentle that is non-intrusive, and then talk them through it, as I did with him.

I will give you another example. A lady was referred to us from the Midwest. She was involved in a terrible car accident and had ended up in a coma for two or three months. When she woke up, she was experiencing severe orthopedic and neurological damage resulting in difficulty moving, ambulating, etc. She was in a lot of pain, and felt very mentally foggy. She had seen her therapist in the rehab center and then at home for a while. A couple of her therapists had taken my Myofascial Release courses and referred her to us. Now I don't mean this in any derogatory sort of way, but she was the typical Midwest housewife. In other words, you wouldn't be thinking you'd be talking to her about "out-of-body experiences." As I worked on her one day, I heard my intuition, The Ancient One, saying,

Ask her if she is out of her body?

I got into this little discussion and fight with myself. "I can't do that," I argued. "She doesn't know what the hell I'd be talking about." I don't believe in thrusting my belief systems onto anybody either, so I tried to come up with a more acceptable label for it. But I've learned to listen to my intuition, so I heard myself saying to her, "Do you think you might be out of your body?" "Oh yes" she said. "I am stuck out here. Can you get me back in?" I was shocked! It was too easy.

I have found you don't have to use the phrase "out of your body." You can use language they won't resist. You can use the words, "Do you have feeling here?" "Do you have awareness here?" "Do you feel numb here?" It is all the same as "are you out of body?" So use some language that they can accept. One of those phrases usually works pretty well.

Back to the story, she said "Can you get me back in?" I replied, "I can try, and I won't hurt you in any way." We went through the routine again; the silver mist image worked fine for her as well. She came down the silver cord into her belly, and we went back and forth a couple times. I usually follow up by giving them homework. I ask them to practice this same process at home for a while. It works remarkably fast for most people. The worst thing that could happen with this process is nothing, so it is worth a try, especially when you are really plateauing with somebody and getting nowhere. Remember that we need our mind, our awareness to be in our body to heal. I really recommend not even waiting. You can be pretty sure most people are having this problem to some degree.

The woman spontaneously began unwinding in the middle of this process, and stopped at a number of still points. She had not remembered the accident from the moment of impact up to the present time. That night, however, during a dream, she had a total recall of the accident. She remembered that she was driving along and was hit from the side at a very high velocity by a drunken teenager. She had been thrown out of the car and she remembers then having an out-of-body experience, where she was way above her body looking down on the entire scene. She saw a couple of the medics walk over to her body, lying crumpled on the grass. They looked down at her and one said to the other, "Oh, she's dead, don't worry about her," and walked away. There is the message that was imbedded in her subconscious! She was so furious that somebody could have been so careless with her life.

The other piece of this was that of a total, obvious fury at the person that had crashed into her, ruined her life, and created misery for her and her family. She had learned that it had been a drunken male teenager driving the other vehicle. How could he have been so careless? She was having great difficulty expressing that fury, or even acknowledging it for a while, because she felt so bad that he had died in the accident. She actually felt guilty. She had also been taught that it was not nice to express anger. "Was it your fault?" I asked her. She replied, "No, not at all." So I suggested, "If it would help you and your family, and it wouldn't hurt him, don't you think it might be okay if you allow yourself to feel the rage, the fear, the sadness? If it would help you to let go of this?" She acknowledged it would be alright. So, with her permission I encouraged her to feel the rage. We gave her a pillow and she started to yell into the pillow and hit it. "Look what you have done to me! Look what you have done to my life! You have ruined my life! You have ruined my family's life!" So she just kept expressing that rage and sadness until a lot of tears came up.

She came in the next day with most of her pain diminished. She will always have some neurological damage, but she was moving and walking much better. It is so important that we be in touch with our feelings. We need to get in touch with a lot of these memories that our linear consciousness has no access to.

The moment you accept what troubles you have been given, a door opens!

Keep in mind the principle that when a person unwinds, they will hit various positions in space that we call "still points," where they stop moving. What it feels like when they stop is that the body is moving

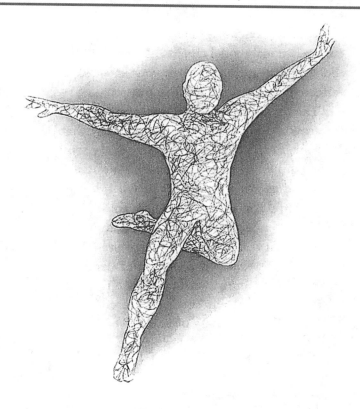

along and all of a sudden it comes to a dead halt. During a still point they also become a little lighter. It is like suspended animation. Reorganization occurs at some level, and when they come out of the still point, there is that sense of softening. Energy comes back in, motion returns, and they become a little heavier. They move again until the next still point. We simply hold them there during the still point, waiting until they begin moving again. When they stop on their own, our job is to support them in that still point. There are times, however, when their left brain will get in the way because it hates the pain and memories within the still points. You may notice a change in the quality or the velocity of the motion. In other words, they will be going along smoothly and all of a sudden you will feel them breaking. You will feel their intention come into the system. In Myofascial Release I, I taught you about analyzing tissue texture. I am now teaching you about the texture of motion. There is a very distinct feel between when one is voluntarily moving, which is a very gross feel that is full of intention, versus true unwinding, which is more of a soft float. The change in velocity may also feel like they switched a gear. They are moving along and all of a sudden...bump; there is a glitch in the motion. They whipped by something. This is one of the only times when we get in the way. We hold them lightly, slow them down a bit, and let them go through that motion pattern again until we feel that glitch. This is where we hold them.

Question: Will the still point be where the change in quality or velocity occurred?

Yes, it will be right there. The change in velocity or the quality of motion is the left brain trying to get the hell out of there. So this is the time we hold them, and mechanically move them. All of a sudden it is like a combination lock that falls into place, and you will feel stillness. The moment we go into the still point every physiological sensation, every physiological event, every emotion, and all the pictures necessary for us to feel or see come billowing forth from the subconscious. We are put back into a position of choice because now the experience is completing itself. We are getting "the message," that interpretation that we made about that particular event or person. So, as we go through various traumas, we go into shock because of the pain or because the fear was so intense. We go into a survival mode, and the experience of the trauma gets shoved into the subconscious. Because we stay locked in fear, the conscious mind no longer has access to that experience after a while. This is why myofascial release is so valuable. This is why talk therapy doesn't always work, because the problem or memory is not on the intellectual, verbal, or conscious level. It is buried in your gut, it is buried in your tissues, it is buried in the subconscious, and it is only accessed by these particular positions in space.

Myofascial release is totally revolutionizing health care. This is why we can't just lie people on tables, why we can't just talk to them, and why we can't just put hot packs on them. All of those techniques have value; but until we find these positions in space through treatment of the fascial system via its unwinding motion, complete resolution of the problem will not occur. The unwinding motion is actually the mind moving the fascial system. This allows for authentic healing.

Question: How do you feel the still points when they are moving wildly?

You are not going to worry about still points too much at that point. You are going to let them express the rage, emotion, wild movement, or whatever they need to do. You are going to let them get that enormous energy out and after it has been expressed, then the system will be quiet enough that you can start to feel still points also.

Question: How do you tell the difference between voluntary conscious motion versus unwinding motion?

Conscious motion is very purposeful; it is full of intention; it has a grosser look and feel to it that is rougher and more mechanical; it is a voluntary motion. You are going to notice that the unwinding, whether it is fast or slow, has a definite smooth, floaty quality. You may miss it for a while, but you will develop a sense of the difference of the feel. It's a very different feeling, one which is learned through experience. And, remember, if you make a mistake, nobody is going to be injured.

Question: Will they ever be injured while unwinding?

If the body is truly unwinding, it will not injure itself, though it will bring up therapeutic pain and fear. If you are voluntarily moving it, or somebody is voluntarily moving you, like through traditional exercise or mobilization, then that pain could be injurious. But when somebody is truly unwinding, they will go into intense pain or fear at times that is tissue memory pain and fear. That is what they need to experience. Then the restriction will melt; this is why it is so important to develop the feel. The two distinct feels of a still point are basically when they just stop and everything is quiet versus the "freeze response," which looks like "the deer caught in the headlights"; their whole body will freeze in tension. This is when it is helpful to say, "Now just feel it, stay there, soften into it, feel it, breathe with it." Then it starts to release. As the freeze response begins to thaw and the energy starts to flow, they might start shaking.

It is important to say to your patients, "You don't need to figure this out and you don't need to understand it. Your mind-body wisdom knows exactly what you need. If you need to know, it will come up in the form of an insight during treatment, after treatment, in a dream, even a couple of days or weeks later; you will have an "ah-ha" experience. But sometimes you will never know on a conscious level. Maybe all you needed to do was get into a certain physical position, or feel a certain emotion, or make certain sounds. Trust that the deepest part of you knows what to do. Take off your brakes, don't try to figure it out, and simply allow your mind-body to do whatever it needs. I will be here to help you and will not allow you to be injured. So, just give up that need to understand, and see where it takes you."

Then there is a series of things I tend to say to people, and you can modify it any way you want. It is never going to injure anybody. After they have been through something, especially something pretty deep, as they are quieting down, I will encourage them to repeat the following to themselves mentally. Don't say it to them, because if you say something to somebody, they go into resistance. They need to say it to themselves. It can be said mentally, because they might be a little embarrassed to say it verbally. It can be verbal, but most of the time, mentally is fine. So, I have them close their eyes, slow their breathing, soften, and I will say, "Say to yourself mentally, repeat after me, 'I survived! I am okay now! I give myself permission on whatever level necessary to learn from this, so I can truly let it go.' Say this again, say it clearly—"I survived! No matter what happened, I love me and I give myself permission to heal. I give myself permission to be fully present, fully aware, fully powerful. I give myself permission to be fully me. I allow my beautiful luminous essence to fill my body, into every aspect of my being, filling myself with love and light."

Over the years I have honed this down and I have found that this is a series of thoughts that work quite well for most people. We all need to hear this on some level. And again, the worst thing that could happen is nothing. There is a part of you that needs permission to come back in— and no matter what happened to you, whether you fell, were hit by a car, were molested—there is a part of you that may have also interpreted that you were wrong, bad, or stupid, and you need to give yourself permission to love yourself again. We have all been much too hard on ourselves.

Question: John, you aren't telling us everything that you know, are you?

I don't consciously know everything that I know, and in myofascial release I "sugar coat" many concepts. My style of teaching is oblique; I leave clues, I open doors. I don't believe in forcing people to believe what I believe, nor do I believe in teaching with a silver spoon. One's struggle to understand has value to help them find their own unique path. I view myself as a catalyst, as a guide to help you help yourself, to assume your own vision, your own way, and your own authentic power.

A THERAPIST'S PERSPECTIVE

Gymnastics was my life (starting at age three and competing until I was twenty-one). The flips, the falls…an everyday event. "Work in the overload…get up and brush it off….You're strong enough to handle it."

While attending the Cervical-Thoracic Seminar, I remember talking to John on the first day, saying that "I would like to have you demonstrate one of the techniques on me but I don't know which one." John's response to me was, "It'll come to you." I think it was the second day when John was saying, "The next technique will be the sternum release. If anyone…" At that moment I stood up and was on the stage and then on the table before he could finish saying…"would like their sternum released, you're welcome to come up."

As soon as John put his hand on my sternum, I could feel the connection immediately…holding my heart safe while my body went through one of its "routines." (In gymnastics, as in many other sports, the training can be so involved and intense that you become "the routine.") Arms and legs extending then contracting, my solar plexus erupting like a volcano. There was no hurry, no time limit; the process came full circle. It ended with me prone and crosswise on the table and John saying, "And that's the sternal release," and everyone laughed!

What had just happened was love and trust enabling a release of a held pattern. Fear was eliminated for the moment, used as fuel. John asked for my comments but I couldn't speak yet. I had "forgotten" that I cracked my sternum and injured the xyphoid process. It wasn't until I left the stage and sat for a few minutes that I recalled the past injury of landing on the lower bar of the uneven bars.

When I shared that with the group, a therapist asked me, "How old were you when that happened?" I replied, "Oh, maybe twelve or fourteen." She commented, "While you were unwinding up there, you looked like you were twelve years old."

Interesting, don't you think, how the tissue memory maintains or freezes in that space and time?

A THERAPIST'S PERSPECTIVE

Before myofascial release, my true self, my essence, was buried under the rubble. Rubble consisting of numerous fascial restrictions tangled with pain, fear, anger, sadness, a little bit of joy, a whole lot of love, and total confusion. Torn between the East and West. Tormented with useless belief systems, disappointing religious background, and highly demanding social and cultural expectations.

The Myofascial Release Approach has taught me to truly love myself by learning to accept and embrace the dark side of me. I have clarity of thought. I sense a meaningful purpose in my life that brings me immense tranquility and joy. I have a more fulfilling relationship with The Divine based on love and trust. No more *fear.*

John's advice was to stop doubting myself, stop being so hard on myself. His words echo in me every time I come close to falling in that trap. I ground myself by loving even that self-doubting part of me, and by renewing my faith in the infinite power of my mind. His witty responses to our comments and questions, his endearing sense of humor, is a constant reminder to loosen up and let go, and enjoy living every moment.

◢

$$E = mc^2$$

For over three hundred years scientists have mistakenly thought that the human being could be fragmented. This erroneous perspective gained momentum over the years, and this myth was accepted as a truth. So, unfortunately, the various healthcare professionals came to view the human as a slab of meat; flesh without a mind or emotions. When problems occurred in this mindless machine, we were taught that we could fix it by medicating it, rubbing it, running an ultrasound machine over it, electrifying it, talking to it, or surgically removing a part of it. Today's healthcare system has dehumanized us. Certainly, medicine, surgery, and electronics have great value when used appropriately. However, it has been estimated that medicine, surgery, and traditional therapy is only effective approximately 10% to 20% of the time. What about the other 80%? It is time that health professionals join hands and work together cooperatively and intelligently for the good of all.

In 1905, Albert Einstein, the century's most influential scientist, developed the special theory of relativity, and in 1916 came up with the general theory of relativity. As these incredible views were proven, they changed man's understanding of the universe—except for the traditional medicine and therapy perspective that still views man as a slab of meat.

Einstein's theories contend that light always moves in a straight line through space and always at the same speed, the universal maximum velocity. As a result, strange things happen to time and matter; time slows down the faster someone travels, mass increases the faster someone travels. Thus, Einstein says mass is just a form of energy! $E=mc^2$.

In other words, mass is only apparently solid. When one chooses to look below the surface, mass is actually vibrating energy. The frequency of vibrations of energy determines the solidity of mass. Mass is an illusion! Traditional medicine and therapy got caught up in this illusion and accepted it as fact. It's important for healthcare professionals to wake up and see beyond the illusion. As I have said, "Reality is a figment of our imagination."

As myofascial release therapists we recognize and utilize this illusion, the mass of the fascial system, as a handle that allows us to use physical "reality" to reach into the depths of the human being. As we release the myofascial system, we also have a positive and profound effect upon the Golgi tendon organs, the muscular component of the fascial system, the nervous system, the vascular system, the lymphatic system, the neuropeptide system, the acupuncture system, the osseous system, the fluidity, the electromagnetic field, the vibrations and functioning of the mind; everything!

Time magazine, in its issue of December 31, 1999, chose Albert Einstein as the person of the century. Neil L. Rudenstine, president of Harvard University, said of Einstein, "This man embodied the power of scientific imagination and genius stimulating a century of the most remarkable research and discovery in human history. Equally important, he did so in a way that indicated how science could be humane in its spirit, wise in its uses and moral in its purposes." Unfortunately, traditional medicine and therapy choose to ignore this! This reminds me of the ostrich that buries its head into the sand to fearfully ignore what is to maintain the status quo. Maintaining the status quo is fine, if it is working. It is not! Desperately clinging to the status quo serves no good purpose. Change is inevitable. There is always the possibility of the new!

As I mentioned earlier, Max Planck, the father of quantum physics and one of the greatest scientific minds of all times, said, "Science progresses one funeral at a time." In the later years of his life, Einstein struggled with trying to discover the equation that would establish an underlying link between the seemingly unrelated forces of gravity and electromagnetism into a unified field theory. The laws of classical physics, which traditional healthcare is based on, appears to be in opposition with the theories of quantum physics. Classical physics has developed an entire set of theories for the big world, the macro-world. But, it turns out that you and I weren't given the rules for the micro-world. We were given an incomplete set of rules to understand the universe, for in the micro-world, on extremely fine scales of space-time and thus reality itself, the world of cause and effect breaks down.

Reductionists have argued that one has to be right while the other is wrong! Could they both be right but on different scales? Interestingly, a set of new theories, the "string theory," may tie together these two great irreconcilable ideas of twentieth-century physics and add even deeper and unimagined new dimensions and understanding to our existence within the universe. The string theory postulates that the smallest indivisible components of the universe are not pointlike particles, but infinitesimal loops that resemble tiny, luminescent vibrating strings. The string theory also suggests that beyond our conventional view of the familiar height, width, length, and time, there might be seven previously unrecognized other dimensions, an eleven-dimensional world! This information on the string theory was paraphrased from a fascinating new book called *The Elegant Universe*, written by physicist Brian Greene from Columbia University.

As I understand this new information, our universe is being described as multi-dimensional luminescent vibrating strings that are the basic building blocks of our visible mechanical world. My experience has suggested that from the most finite level to the largest level we are love and light; another word to me would be God. Luminescent vibrating strings!

What happens when you pluck a guitar string? It vibrates and produces perceived sound. Is the string theory saying that we are essentially light and sound? Could light be information? Could sound be love? Could this be interpreted as a vibrating universe of love and light of different frequencies? Could disease, pain, and agitation be disharmony, and health, clarity, awareness, and joy be harmony?

Our goal with myofascial release is to discover the vibrations that are out of synchrony with the whole and attempt to encourage a return to harmony. Our goal is to help the person move through darkness (low-dense frequencies) into the higher and finer frequencies of love and light. If love is indeed sound, maybe that is why Cupid played the harp! (Just trying to lighten us up on the subject of love and light!) I find all this theorizing very interesting. I feel it needs to be pursued. However, the bottom line is that while these theories may turn out to be correct or incorrect, following the principles of myofascial release will profoundly help many people, even those who have responded to nothing else.

The crashing of the obsolescent healthcare system in the late 1990s created turmoil, but it also created the opportunity for change and growth. These massive shifts in awareness made people stop and examine what works and what doesn't work. Let us now continue to explore what works.

The research of Dr. Candace Pert, Ph.D., the discoverer of the endorphin theory, has found that every cell of our body has intelligence, memories, and emotions. This is another way of describing our mind, which is in every aspect of our body and beyond it. Are we a body with a soul? Or a soul with a body? Maybe our body is the densest part of our soul. As we have said, another label for our mind could be our electromagnetic field, or consciousness, awareness, feeling, or love. I believe another word for our mind is our essence, a beautiful luminescent mist that interpenetrates our being and goes beyond.

The fascial system is our handle into this deeper dimension of our being, the interface of the physicality and this subtle energy or essence.

The subtle energy of our mind-body complex can be viewed as a powerful river, flowing throughout. A person's myofascial restrictions can be seen as boulders in the river diverting the flow of energy. These blockages create chaos, disharmony, friction, heat, vibration, or turmoil. The eddies and chaos in the river caused by these blockages can be felt by the highly skilled myofascial release therapist as thermals or heat in and beyond the body, as vibrations, or as an electromagnetic feel. Once trained properly, the therapist can then easily and accurately use this sensory information to ascertain where the myofascial restrictions are and apply appropriate myofascial release techniques. As the myofascial restrictions soften and release, it is the equivalent of a dam breaking. The system goes into chaos (an opportunity to change). The system shakes, shudders, and twitches; as the restriction releases, the patient softens and there is a sense of melting as the energy begins to flow. So, as we facilitate the "breaking of the dam" by sustaining pressure into the myofascial restriction, the enhanced flow of bio-energy initiates the healing process. In other words, that which was hard, tight, solid, and dark becomes soft, open, flowing, and enlightened!

There are some key areas that we can touch to access and treat the subtle energy of our bodies. As you are unwinding somebody, you may touch any area that you see that is hot, tender, or red. This "fascial voice" or body-language experience is telling you that this area is ready to release, but it needs some stimulation. As you touch them, encourage them to bring their awareness, through feel, into this area. It is important to make sure they understand that when you say awareness, you mean feel, not thought. When you say awareness, they'll think you mean "think," and they'll think about it. You want them to feel! It is through feel that their mind melds with your mind, creating a deep and profound connection and communication.

Go anyplace that your hand is drawn to. It may appear to have nothing to do with their symptoms. Don't think about it, because by the time you think about it, the moment is lost. Touch any place that is vibratory. Now some key areas that you can touch for assessment are the pelvic floor areas. This would have a lot to do with pelvic and/or lumbo-sacral pain and tightness, sexual abuse problems, sexual problems, menstrual problems, and digestive/elimination problems.

A THERAPIST'S PERSPECTIVE

John, after you treated me in Paoli, Pennsylvania, for my pelvic and back pain, I knew that the impacts and traumas from numerous falls off horses, skiing, and car accidents had created my frequent urination and urgency problems. I know that the symptoms were actually huge restrictions throughout my body. After four years of marriage and knowing we wanted to have children, I knew my body had no place to hold a child and told my husband I could not live with this level of pain and carry a child, nor did I think I would get pregnant without treatment. Three and a half years from when I attended Myofascial Release I, I went for a week of the "Therapy for the Therapist" treatment program. This week was a life-changing experience! My first session was with John, and I unwound instantly and landed in a heap on the floor. I stood up and hugged John, and that was just the beginning. Even though his hands were never on me before, I intuitively trusted and let go and felt safe with his touch.

When I came home my husband could not believe the wonderful transformation. I moved and looked different, and had insights beyond imagination. I am thankful that I am now living and experiencing life fully... restfully, peacefully, sexually, completely. And yes, I got pregnant three months later. I feel myofascial release has made me so much more in touch with myself. With John's touch, layers of tissue memory emerged and took me many places, many dark places. I never got lost in the darkness, though, and always came through it into the light. I continue to release myself regularly and unlike many, have had a pain-free and enjoyable pregnancy.

It is important to be genuine with each of your patients. Truly connect with them. They will know otherwise. I believe each encounter in life is about connecting in a loving way.

Many people have had tightness in the pelvic area that has become a chronic, unrecognized holding pattern. These restrictions can cause a multitude of seemingly unrelated symptoms and behavioral problems.

A Patient's Perspective

I would like to share something very personal. Although I am a very private person, I feel this is important to express. I think the major importance with this myofascial release concept (myofascial release helping clear up sexual issues to assist sexuality to blossom) is that restrictions in the body can keep a person from truly being. I thought it was my upbringing, my attitude, my body, and my husband (you name it) that was preventing me from enjoying a sexual life only read in books and seen at movies.

A restriction can also manifest itself in our bodies from our belief systems. I was brought up in a very rigid religion which taught me that being sensual was bad and that it is not right to enjoy yourself. I felt very guilty when I felt good. Initially, myofascial release represented everything that was wrong for me. It went against what I was brought up to believe; it seemed to go against my religion. With the release of my physical restrictions, I began to feel sensual. I started to enjoy myself, feel freer, and the ultimate, I think, was that I found a voice. I have become a being. I am not a product of a closed-minded family anymore. I am free to be me!

Being a Christian at first held me back from embracing John's work, my emerging sensuality, and me. I can see a clearer picture now through the fog, that this work only enhances one's religion! There is something very old and spiritual about myofascial release. Religion was not meant to instill guilt and fear, but to instill love and acceptance. Restrictions and upbringing hold the guilt and fear. I continue to battle with the guilt, especially when I start to enjoy myself. Upbringing (restriction) is very strong in me. Myofascial release takes away the restrictions, lifts the spirit, and can create sensual beings. Beings who can feel love, and embrace the freedom to experience.

I've seen this therapeutic process help so many people get in touch with their inner selves. It allows us to break the mold of who we were told to be, what we should think and should say. We relearn how to be "real" and genuine.

Let's move to the psoas area. Always check this area because this is where we hold so much of our emotion. Most people are hot, vibratory, hard, and tender here. Always touch them lightly, but if the psoas area needs a little more facilitation, go in with deeper pressure and stimulate them. Years ago I was invited to a convent. This wasn't my normal place to hang out, but I'll tell you an interesting story about it. One of the sisters had taken my seminar and felt many of the sisters in the convent could benefit from this form of treatment. So, I set aside a weekend and scheduled appointments for the sisters at their convent. As I entered the treatment room one of the nuns was sitting on a table glaring at me. This brought back old memories for me, because I had attended Catholic school and the sisters were my teachers. She said to me, "I'm going to give you a hell of a fight." I thought, oh boy, at least she warned me. I put my hand on her back and her head and she sat there like a stone. She felt like a statue. Have you ever seen the statues on Easter Island? That's what she looked and felt like, and I knew there was no way this woman was going to unwind. I had been informed prior to her treatment that she had not expressed an emotion in over thirty-five years!

I have found that when I don't know what to do, I just quiet down and ask. I then just go with my instincts. It works well. So, I asked her to lie down, and as I was slowly walking around the table I noticed that my body language was changing. I heard myself saying to myself, "You are stalking this woman." Then, all of a sudden, I dove into her psoas! Well, she went airborne...punching, kicking, and thrashing. When some-one becomes violent, go to the center of the action just like when you are in a fight. And remember this always, stay above the knees and above the elbows! I don't care how strong you are. If somebody's unwind-ing, there is adrenaline flowing through their body, and something else is happening on an energetic level: they become very powerful. The extremities can generate too much power and momentum to control, so as my karate experience taught me, go right in to the center. So I went right into her center. She then taught me another lesson: watch the head! She started to use her head as a battering ram! The sister explained after her treatment that my pressure into her stomach recreated the experience of being attacked as a little girl. She had shut down emotionally since that trauma as a way to protect herself from the overwhelming fear and pain of the incident.

So with the psoas, it is best not to dive in like I did. Start off slowly, and then go in a little deeper at times, if needed. There is a phenomenon called the "dead dog syndrome," where the deeper pressure is needed. Some people have extreme difficulty letting go of control. When this type of person unwinds there is no energy; no one is home. This is when we need to stimulate the psoas. They'll get ticked off at you, so beware, but this will take them into another realm of feeling. They are feeling what has been buried. It is difficult for them to let go of control, because it will usually uncover a powerful source of rage and it can be very frightening to confront this. But that's exactly what we need to do, confront it! Otherwise, it eats away at us and eventually manifests in erratic behavior, pain, or disease. So if you get a "dead dog" on your hands, if they become very passive, like a heavy rag doll, this is when it can be beneficial to go in and tickle their psoas with heavier pressure. Always do this with awareness. This will wake them up.

A THERAPIST'S PERSPECTIVE

John is truly a catalyst and tends to "stir the soup" and encourages others to stretch their imagination, to reach the depths/core of our beings, even out into the cosmos, to bring us to a clearer level of consciousness. The microcosm and the macrocosm. I felt that I could never totally express, in words, the impact that John's touch, presence, and energy have on my mind-body-spirit. I had initially no clue of who John was. However, there was a knowing in his voice, and his ability to express that knowing, so eloquently and on many different levels, struck my intuitive chords. There was no doubt that I had just met a teacher who had attained a level of mastery surpassed by none. Myofascial release was truly the "missing link" that afforded my clients the opportunity to participate in their healing. It's quite an adventure.

I am "triggered" by John's presence/energy in countless ways. The first time it happened, I was in Paoli, Pennsylvania, for the Skill Enhancement Seminar. On the third day, John and two other therapists and I were in the treatment room with one of John's patients. As he pressed into her right psoas, my body started to unwind, as though it were my psoas. The second time was during Myofascial Release III. It was the last day and the last technique. You guessed it, psoas. John asked everyone to step in closer to the treatment table, which really intensified the energy field. Once again, as he reached for her psoas, my body doubled over, feeling the intensity of her/my psoas. The third time was also in Sedona during the Advanced Myofascial Unwinding Seminar. John was demonstrating the "slap" technique. As soon as the sound occurred, although I was in the back of the room I felt an impact, and immediately started crying. I was thrown into the emotional trauma of a car accident that my children and I experienced.

In the Advanced Myofascial Unwinding Seminar, John teaches the "slap" technique. The therapist's hand is cupped and the patient is lightly tapped. This impact is felt down to the cellular level and can mimic the impact of a previous accident. It is a very powerful but gentle technique that never injures, that takes the individual under the holding patterns, and frees the "stuck" energy pattern. John calls this "shocking the shock!"

After my spontaneous unwinding, my psoas released and I felt soothing peace and calmness within.

Back now to the key areas. We have covered the pelvic floor and the psoas areas. We will move on to the respiratory diaphragm and the solar plexus. This is where your inner child lives, or your emotional brain—whatever you want to call it. We hold so much fear here. We are all so shut down in the solar plexus/respiratory diaphragm area. The fascia has solidified like a hard ball. We can't feel and have no power. We're being drained of our power. This tightness can eventually lead to a forward-head situation where the person is walking around with headaches, and neck and back pain, and some traditional therapist is putting hot packs and ultrasound on the back of the neck. I did that for years. I could never understand how that really helped and kept thinking, "I went to college for this?" Well, the problem is actually in the front, and the solar plexus and respiratory diaphragm is a key area. The solar plexus is considered to be the "emotional brain," with more neural connections than any other area of the body except for the "intellectual brain" in our head. Restrictions in the solar plexus and respiratory diaphragm area can create physiological dysfunction and disharmony throughout the mind-body complex.

A THERAPIST'S PERSPECTIVE

I am a pediatric occupational therapist and have found the respiratory diaphragm area to be important in the treatment of both adults and children.

I took my first Myofascial Release Seminar in New York City in the late 1980s. I believe that there were at least two hundred students taking the seminar. The first thing that was so impressive was John's lecture. Everything he spoke of made so much sense. No one else had ever talked about the fascial system before. During the lab sections of the seminar, I could feel my own fascia changing and releasing. It was both so simple and so profound.

Then I started practicing the techniques in my practice, and the results were incredible. I had a little girl with severe seizures and cerebral palsy. She was eighteen months old. She cried most of the twenty-four hours in the day. I did a respiratory diaphragm release and she stopped screaming. Her parents and I were in awe. For the very first time in her life she quieted herself and stopped arching her body. I believe that her vagus nerve, which passes through the respiratory diaphragm, was trapped, fascially restricted, creating a situation of constant vagus nerve irritability.

My next client that same Monday after the seminar was a two-year-old hemiplegic cerebral palsy child. This child did not like to be handled and he was very tactilely defensive. I did arm and leg pulls and transverse plane releases. Two days later when he returned for his next session, he laid down on his therapy mat and handed me his hemiplegic arm. After these two responses in the first week after Myofascial Release I, I was hooked on integrating myofascial release into my work. I then proceeded to take all of John's seminars, with the full support of all my clients. John talks about being focused and fully present when working with his patients. I said to him, "Someone can actually be focused and tune out their own internal chatter?" I was baffled, I could not imagine anyone, especially myself, being focused 100% of the time. The concept about being fully present and aware of one's intent was absolutely foreign to me. Astonishingly, I now can easily deeply focus and be quiet, calm and centered.

Initially most have a very difficult time quieting their mind. This is why I feel it is important for all therapists to receive regular treatment from a highly skilled myofascial release therapist. Your restrictions, your pain, your hidden, unresolved emotions keep you in a state of agitation, and it is almost impossible to remain quiet and focused for any length of time. As you receive a series of treatments, you will return to your natural, comfortable, tranquil way of being.

Another key area is the heart. We hold a lot of our sorrow here. The heart is where we are restricted from a perceived lack of love. We have a difficult time loving ourselves. If we don't love ourselves, how can we ever love anybody else? It is necessary to open up to our own self-love, our own self-worth, to give and receive love with others. Love for most in our society is just a word. Feel it! Experience it! Bring it into your body!

A Therapist's Perspective

John has stated that scoliosis can be from birthing injuries or early childhood falls.

I had told John when he treated me that I had been abused as a child. He stated that the emotional turmoil and problems with self-image can twist the emotional body, which then over time twists the structure; hence, scoliosis. An abused person can feel "twisted" and can be out of their body from the past trauma and/or abuse. So, the subtle energy is not aligned or properly supporting the body and its physiological functioning.

I had scoliosis when I was a child and wore a back brace for ten years. I had a significant leg length discrepancy, and during my first myofascial unwinding seminar I felt the floor for the first time with my shorter leg. During the four-person myofascial unwinding I felt and experienced old traumas and situations that I thought I had already resolved. This concept that my body/tissue had memories and could be accessed was actually happening. The journey to being free from the hold that these tissues had and still had on my life was unfolding, unraveling. I was unwinding, and my mind-body was really letting go all the way down to the cellular level. And each time my left brain would become quieter, my proprioceptive senses through my hands and beyond would become softer and deeper and more intuitive. Somehow, each time I was involved in an unwinding as the therapist or assistant instructor, something within my soul and essence would open up, awaken. I actually felt myself take a quantum shift to being fully present to another human being. It was a life-changing experience!

Question: John, so many changes and growth occur with myofascial release. Doesn't this change impact negatively upon one's relationships?

It can. Don't expect everyone to be jumping up and down with joy because you are growing and evolving. Change can create chaos and fear in others. As with the principles that you have learned with myofascial release, be patient, don't force, accept what is. Your change produces chaos, and through your positive example, a real improvement is possible in a relationship. Remember that we must establish a loving relationship with ourselves before we can truly have a deep loving relationship with another!

Myofascial release can change your life. In workshops, in therapy sessions, at home, tissue releases from restrictions can produce powerful results. You can go from being insecure, fearful, and pain-ridden to a totally free individual with a new lease on life. Even though this sounds wonderful, not everyone will follow you on this path. It becomes difficult when a close friend or spouse is not quite ready for the new you, or not ready to become a new person for you.

It is difficult to grow when your partner has not. Some seem unable to wait, and move on too quickly. Some stay with that partner and become disillusioned and unhappy. Change can be difficult, but through the darkness you will see the light. If one remains centered and focused, change can occur within one's environment and extend to those individuals closest to us. Relationships can become deeper, richer, and more loving, not because the partner has changed, but because *you* have changed. These experiences can enhance old relationships or partnerships and can also deepen understanding of who you are and who you have become, thus enhancing a relationship.

Let me share with you a letter that I received from a husband and wife on how myofascial release has enhanced their love for each other.

A Husband's Perspective

When I initially took a holiday series of courses of Myofascial Release I, Myofascial Unwinding, and Myofascial Release II in Orlando, I assumed that it would offer me some unique treatment tools to add to my clinical skills. I had done extensive post-graduate work in mobilization and manipulation training. The reason for taking the Myofascial Release Approach was because it was apparent to me that mobilization, manipulation, and strengthening was not taking my patients as far to recovery as I felt possible.

A number of things happened during my coursework. It became apparent to me that my overall education was sorely lacking in terms of overall comprehensiveness. As well, I found it quite odd that during this most peaceful and calming course I was experiencing something odd in the pit of my stomach. Despite having a great course and having a wonderful holiday with my family in Orlando, I was uncovering tension within, of which I had been previously unaware.

Following this wonderful course in what was the ultimate mind-body approach, I was quite unsettled when I came back to my regular job. I am a partner in a large and well-respected private practice in my home province. However, the treatment philosophy that clinics have voluntarily undertaken in order to make money was starting to cause me considerable grief because I no longer wholeheartedly agreed with the functional activation approach that was being advocated by the major insurers. Patients were getting stronger and being sent back to work even though the treatment was making them biomechanically worse and increasing their symptoms.

As I struggled with all of this, my only time of peace and calm was when I had the opportunity to spend time with my wife and my two children. My marriage and family relationship has always been my top priority, and likewise that of my family.

As time progressed, I was working through past anxieties that had been long since forgotten. But the time I was spending working on my patients was starting to open up to me the fact that myofascial release work goes deeper than just mind and body, and very much into a spiritual realm. I have always been very closed spiritually. This has been hard on my wife, because she comes from a strong spiritual background. The basic agreement that we had made was to refrain from going into discussion on spiritual ideas because this is where we had absolutely no agreement. Consequently, this was always avoided in our relationship. Otherwise, it was as close to perfect as a marriage and family relationship could be, because our main goal has been to really focus on love in our family.

As the months were going by in my MFR journey, and I was beginning to understand the spiritual aspect of it, I started treating my wife with MFR and showing her how to treat me. This started to open up what I had already considered to be a good relationship and we have felt our love towards each other grow in quantum leaps. Our family unit is much closer now than it was. I had not considered it possible to become closer than we already were.

As well, I will be leaving the partnership that I am presently in. We will be opening up a small practice. She will be the clinic manager and I will treat patients. Our goal is to have more time together as a family and we are quite excited about the prospect of working together.

In November of 1999, we spent two weeks in Sedona, Arizona where I had the opportunity to take Skill Enhancement Seminar and "Therapy for the Therapist" with John. During my first week, my wife came out on the "Therapy on the Rocks Day" with the group. It was a profound experience and we felt our love increasing further. John Barnes is a remarkable, loving individual who has had a profound influence on our lives. We cannot wait to spend more time with him and all of the MFR people at his clinic.

A Wife's Perspective

From a very young age, I have loved my husband. We grew up together through our dating years and have always had a "special connection." Our religious backgrounds are different. I grew up with a true sense of God and spirit whereas my husband's spirituality was limited to one of skepticism and philosophical questions and answers. Early on I made the decision to concentrate my energies on our relationship and put my spirituality to the side except in times of need. I felt that the religious differences might somehow stand in the way of us realizing the full potential our relationship had. After having children, my husband became more open to the idea of a divine being. With childhood illness plaguing both of our children quite seriously, prayer and answer to that prayer opened our hearts to more spiritual searching.

When he started taking some Myofascial Release courses and was practicing breathing and meditation exercises, I did them as well. This was not hard because I have always felt that the more we experience life together, the better it is for our marriage. Making time to begin focusing on God and Spirit, the Bible, and my inner self made me feel more whole than I have for a long time. I did not know I was missing anything. I thought I had it all. I never knew I could love my husband or my children more than I already did. I was wrong!

My husband and I began unwinding sessions together along with our breathing, releasing, stretching, and individual devotional time. We went to Sedona and he was on a Skill Enhancement week. I had booked a one-hour myofascial release treatment session and an afternoon "Therapy on the Rocks Day" experience.

Our time with John on the red rocks was an unforgettable experience of love and inner peace. Making the journey together has been remarkable to this point. I am devoted as a wife and mother and now also devoted to strengthening my inner spirit. Myofascial release has given us the medium to discover and uncover new potential to our individual lives and our relationship. Thank you once again for your love and friendship. Looking very forward to our next encounter and the continuation of our journey.

I have found that it is very helpful and rewarding for both individuals in a relationship to be treated. This enhances the speed of growth and encourages closeness, understanding, and intimacy.

A Therapist's Perspective

John has treated me as well as my husband, who had a severe spinal cord injury.

My husband describes a return of internal energy with myofascial release treatment, a sense of awareness in parts of his body that he usually tries to or has to shut off for lack of physical motor function. Pain of the "slipped disc" is virtually gone since his Myofascial Release Intensive Treatments with John and his team in Sedona, Arizona, after months of unsuccessful chiropractic work and traditional physical therapy.

Overall, life has lightened. We now have a path, a way of health and feeling good. Most importantly, we have our energy back, as individuals and as a couple, which is more than words could possibly describe. And I have a passion for my profession as a physical therapist that I never thought possible.

Sure, myofascial release doesn't cure or reverse paralysis, but I can honestly say that it has given my husband his energy back, the light in his eyes, the calmed expressions on his face, a return of his unparalleled love of life, so often ignored by those so much more physically fortunate. If that's not true healing, I don't know what is. No words really can do myofascial release justice when it comes to our lives. Thanks, John.

Let's move on to the throat area. How many people are always getting red in this region, even when you are doing J stroking on the back? Because of the continuity of the fascial system from head to foot, treatment in any area of the body will commonly trigger a vaso-motor response in another part of the body. A vaso-motor response in the throat area can reveal unexpressed sounds of pain, thoughts, and emotions, which over time can become myofascial restrictions. Often times this response reflects a need to communicate something important. Some children were told to keep quiet and not tell.

A THERAPIST'S PERSPECTIVE

Opening up my throat area has been very powerful for me. I was abused as a child and told not to tell! I won't go into the details but since myofascial release, I have come a long way. I am a different person now. Myofascial release has helped me do it. I can make eye contact and stand up for myself and most of the time, I am not afraid of people. I still have my moments, but life is so beautiful and each day is a new experience to live. I am so thankful to the Myofascial Release process, John, all the therapists, and staff at the Myofascial Release Treatment Centers, and seminar instructors. You are all wonderful people and I thank you all for helping me get my life back. I hope that in some way, I can give back to others what I have been given.

A THERAPIST'S PERSPECTIVE

After the Myofascial Release Seminar series in Dallas, Texas, I came home and treated my three-year-old daughter. John had suggested that I start with a light thoracic inlet release and then progress up through the hyoid area, masseters, TMJ area, temporal and other cranial areas.

I used cranial techniques on my daughter who had a total bilateral blockage of her ears from acute media otitis. She was scheduled in the following weeks to receive a second tympanoplasty. After five days of twenty-five minute sessions, her ENT cancelled the surgery! He couldn't believe it. John I thank you a thousand times over, because without your vision, love, and courage, none of this would have been possible. I love you!

A THERAPIST'S PERSPECTIVE

I am a therapist and have been treating children from the ages of seven to nine and have performed myofascial techniques and some unwinding on them. I was hesitant to do "rebounding" on these little ones; however, I must say that it really is worthwhile. Upon utilizing the rebounding techniques...at first they giggled, then grunted, then got frustrated and they seemed to go into some sort of "zone." After that, I could see the emotions and movements come from "within," deeper than they ever had before. Two children I treated are on Prozac and Ritalin, and they had a new sense of calmness to them. After three treatments, their dosages of these drugs have almost been cut in half.

I view the Myofascial Release Approach as a "Triad": myofascial release, myofascial unwinding, and myofascial rebounding, and utilize all three gently with children. The myofascial therapist provides a rhythmic, oscillatory motion into the ground substance and fluids of the body, creating a fluid wave within the patient's mind-body that powerfully energizes the entire fascial web. This rhythmic, fluid wave erodes deep restrictions and unleashes deeply held feelings that have impeded the patient's progress.

A THERAPIST'S PERSPECTIVE

I am a physical therapist who treats disabled children, mainly with cerebral palsy and spina bifida. From the instant I begin rebounding them, they change from having a glazed, far-off look to giggling and deep laughter. The deepest laughs come from the most severely affected children.

Rebounding seems to reach them in a way that nothing else does. The ones who are capable of doing so will request to be rebounded. The best part of this treatment with the children is that it is really fun, as well as being therapeutic.

Myofascial rebounding produces incredible releases gently, with both adults and children. It is so important to treat children. Myofascial release has the potential to change their attitudes, behavior, and lives for the better. Children are so willing to heal; they haven't yet been told they can't.

Let's now move our attention to between the eyebrows, the location of the "third eye." Place your finger between the eyebrows lightly, and this will stimulate their insight.

A THERAPIST'S PERSPECTIVE

Earlier, I had mentioned my life-altering experience with John in Sedona after my car accident, and how I was studying for the bar exam to become a lawyer. John stimulated energetically my "third eye" between my eyebrows and deepened my insight and intuition. I studied and memorized that week in Sedona in between sessions, while walking on the rocks, while continuing to unwind, even while sleeping. And I decided that my own health was worth more than passing the bar. After all, the bar is offered twice a year, but this time at "Therapy on the Rocks" was a gift of a lifetime!

So I decided to use the first take as a practice and redo it in the summer. Nevertheless, I am not one to waste time, God forbid! So I sat outside the hotel conference room where myofascial release was being taught inside. I figured the energy felt good in that space, and what could it hurt? John came by one early evening on his way back in the classroom after the break. I was sitting in my customary corner, hammering away at obscure corporate law, which I could not understand. John stopped and told me to rest my eyes a second. I did. I felt his finger touch my forehead, so very warm and gentle, yet deep—it felt like his fingertip went into my head. I kept my eyes closed and enjoyed the warm feeling and relaxation. I felt very rested, but I did wonder how long he planned to hold his finger there. I snuck a tiny peek through one eye. Imagine my surprise to find the hallway deserted. I opened both eyes and saw that the doors to the classroom were closed. I could hear the class. How long had he been gone? I'll never know. But what I do know is that the exact complex, corporate law I had been struggling with when John touched me, was on the bar exam, and I had total recall and answered with ease.

I went to the bar exam totally at ease. After all, this was practice time. I stayed away from the other anxious souls looking so strained. I said a prayer for them and enjoyed myself. I didn't want the myofascial release afterglow to be gone too soon. Imagine my absolute astonishment in April to find a letter of congratulations on passing the bar exam and inviting me to be sworn in the following month. I heartily recommend myofascial release in conjunction with studying for the bar!

You are certainly a beautiful example of the awesome power of developing and blending the left and right side of your brain. Intellect and intuition, that is true genius. This combination gives us the ability to reach our potential and be fully human.

Finally, touching the top of the head, the center of higher consciousness, can be very helpful and powerful.

A THERAPIST'S PERSPECTIVE

I had a very special experience recently while assisting at a Myofascial Release I Seminar. My future husband arrived early to pick me up on Saturday afternoon. He had not been exposed to myofascial release and was sitting in the back of the room, at least thirty feet away from the participants. The lights were down low, and as the group began a very gentle cranial and cervical distraction technique, I heard sobbing. Thinking it was coming from my group, I began to circulate through the tables to see if I could assist. I was puzzled when I found no one, but assumed it was coming from someone at a table outside my group. I headed back to the instructor table where I had been doing some computer work for the seminar. Suddenly, I saw my future husband, head in hands, sobbing in a chair near the projector. I approached him, and asked if he wanted to wait in my hotel room. When I joined him an hour later, I asked if he wanted to talk about it. He told me that while his previous wife had been dying of cancer, the only relief she obtained from her excruciating pain was when he would touch the top of her head and put gentle traction on her neck. So, what I gained from this was further validation of what I had chosen to do with my life. Myofascial release can have very far-reaching effects, and I have never known of them to be negative.

A THERAPIST'S PERSPECTIVE

The phrase, "myofascial release has far-reaching effects" triggered me to tell you about my experience a couple of months ago.

Three words come to mind to describe myself prior to attending the Myofascial Release Seminars. The words are closed, protective, and judgemental. Not only of others, but mostly of myself. Fear of not being good enough has always been a biggie for me. I am one of those people who tries to please everyone but myself. So I have made some lousy decisions just to please someone else.

At the end of Myofascial Release II, John said to me, "Let go of the fear." I felt that he was able to touch my soul, see what was there, and say the words that would help me grow. I not only hear John saying those words; I let myself feel the meaning. I am finally starting to believe it in my soul.

Several months ago, I had an appointment with John's son, Brian, in San Francisco. Brian told me that he would have to catch a phone call, as he was expecting his dad to call him regarding a question he had. He stepped out at about the time John was supposed to call, but missed the call. Brian brought the portable phone in the treatment room with him, and asked if I would mind if he took the call when John called. Of course not. Brian was doing the cervical stretch technique on me when John called back. Brian told John that he was treating me, and just then my neck and head started to uncontrollably unwind. This went on for three or four minutes. About the length of the call. John's energy reached through the phone line, through the portable phone!

When Brian hung up the phone, he said something to the fact his dad had treated me (long distance) through him. I knew it even before Brian said anything. At John's Cervical-Thoracic Myofascial/Osseous Release Seminar in Minneapolis, I spoke to John regarding this event, and he said "Oh, that was you?" And he kind of chuckled. Thank you John Barnes, for having the courage to give myofascial release to the world. I sincerely thank you from my very essence. It keeps growing and glowing brighter.

How these things happen, no one really knows. I believe that we all have these latent talents that can be developed. Einstein found that time/space, matter, and energy are relative, $E=mc^2$. He discovered that the solidity of mass is an illusion, and our concept of time and space are illusionary. Another illusion is our personality. Our personality is but a small part of the much vaster being that we are. Identification with your personality, the false ego, consumes your vital energy. "Persona" means mask. Most identify more and more with the mask, the personality. We forget that we are acting and become the role. As you become lost in becoming the mask, your essence withers. Your essence is your "vital spark of life!" You need to rediscover and reconnect with your essence, then nourish, love, and cherish it and your uniqueness. Identify with your essence!

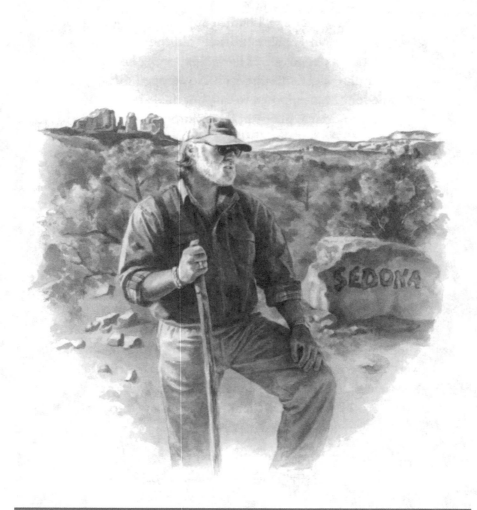

N

A PATIENT'S PERSPECTIVE

As his patient, you feel John's powerful, yet loving energy engulf you and you are swept away into an indescribable dimension of healing. John's "presence," his essence, guides you into reconnecting with your essence. The depth of his confidence instills a sense of safety and hope, so that you can let go, and flow with the experience. He sweeps you up and takes you back in time to a place you have been to before, to heal ancient wounds.

A THERAPIST'S PERSPECTIVE

There is something else. He is big and strong. He is so calm. There is an ease about him. He is deep, wise, and his humor disarms you, taking you to another level of understanding. But, there is something else…you leave your first Myofascial Release Seminar realizing that you have just encountered the most impressive human being that you have ever experienced! Then as you take the advanced Myofascial Release Seminars, John's mastery continues to unfold revealing more and more of his incredible depth and talent. He inspires you to reach for your own inner strength and wisdom. His example and encouragement lifts you to new heights and you hear your inner voice saying, "I can do this!"

I want to be very clear that I don't have any special talents that you can't develop. It's important to learn the proper therapeutic principles, learn to center yourselves, develop your sensitivity and clarity, and your therapeutic artistry will develop and expand. You all have the potential to open your hearts and become loving healers. You are all more expansive and powerful than you may realize!

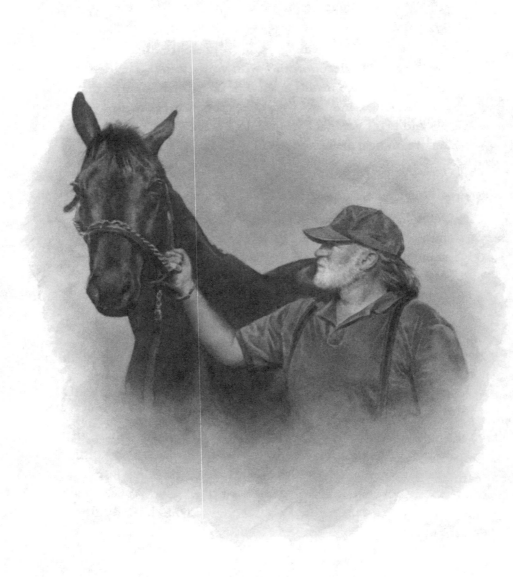

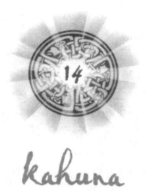

kahuna

When I was teaching myofascial release in the late 1970s, a physician approached me at the end of the day and said, "Do you realize that you are teaching Huna? You are a Kahuna!" I had never heard the terms before. This physician piqued my curiosity and I have since studied Huna philosophy deeply. It is an intriguing ancient healing method. Its one tenet is "Hurt no one!" Huna utilizes techniques that include deep physical pressure as well as visualization techniques coupled with subtle energy-flow techniques, administered with a tough-love approach by skilled, highly evolved and centered Kahunas. Huna means inner knowledge or secret. A Kahuna is a healer and "Keeper of the Secret." There is also a deep respect for our intuition and animal aspect, or instincts. Huna is based on love and respect for oneself and all living beings: human, animal, and nature. As you delve into your inner love, power, and knowledge, maybe you will discover that you are a Kahuna.

I have always loved animals. Treating animals in pain has been a very special experience for me. They are so appreciative and full of love. They help us to learn a true "heart to heart" connection. I believe that with myofascial release we are treating the "being" of the human being and the "being" of our animal friends. This is what enables us to communicate with them without the need for words.

Question: I understand you have treated racehorses. Could you tell us how you got involved in treating animals?

Years ago a friend of mine who had some racehorses called me. He had this two-year-old horse that had wonderful conformation, with great potential. Every time they would run this horse, it would go lame within one hundred yards or so. My friend was an interesting guy who had a very successful business where he had picked every one of his employees based on their astrological charts. You wouldn't have thought their talents had any relationship to the business, but whatever he did, it worked for him. I was up at his ski house one time, and most of the time he had his head buried in this magazine. Eventually I said to him, "What is it you are reading?" He said that he was looking up information on horses, because he was going to buy a racehorse. I said "Well, do you know anything about racehorses?" and he said "No." I said, "Aren't they rather expensive?" and he said, "Yes. I'm going to pick my horse by his astrological chart." Oh right!

He paid $19,000 for this horse. One day after the purchase of this horse, he called me and was very upset about this horse's performance. It wasn't doing well. He had taken it to New Bolton Center, which is one of the leading veterinary centers in the world, based out of the University of Pennsylvania. The vets had done everything they possibly could, and eventually told him, "there is nothing else we can do for this horse. If you keep running him, he is going to be destroyed. The only thing you can do is put him out to pasture."

So certainly this was a huge financial problem for my friend. He loves animals and really cared about this animal, so he called me and told me the situation and asked me to treat his horse. I told him I didn't know anything about horses, but he kept after me. And I kept telling him I didn't know anything about horses! He was very persistent and eventually he said, "Listen John, I read your chart last night. Do you know you're a healer?" I said yes, and he added, "But I mean for animals too." I knew I was sunk, so I said okay, and made arrangements for him to pick me up the next morning. After I got off the phone, I quieted down and asked myself, what was this horse's problem? I got a picture of the left forequarter of a horse with a big red swirl on the left shoulder and another one down near the hock.

On the way to the stable the next morning I asked where the horse's problem was and my friend said, "The left forequarter." Interesting, I thought. We took a couple other people up with us, and when we got to the stable they brought this magnificent animal out. Now here I am looking at this horse, and this horse is looking at me, and I'm thinking, now what do I do? So I thought, well, I know something about the energy system of a human being, maybe I ought to check this horse's energy first. So, in those days, the only thing I really knew about horses was that the front end bit and the back end kicked and did other things. So, I made a big sweep around the ends. I started to feel the energy on the right side and eventually got around to the left forequarter. Sure enough, right where I had seen this red swirl, I felt a tremendous amount of heat pouring out of him. I also felt a lot of heat on an area called the hock, which is just above the hoof. I then started to check the tissue texture and I felt all this hard, gristly buildup in those hot areas. It was very similar to what I had felt with human beings, but a much bigger version of it. The trainer was holding the horse by the bit, so I started doing some elbow work and some strumming-type techniques on the horse. We had somebody on the other side of the horse to help stabilize and to be sure the horse wouldn't move away. I eventually decided I would do a crossed-hands release over the shoulder area. As I was quieting myself and leaning into the horse, I heard myself say, you don't know what the hell you are doing! And my intuitive voice, The Ancient Warrior, said, "Shut up!" So, I quieted down again and the instant I did, the most amazing thing happened. My awareness fell into this horse and I "got" instantaneously where this horse's problem was. The moment I quieted down, everybody that was watching said, "He's leaning into you." We had made a connection!

The release was very similar to a human's also, except again a much bigger version. This is why it's helpful to learn on horses, because the release is so big you really can translate it easily back to a human experience. I then decided to do an energy technique. The trainer was holding the horse by the bit; I had somebody put their hands between the ears over the parietals, somebody else above the hoof, and I put my hands over the shoulder area and upper back. I closed my eyes and started to quiet down again. I started to feel this motion. I was thinking to myself, gee, that feels familiar, and all of a sudden it hit me. Oh my God, *this horse is unwinding!* Here I have twelve hundred pounds of horse coming at me, coming at me, coming at me, and I'm thinking, now what do I do? Then I hear the trainer saying, "He's falling asleep, he's falling asleep." The horse's eyes closed, his ears went down, his head started to rear back, and his left forequarter went into hyperextension. Zap! He hit the position of injury in space, the still point, and at that moment his eyes opened and became bright, his ears straightened up, and we all felt a lightning bolt of energy go through his body. At the same time his hoof thumped into the ground loudly and he just about threw us all off his body. I had never felt such a powerful experience! It was unbelievable!

After we finished, I asked the trainer if he would take him out and run him again. He took him out and the horse ran a mile for the first time in his life! The owner told me that when he went back to the stable a couple of days later, the trainer came running out of the stable exclaiming, "Who was that guy? I've been a trainer for thirty-five years and I have never seen a horse turn around like this in my life. He just ran three miles, and in good time!" With only three months of training, he broke and shattered the record at Belmont Stakes Park, which is one of the most important racetracks in the New York area. Within six months from the time of purchase, this horse had won over $600,000!

It has been my consistent experience with horses that they make significant improvements, returning to racing and shattering records. They love treatment! They lean into it, many times using you as a fulcrum to correct themselves. Once you've treated a horse they'll come running to you, as soon as they see you, as will other animals. Every time that I have ever unwound a human being and there has been an animal in the room, like a dog or a cat, they will get up instantaneously and move right into the energy field and participate. Dogs unwind, cats unwind, and I have even treated birds.

Question: How do you treat birds?

In Chicago a couple of years ago, a therapist who had taken a lot of my seminars called before the seminar and asked, "Is there any way I could bring my bird, Kahuna, in for treatment while you are in Chicago?" I receive a lot of strange requests. Kahuna was a beautiful cockatoo, six or seven inches tall with orange and white feathers. Kahuna was absolutely gorgeous! Cockatoos live to be eighty or ninety years old.

The therapist went on to explain that she had decided to take a week or two vacation when Kahuna was less than a year old, leaving the bird to be cared for by somebody else. It was the first time the bird had been left alone. When the therapist returned from vacation, Kahuna was self-mutilating. It was picking all the feathers out of its chest, to the point where the skin was raw. It had continued to do this for a couple of years and had to wear a cardboard collar to protect itself.

Kahuna had an open raw area on its chest, where it had picked away all the feathers. The woman had taken Kahuna to many vets, including holistic vets and even to crystal healers. Whatever you can possibly think of, she had tried. Finally, she took it to a veterinary surgeon, who decided to cut out the dead tissue in hopes of stimulating new growth. Well, he very honestly said to her after the surgery that he was sorry he did it, because he didn't think the wound would ever heal up and if it did, it would probably take three years or more. The size of the wound on the bird, if it was equivalent to the size in a human, was about the size of a football. I agreed to treat Kahuna to see what we could do for him.

So, she brought the bird in and she held it while I very slowly approached the bird's energy field. I waited there a while until Kahuna invited me in. I slowly felt the energy drawing me in, until eventually Kahuna let me hold it on the outside of its wings, which the owner said birds never do because they feel very vulnerable that way.

In a short period of time, Kahuna started to unwind. The motion felt like a roller coaster track in the air; that's also the same way it feels when you unwind an infant. Eventually the bird went upside down, with its head all scrunched around and stopped in a still point. Now I don't know whether or not the bird had fallen or been hit but it looked something like that might have happened. I held the bird in the still point; then I decided to do what is called an "energy chain" technique. I had the rest of the people in the class connect hands and form a circle around me. The two closest to me put their hands on my back to complete the chain. I don't usually sweat very much, but as I was quieting down, I began to sweat profusely; I felt like I was in a blast furnace. All of a sudden, it felt like a dam of energy burst through me, and the energy went into the bird and he screeched!

The bird's owner wrote to me about a month later. She said that on the ride home after the treatment, Kahuna felt physically lighter than she could ever remember, and more tranquil than it had ever been, even before this problem had occurred. That within one week the size of the wound had reduced down to the size of a thumbnail. Within one month the skin had completely healed over and a new feather had just emerged.

So, you can treat any type of an animal. That answers people who say "you set it up" or "it's just the human belief system, a placebo-type effect," or "you hypnotized him." How do you hypnotize a horse or a bird or an infant that doesn't speak? It's not that at all. It's applying sound principles from a deeper awareness and an inner knowledge, power, and love. Could it be Huna?

I've had reports of people treating many other types of animals too. I've had very good results with dogs. My dog Thor was a 220-pound mastiff. When he was about seven years old he started to develop some hip problems. I was becoming concerned. He couldn't run up and down the steps to the house, and I knew I wasn't about to carry this 220-pound dog up and down the steps every time he wanted to pee. So, I took him to the vet a couple of times and that didn't help at all. One day he was lying there looking really uncomfortable, so the first thing I tried was a leg-pull; he didn't go for that at all. Then I started doing crossed-hands myofascial releases over the hip and sacroiliac areas. The next day he was running up and down the steps without a limp. He lived to the age of thirteen, which is quite old for a dog of that size, and had no further problems after I treated him.

Years ago I was down in Jamaica for the Christmas week. I had rented a beautiful villa with a maid and a gardener. The maid had a couple of dogs, a couple of young puppies and one older dog who was limping and couldn't get around too well. He appeared frustrated because he wanted to play with the puppies, but they'd run off and jump up on this ledge and he couldn't jump up there with them. So one day I was up on the veranda reading. This old dog came over and sat down, eventually lying down next to me. I felt really sorry for him, so I slowly brought my hand down toward his body, and I could feel tremendous heat pouring off his hip. As I hit this hot spot off his body, he looked up. He felt me out there. I waited a bit, and eventually got a little closer and closer until he let me touch him. I also touched his head and he started to unwind. His tongue came out, his eyes rolled back in his head, he started to pant, and after a while he jumped up, ran off like a puppy, and jumped up on the ledge that he could never make before. The whole rest of the time I was there, he was chasing the puppies and doing really well. The interesting thing about animals is that when they are done, they get up. They know when they are done and they are ready to move on.

There's a therapist who has taken my myofascial release classes that has a cat, and he told me a funny story. Every morning at six, the cat would be on his chest doing that kneading thing with his paws, waking him up, ready to be fed. You know how cats are. He said he came back from the unwinding class and he unwound his cat. The next morning, for the first time in its life, the cat wasn't there at six. When the therapist got up out of bed he saw that the cat was lying down on his back across the doorway, so the man could not get out the door. The cat was basically saying, "Unwind me again." This is now a new morning routine. He cannot get through the door until he unwinds his cat. Smart cat!

Some cats are easy to treat; others are pretty skittish. So, with any animal, I start slowly by petting them. They then gradually start to unwind. With some cats you might have to do off-the-body work, though, because they are not going to let you touch them. Dogs are easier.

I had an interesting experience with a dog in Maryland. I was giving a Myofascial Release II class, and this therapist came up and said, "I'm having this problem with my dog. He's about eight years old now and has always been a wonderfully relaxed dog. We moved a month ago and ever since then, he's been in a total state of agitation. He runs constantly, he never sits still, he's messing in the house and barking all the time. He never messed in the house or barked before. Is there anything you can do?" I replied, "I don't know, but I am willing to try. Why don't you bring him in at lunch." She said "Okay, but I can't tell my husband, because he thinks you're crazy." I said, "okay." So, at lunchtime she brought him in. There were a lot of people in the room, so I just let the dog do his thing for a while—you know, he ran around sniffing everything. I just sat on the floor and eventually the dog came to me and I started to pet him.

Eventually I touched his head and back and he started to unwind and rolled on the floor for a while. I just got this sense while treating him, and the message I received was "This dog is in a total state of panic because its world has been taken away from him." All that dog had ever known for eight years was that other house, and so it was in a total state of fear and panic. So, I communicated to him visually and mentally, and I gave him permission to be calm. I explained to him that he has a new world to explore and that his parents/owners love him very much and he will be safe in his new home. It sounds stupid to some but it seems to work, so I'm willing to be stupid once in a while.

In any event, the woman came in the next day, laughing, and said, "Well, my husband doesn't think you are nuts any more. The dog stopped messing in the house, he stopped running around, he is not barking any more, and he slept the night through." So, somehow there is this wonderful communication that can occur and it's definitely worthwhile trying. I love animals, and this is a very loving thing to do for them.

Question: Do animals have emotions?

Animals definitely have emotions; I've felt and seen them so much. My son Mark has a successful myofascial release practice in Boulder, Colorado, for humans, and has developed the Equine Myofascial Release Therapy Seminars. A couple of months ago he was treating a horse that was having a behavioral problem. He was difficult to ride and he tried to bite people, and its owner just was fed up. Mark said he was treating the horse and the horse started to unwind, and eventually the horse's head went way, way down and stayed there for a long, long period of time. Then the horse started making a "pfff, pfff" sound. Mark looked down and saw a big tear was running down the horse's face. The next day, the owner exclaimed, "I can't believe the difference. I can ride this horse, and he's no longer biting." Traditional horse training is really barbaric, and I really think that a lot of times they are hurt very badly on a physical and emotional level. I know that you can help them quite a bit with this type of work.

Question: How do you start with a horse?

The first thing I always do is create a communication with the animal. Before I start treating them I want to make sure they can see me; initially I do not go to the rear of the animal. I want to be sure they are not worried about what is going on. I then touch them very lightly. I have treated rodeo horses that were severely abused, and the owners told me that I wouldn't get near this horse and to be careful because they'll hurt you. Within two or three minutes every one of them is just in this calm state, unwinding, and making incredible changes. This is a universal touch and communication. This is why you can treat children, animals, and people that speak other languages. It doesn't matter. This is a loving, universal language of touch that generates safety and confidence, that feels loving and right.

Question: Have you ever been injured treating a horse?

When I'm treating a horse I am centered. What it literally feels like to me is that I am in this energy bubble. This energy bubble protects me. It actually lifts me up and moves me out of the way when needed, so that I've never been injured. I've even had a couple of horses try to kick me, but you can feel it happening in their body before it even happens and you just flow with the energy and move out of the way. They love the tail-pull. They will treat you, also. They will touch you on a very emotional level and teach you.

A friend had asked to go to the stable with me to treat horses. When we got there, I gave her some suggestions to help improve her proprioceptive abilities. We treated the horse and as we finished and we were driving out of the ranch, I looked over and asked, "How was that for you?" She started to tell me that she didn't feel she had noticed or felt much, when suddenly she burst into tears and began sobbing and wailing! She went into a spontaneous unwinding while I was driving down the New Jersey turnpike. I had one hand on her head and one on the steering wheel. We arrived at the tollgate of the New Jersey turnpike and she is upside down, bawling her eyes out. The attendant never batted an eye. He just collected my money and on we went. He wasn't about to get involved. The experience made a significant shift in her. It does with a lot of people that treat animals. Animals love the treatment. I think maybe this is the dimension we are treating human beings on, and that's why it is so universal. There is an instinctual, loving connection that occurs.

The following is a story about a cat named Waldo. This story was posted on our MFR Insight Facebook page. By the way, before I tell the story, I would like to encourage therapists and patients both to subscribe to MFR Insight. It involves therapists I've trained from beginning level to advanced, from around the world. The group also includes patients receiving and/or interested in myofascial release treatment. It is free and your questions and insights are welcome. The website address is www.myofascialrelease.com. To become a member of MFR Insight, search for the group page on Facebook and join.

While written humorously, this is a true story. This experience illustrates the sad and typical medical, veterinary, and therapeutic traditional symptomatic viewpoint versus the "structural/functional" myofascial perspective.

When Waldo was somewhere between five and eight years old, he chose his owner by showing up on her doorstep and refusing to leave. Waldo's surgical history, as assessed by the vet, was that he was neutered and later developed a chronic urinary tract infection and feline urologic syndrome; because of this, the vets surgically removed his penis. (In Spanish, this is called *"El Gato Unhappicus,"* or "unhappy cat syndrome.") Other surgical procedures included a thyroidectomy. Waldo became an inside cat after his owner moved to Arizona, since in Arizona coyotes consider cats to be appetizers (*El Gato Scrumptisioso*). He is now fourteen years old, living inside, and has had no major traumas until a few weeks ago, when he had a tooth removed by the vet. Afterwards he lost his appetite, became listless, and could not flex his neck to eat out of his bowl on the floor. He then began projectile vomiting, redecorating his owner's walls and rugs. After numerous visits to the vet, who was very comprehensive from a traditional symptomatic point of view, Waldo's problem was diagnosed as probable pancreatitis. The solution was intravenous steroids.

When Waldo's owner explained his plight to me I said, "Bull!" and suggested she bring Waldo in for treatment. The surgical removal of a tooth as part of his recent history gave me the clue as to what could have been the probable cause of the onset of his symptoms. Visualize this experience. The cat was anesthetized, strapped down, and his head and neck were probably held in extension to facilitate the removal of the tooth. This must have jammed his occipital condyles. Doing so creates a fascial strain around the jugular foramina and restriction of the occipital condyles, which then can entrap the vagus nerve, producing Waldo's symptoms (nausea, listlessness, projectile vomiting, and limited cervical range of motion).

So the typical symptomatic traditional approach, that so many of us, our patients and animal friends become bogged down in, created unnecessary, prolonged suffering for Waldo. For his owner, it meant unnecessary expenses, and time spent cleaning the house and taking Waldo back and forth to the vet. In contrast with the Myofascial Release Approach, in less than ten minutes I had scanned Waldo's body, and found and released his restrictions. His owner held Waldo while I used a gentle myofascial/osseous release to the occipital condyles, and upper cervical and thyroid areas, and finished with a gentle unwinding with Waldo's head and cervical spine. Waldo, by the way, enjoyed his treatment! The day following his treatment Waldo was able to reach down to the floor to eat for the first time since his surgery, no further vomiting occurred, and he experienced a return of his energy. He's playful and happy and really glad that he's not going back to the vet!

Question: How much knowledge of equine anatomy did you have before treating horses?

Very little. I now have extensive knowledge of equine anatomy and performance. But we have to be cognizant that the anatomy of humans and animals that we learned is inaccurate. Our training was incomplete due to the fact that the fascial system wasn't included in the health professional's education. Assessment and treatment of the myofascial system is performed through the feel of the anatomy by a highly skilled myofascial release therapist's proprioceptive awareness.

Intellectual information alone is insufficient. It is only through the development of our proprioceptive awareness that allows for the sensitive palpation of the multitude of anatomical structures that can provide the intimate understanding of that individual's unique configuration. Most traditional physicians and therapists either have no palpation training or the emphasis has been on only the tactile senses. The tactile senses embryologically emanate from the ectoderm, the nervous system. The training that I provide is a combination of the tactile senses and the proprioceptive senses that embryologically emanate from the mesoderm, which lies in the tendons, muscles, and predominately the fascia. One of the many attributes of our proprioceptive senses is our ability to detect motion and change in our environment with our mind-body.

I emphasize the development of the therapist's ability to be in silence at the center of the cyclone. When the therapist quiets themself physically and mentally and touches another for a sustained period of time, that other person or animal becomes the therapist's environment. This enables the highly skilled therapist to feel deeply and accurately into the body, to "know" exactly where the person's or animal's problems are, and then to be able to feel when a release occurs and when a correction has been accomplished. Myofascial release takes the "guesswork" out of health care.

The therapist uses their proprioceptive awareness to ascertain where the fascia has lost its fluidity and has solidified; where there is restricted motion within the system; where there is a bio-energetic blockage that is leaking thermals and creating vibrations that are out of synchrony with the whole. In other words, the myofascial therapist doesn't just feel with their hands, they also feel and perceive with their minds!

When one is thinking or talking, they are in a state of disassociation, always one step away from the action. They are putting out energy and not capable of receiving the information that is critical in making proper analytical decisions. We never learn when we are talking or thinking. So, without feeling, intellectual decisions are all guesswork.

Thinking and talking are like static on a radio. Nothing is being accurately perceived or heard. It is only when we are in deep stillness and silence that we are capable of receiving the information we need to make proper analytical and intelligent decisions. This is wisdom—one being's mind-body wisdom communicating with another's mind-body wisdom. It is this deep communication that allows the therapist to accurately perceive what a person's or animal's unique problems, dysfunctions, and potentials are, and then make accurate therapeutic decisions moment by moment to enhance their performance, health, and well-being.

As a patient, when you are being treated by a myofascial release therapist you are encountering a very unique individual, one that has extensive and very special training and talents, a person who has expended a considerable amount of time developing their skills and awareness. They have done everything that they will be asking you to do and feel. They are interacting with you from an extensive knowledge base and extraordinary personal and professional experiences. They have had the courage to feel their own pain and face their own fears. They have already been to where they will take you for your healing to occur. We believe that you can only take your patients as far and as deep as you are willing to go yourself!

When you are with a myofascial release therapist you are in the hands of someone who has internal strength, courage, integrity, and incredible awareness. You will sense the gentle, yet powerful feel of their essence when they are near you and as they touch you. Allow their presence and the luminescence in their eyes to inspire you and reconnect you with your essence. We know that you have these attributes also, and we will help you reach your full potential! We will help you reach your goals as long as you are willing to help yourself. What you will get out of myofascial release is what you are willing to put into it! Your myofascial release therapist's formidable skills, inner calm, and confidence will help you peel away myofascial and emotional barriers that have blocked the full expression of your true self, to rediscover your own tranquility, strength, mental clarity, and awareness. Re-igniting your "spark of life" will return you to a natural, joyful, healthy, and pain-free active lifestyle!

1703

Question: Would you relate your experiences with the first patient that went into a past-life experience?

I had been asked to speak to hundreds of physicians at a large international conference on pain. The conference was held in a beautiful beach hotel overlooking the turquoise waters of Bermuda.

After my lecture, a number of physicians were congratulating me and asking me questions pertaining to their particular specialties. I noticed one man standing off to the side, obviously waiting for me to be alone. As the crowd around me wandered off, he approached me and asked for a minute of my time. He said that his wife has been having terrible problems for years. She has been suffering with chronic pain, headaches, menstrual difficulties, and fibromyalgia, and despite being a physician, he has been unable to help her. He went on to say that she also struggles with dizziness and vertigo whenever she rides in a car, plane, or any moving vehicle. The dizziness is so extreme that she has panic attacks, becomes nauseous, throws up, and is left incapacitated for days afterwards. They knew that flying to Bermuda would be stressful for her, but they had not been on a vacation without their children in years and wanted to be alone together and rest. But the airplane ride stirred her up worse than ever and she feels like she is going to die. She can't leave the room and only gets out of bed to throw up. "I normally wouldn't bother you, but I am desperate! I was very impressed by your lecture, your command of knowledge and of the audience. I asked a friend of mine, who I trust, about you and he told me that your skills are far beyond that of most therapists and physicians, and that people seek you out from around the world. He told me that you are renowned for resolving complex situations. However, all that considered, I still would not have approached you, if it was not for my wife's determined insistence that I ask for your help. When we checked into the hotel, you were in the lobby. She saw you and had an immediate and strong visceral reaction. She blurted out, 'I know him, his look, his presence, his strength. He has come to help me!'

"As we approached you, you hopped on a motorcycle and drove off. She was shaken by the experience and pleaded with me to find out who you were. One of the people that you were talking with in the lobby said that you were lecturing at the pain conference. So I attended your lecture today, and we are asking if you would please consider helping her. Would you? My wife is not a kook; she is a wonderful, strong woman that is mentally sound and stable. She is in a desperate struggle and has handled this long ordeal with great courage. She is totally exhausted and I don't know what else to do..."

I felt for him and his wife. They were caught up in these terrible circumstances that create such a struggle for so many patients and their families. I said that I would be glad to try to help them. I was committed the rest of the day. The only time I had available would be after dinner that night around nine thirty. We agreed to meet in their room. When I arrived, he greeted me at the door and introduced me to his wife, who was an attractive woman in her late thirties.

She reiterated the story of her problems. As she spoke, I noticed that her complexion was ghostly white, with a light greenish hue. There was no sparkle in her eyes; they were dull and almost vacant. I could sense tremendous agitation in her energy field. I asked her to lie on the bed and I lightly touched her body for assessment purposes. Her husband sat on a chair near the bed.

I discovered myofascial restrictions in her respiratory diaphragm, thoracic inlet, and severe cervical osseous restrictions and occipital condylar compression. She also presented with torsion in both her pelvis and temporal bones and restricted motion of her sphenoid. These are commonly found myofascial/osseous restrictions with someone experiencing chronic pain, headaches, fibromyalgia and/or vertigo symptoms. I could also feel enormous fear in her body and a hot vibration emerging from her upper neck and head. I knelt on the floor and placed my hands lightly on the back of her head. I slowed my breathing, softened my body, and quieted my mind.

I could feel a melding of our energies and began to see a cobolt blue orb of light floating between my eyes. When I become deeply centered and move into a "healing mode," I have a felt-sense of quiet, flowing power and I see a beautiful cobalt blue orb with a pulsating orange corona around it in my mind's eye. I then sink into the felt-sense of the energy, become the color and flow with the power.

Her head and neck began to move and unwind slowly. I became aware of The Ancient One's presence. He didn't say anything. The atmosphere of the room became highly charged and I could feel this enormous power burst through me and into her! She started to shake and then move on the bed. She said, "I feel so cold. Why am I moving like this?" I said, "Don't worry, trust your body and instincts and allow yourself to let go. I will take care of you. I will not allow you to be re-injured. Just take off your brakes, trust, and let go."

I quieted down and moved into a deep stillness. Another strong charge roared through my body and into her. She jolted and shook violently. With a quivering voice she said, "I feel so afraid inside and so cold. I can't stop shaking!" After a few minutes, I turned to her husband and assured him that she was safe and releasing. "Trust me and I will explain later." He had a very worried look on his face.

I could sense that her consciousness was shifting to another time. She felt like a different person energetically. She said, "I'm confused, where am I?" The tone of her voice, while still quivering, had shifted dramatically. "Who are you?" I asked her. "What year is it?" She replied "03." 03? I was shocked! She was about thirty-eight and we were presently in the mid 1970s. I calculated and wondered how could it be 1903? I asked again, "What year is it?" She answered "1703"...I was stunned!

Do not distract yourself with disbelief. Focus. Ask her to look around and identify her surroundings.

So I asked her to look around and see what she could see. Her eyes went into rapid eye movement and her head turned as if looking around. She reported, "I am lying on a stone floor, cobble stones, and there are stone walls with a little rectangular window. I am very cold and the room gets very bright and then very dark, very bright and then very dark. Where am I?"

I asked, "What do you feel?" She replied, "Cold and fear!" I asked, "What are you afraid of?" She said, "Of him!" "Who is the man you are afraid of?" She said, "I don't know, but I am in a panic." I encouraged her to go back in time a little further and see what had happened to her. Her eyes fluttered again, her body arched and she began to fight violently and she yelled, "Stop! Don't!" More wild fighting ensued and then running motions with her arms and hands with heavy, loud breathing. Then all of the sudden, she stopped and went totally silent and her body went limp. She was quiet for a while and I looked over at her husband, who at this point was in a total panic seeing his wife thrash around. I put my finger to my lips using body language to keep him silent and not disturb this very unusual, but important healing experience.

Her eyes opened and looked dreamily up with a faraway look. I asked, "What are you seeing?" She replied, "I am watching beautiful clouds float by. I am lying on my back on the grass." Suddenly, she shrieked and added, "Oh my God! I passed out, but he is still after me! I've got to get away! There's the windmill, I'll hide in there." Her body started running again and she collapsed on the floor of the windmill. She gasped, "He tried to rape me! I got away, but he is still after me, I can't stay here!" She ran outside down a path by a canal where a boat with one sail on it went by. She began running as fast as she could down the trail by the canal and then into the woods to hide. She lay there panting, trying to catch her breath. As she eventually quieted, I heard her mumble, "I'm free. I got away. I'm safe! Thank God!"

After a while, her consciousness returned from 1703 to the present time. She looked at me bewildered and then started to sob. "Oh thank you, John, thank you! It's over! We did it! My nightmare is over! You were with me the whole time." She looked at her husband and I waved him over and asked that he hold her. She collapsed in his arms sobbing. I quietly left the room so that they could be alone in that very special moment of togetherness.

The next morning, I was in the dining room having breakfast with a few of the physicians speaking at the conference. When I looked up, the physician and his wife were walking towards me. I got up and moved away from the table so that we could talk privately.

I was looking at a totally different woman. She was radiant, eyes sparkling, rosy complexion, with a jubilant spring to her motions and walk. She hugged me tightly and warmly, saying, "Thank you, you saved my life! You brought me back. I will never forget you and your kindness. Thank you!"

Her husband shook my hand, and said, "You have changed our lives forever. If I had a pot of gold I would give it to you gladly. You brought my wife back. Look at her! No pain, no headaches, no nausea, and no vertigo. She is so beautiful! Thank you!" He continued on, "We are strict Christians. If you had told me about this beforehand, I would not have believed you and would have considered it the work of the devil! But anything this powerful that can help my wife this positively and dramatically has to be God's work. The test will be on our flight home. Let's pray that it doesn't start all over again." They thanked me again and left, arm in arm.

I went out to Bermuda's turquoise ocean and listened to the water crash into black volcanic rocks. I had never believed in past-life experiences before. This experience had a profound impact on me and took my awareness and skills to a totally new level; a quantum leap! I opened my focus and absorbed the beautiful surroundings. I thanked The Ancient One for his help and told him, I couldn't have done it without you.

I am you! You are me! You are more powerful than you can possibly imagine. Everyone is! Our mission is to help others become aware of their own loving power, so that they can heal and live life fully. When you want help, quiet yourself, ask for help, and let go and flow with the action.

I have followed that advice, with ever-increasing results, throughout the years. You know, when we are young, growing and maturing, we make a lot of mistakes. We take a lot of zigzags, lost in the confusion. As I look back over my life, I realize that I have been blessed. I have been guided by a higher power, God.

I have trained a multitude of therapists and physicians, who are healing millions of people with myofascial release, and nobody has ever been injured. So, it certainly is not the work of the devil. My intuition, The Ancient One, has a strong, loving presence. God may work in strange and mysterious ways, but however it may unfold, it always produces a loving and positive result.

About a month after I returned from Bermuda, I received a present in the mail with a letter from the couple that I had helped. They were thrilled that she continued to improve. Her pain and headaches are gone. She had no vertigo or nausea on the plane ride back home, and none while driving in cars. She went on to write she feels better physically, mentally, and emotionally than she has in twenty years. She wrote that she realized that her 1703 experience was in Holland and the reason that the room kept switching from very bright to very dark was that she was lying on the cold stone floor of a windmill. And every time the windmill blade would sweep past the window, it would block the light and darken the room. As the windmill blade would pass the window, light would flood in again.

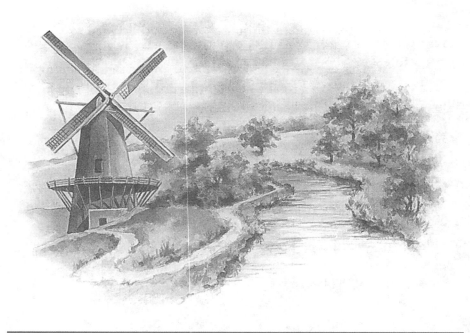

Fear is gone from her body and she feels lighter as she moves. In the past, she was never comfortable with her sensuality. She now feels naturally sensual and is enjoying a deeper sense of intimacy with her husband. She realizes that the attempted rape had left her in fear of men and sensuality. Since the 1703 experience, she feels the pattern is broken and feels free; free from the past fear and now, free to be herself!

She had expressed clear goals for her treatment session. She wanted to be free of pain. She had wanted to eliminate the vertigo and nausea and the fear of driving and flying. I had asked her to see a picture of herself smiling, radiant, and pain free, and to feel what that would be like…and to expect it to be her new reality, and then take off her brakes and trust. I had encouraged her to let go. It is helpful to ask your patient what they want, what their goals are, what would be meaningful to them. Ask the patient to tune into their intuition, become quiet and ask what would be in their best interest.

Question: Can you give us some hints on how to develop our intuition?

Scientific thought is important, but never sufficient. In school we were taught about the art and science of therapy. After leaving school, we heard a lot about the scientific aspect and almost nothing about the artistic aspect. In fact, our intuitive side was ridiculed in school, and it was emphasized that the only valuable form of thinking was our analytical thought process.

Although our schools pay lip service to the idea of using both hemispheres for complete balanced thought, in practice we suffer from a pandemic of half-witted thinking. Unfortunately, our educational system, as well as science, tends to neglect the non-verbal form of intellect. This neglect may be why the healthcare system is in such chaos now, by its insistence on just myopically treating symptoms. We were taught in school to just treat symptoms, the tip of the iceberg of the total problem.

We lose our way when we just use our analytical side and don't also combine our thinking process with our subconscious, intuitive side, which gives us the big picture. Neuroscientists estimate that your subconscious database outperforms the conscious analytical side on an order exceeding ten million to one! The subconscious is the source of your creative potential. This is why only using your analytical side is considered half-witted thinking.

Albert Einstein, one of the world's most prodigous geniuses, said that most scientists are mere technicians. He felt that most scientists only rely on the analytical side of their brain and simply memorize the thoughts of others, who had memorized the thoughts of others, thus passing on limited, *mis*information from generation to generation. Einstein said that all of his great ideas came from his intuition. He said that he didn't just sit down and analyze things or try to think things out. He described how he would get an intuitive flash, a total picture of the solution to a problem. Then from this intuitive picture, he would utilize his analytical abilities to break the total solution into pieces, so that he could communicate it to others.

I teach techniques to bring out your inner wisdom, allowing you to make more accurate analytical decisions. Combining rational thought with intuition is essential for the therapeutic process to be successful. Here are some ideas on how to expand your creative abilities:

Quiet your mind. The endless left-brain chatter is like static on a radio. This constant internal dialogue is a distraction. Ask yourself a question, then don't try to figure it out. Quiet yourself and wait. Your creative side needs time to process. Sometimes it helps to go and do something pleasurable. Many times, the answer will just pop up in the form of a thought, picture, feeling, or symbol during another activity.

Ask dumb questions. Dumb questions lead you to a deeper truth or reality. They can show you how to look at old things in a new way. Become immersed in the moment, so that you *become* the moment. You will increase your focus and concentration by becoming lost in the task.

Destroy judgement, and create creativity. Judgement is a criticism whose function is to slam the door shut on further discovery and curiosity. Love what you do! Best results occur when you enjoy what you are doing. That means enjoy it all, the hard work and tedious aspects as well. Follow your intuition rather than logic.

Develop a relationship with your intuition, and allow it to grow at its own pace. Visualize your intuition as a separate being. This will help you connect with your inner awareness on a deeper level.

Try to refrain from judging or analyzing. Your visualizations do not need to be understood or make analytical sense. Invite your intuition to come to meet you. Open your mind and heart; allow your intuition to assume a form. All you need to do is remember how it felt to be there. Create an open space, a fertile "not-knowing" space, and wait. Pay attention to what it physically feels like when your intuition communicates; it may be in words, pictures, colors, symbols, or emotion. Remember, what was the felt-sense of it?

Remaining in the open focus of the present moment takes strength and courage, for your powerful true feelings, both good and bad, will rise to the surface. We tend to avoid our feelings by slipping into thoughts of the past or the future. Discipline yourself to overcome this tendency to slide away from the "now." Take responsibility to be in the present moment, to be centered in the eye of the cyclone.

Doing things, doing things, doing things... and while they are doing things people are frantically thinking about what to "do" next. Rarely are people flowing in the present moment. They have given their power to the past and future. They are in a state of severe abstraction, always one step away from true meaningful experience. Their lives revolve around being worried about what happened to them in the past or fretting about the future.

Your clarity, tranquility, and power lie within the "now!" The present is the timeless, spaceless dimension of eternity. Reclaim your power! Live and flow in the present moment!

Ask your intuition, "What is my mission? What is my purpose in life?" Without awareness of your purpose, time is wasted, energy is scattered, and there is a felt-sense of internal anxiety. Once your intuition has helped you discover your life's purpose, your life will have a powerful focus that will have an enjoyable flow to it.

Develop the genius that lies within you!

The following is an example of not trying to figure it out, and intuitively going with the flow. A therapist brought his wife to me for treatment; she had, years before, fallen in a ceramic shower. She fell on her tailbone and severely injured herself. She had not been able to sit for years, had constant back pain, neck pain, and coccygeal pain, hadn't been able to make love; her life was miserable. So, he brought her down to Paoli, and I treated her. She unwound and we went through the shower accident pretty quickly, but there was still some pain left. One day, her unwinding took her back to a time, when she was around three or four years old; her body flipped up in the air and she came down on her tailbone. She remembered that when she was a young child, she had been on a farm, visiting an aunt and uncle. As she walked out past the fence, a bull hit her in the butt and flipped her in the air. So that was the problem. How would she have ever known? After her unwinding, her pain went away and she is leading a normal life again. She logically thought the problem was the fall in the shower, when in fact the fall in the shower just took her over the edge. So, don't predict where you should be or go; trust. Your essence will take you into some of the most interesting areas you could have ever imagined. Trust, because your inner self is totally impeccable and will take you where you need to go, if you just get the logical, left brain out of the way.

Saying you should be doing this, you should be doing that, I know it sounds easy for me to say, but believe me, I have been there. Whatever happens, go into it, and go into it as deeply as you can, without restricting whatever naturally happens.

Along those lines, the other thing that can happen is when you hear the person say, "My God, I went home and cried for hours; I couldn't stop." What you say to them is, "That's because you were *trying* to stop. Cry now, and I defy you to cry for more than ten minutes." They'll be over it in no time. It's our resistance to things that causes our suffering. It's our resistance to what *is* that prolongs our suffering and gets in the way of our healing. Accept what is, and make the best of it!

We have to keep getting out of the way and it's really hard, because it's so familiar to us. It's been our way of life, all of our life; even though it hasn't worked for us, it's familiar. Your patients may hate their pain, they may hate the fact that they can't move well, but this is why it's helpful to have a goal. Nature abhors a void, and even though you make progress, if you have no goal, no vision—and it has to be a picture—you're going to slip back into the familiar again. Although we're recording everything that ever happened to us on some level, we seem to have hung onto the things that we have resisted, or those events that had a high emotional content to them.

Question: What if the patient triggers you?

If something really gets to you, they have just done you the biggest favor; they've just mirrored something for you. So give yourself permission to go take care of yourself, and cry, or beat up a pillow. You don't have to even know what it's all about; whatever emotion is there, whatever sensation is coming up, go into it deeply. We all have to keep clearing out for a while, because we've got a lifetime of stuff in there now. The thing that I hear a lot from therapists is, "I'm glad I got into this, but I've got so far to go." Or a lot of times, they will come to the advanced seminars and I hear them say, "I thought I had it all together, I thought I knew it all, and now I realize that I have all this other stuff to learn now." And what I say is, "You know, life's a journey. Don't worry so much about the destination, just enjoy the trip. At least we're all heading in the right direction now!"

If you find yourself always being triggered by your patients, you're not grounding, you're not centering yourself, and that's why you're picking up their stuff. That's why it is important that you learn to center yourself. My audiotapes, *The Inner Journey*, are an easy and effective way to center yourself. It doesn't have to be *our* tapes; get any good relaxation training tapes. Give it a little time, be quiet, listen to the tapes often, and eventually you'll get a feel for it.

You should walk away at the end of the day with a sense of energy, a sense of achievement. At the end of the day, you should feel exhilarated, versus wrung out like a washrag. When you're wrung out like a washrag, you know you're not centering, you're trying too hard, and you're picking up all their stuff. We have enough stuff of our own, let alone dragging everybody else's stuff along with us too. So try to center yourself—that's the key!

Question: What do you do when the client says they're nauseous?

You know when somebody says they're getting sick, it's usually an avoidance issue. What I will do is pick up the trash can and say "Go for it!" They never do. Once in a while, if they are really sick, that might happen, but usually it's an avoidance issue. And speaking of avoidance issues, watch their patterns. If they are always going in the same physical motion pattern, let them do that for a while, but after a number of cycles, this is when you need to get in the way and break them out of that pattern; otherwise you are just perpetuating that pattern. If they're always crying, let them cry for a while; there's a point where that's an avoidance issue. Or maybe they always laugh, or maybe they're always quiet, or maybe they never move. Watch these patterns of theirs, and then you do the opposite. If they're always crying, say "Let's go under that and see what you feel." It's like a switch; all of a sudden they're into something very deep. If they are always moving, say, "Be still." So just watch the patterns, let them go on for a while. Maybe all they needed to do is go through the pattern for a while. But over a period of time, then it's time to have them change the pattern and get under it somehow, do the opposite.

Question: Does tissue memory feel real?

Tissue memory can be very intense. There'll be times when you're touching somebody very lightly and they'll be screaming at you, "Take your hand off me! You're breaking my arm!" Now, you know if you're touching that lightly, you're not breaking their arm. Or they'll say, "I'm choking, I'm choking, I can't breathe." Now they're talking to you, so you know they are breathing. Sometimes they're going to start coughing up stuff. Give them permission to cough it up. Give them some tissue, and even if nothing comes up physically, symbolically trying to cough it or spit it out can really help. Old anesthesia memories will come out, so just give them permission to do whatever they have to do.

Question: Do you always get what you ask for?

I'll tell you a really funny story about asking for what you want. Be careful what you ask for. I was in Santa Barbara a couple of years ago doing a Myofascial Unwinding Seminar. On the second day we did the multiple-person technique, and the lights were low. There were four or five people each unwinding each other, and there was a lot of crying and screaming going on. The lights were very low, and all of a sudden the door swung open and light poured into the room. This business-type of guy with a coat and tie came storming into the room screaming, "Control yourselves! Control yourselves!"

I had just spent two days trying to get everybody to *let go* of control. Then he screams, "Who's in charge here?" I raised my hand, and he came at me like he was going to try to rip my head off. When he got to about ten feet from me, I projected my energy out. He hit my energy field and went FROOOMP, slumped, shook my hand, smiled weakly, and walked out of the room.

It turns out they were having a business meeting next door, and you can imagine what they were hearing and thinking with all the screaming and ranting and raving. Some of the ladies in the audience said it was perfect, because he reminded them of the creeps they had just divorced, and they were able to get it out of their system. We continued, and a few minutes later one of my instructors came over and said, "John, I think I smell poop." I said, "No." She said, "John I know what poop smells like. Come here." I followed her over, and sure enough, there was a line of this stuff all the way out the door and into the ladies' room. The cleaning service was really happy with us. The therapist was very brave, and told on herself. She said, "That was me that made that mess and I'm really sorry, but it was the most wonderful thing in the world for me. If you remember the first day, I was up on the table, you were treating me, and you saw a greenish yellow streak on my belly. I said that my goal was to get rid of my shit. So, watch what you ask for...you may get it."

A Patient's Perspective

I have TMJ and fibromyalgia and myofascial pain syndrome. I had TMJ surgery back in 1981. For almost a year I have been seeing a chiropractor, who introduced me to a myofascial release therapist. That was last April. I have had an awakening!

How was I before myofascial release? I was angry, rageful, in pain all the time. But since I have seen a myofascial release therapist (who, incidentally, is the most compassionate, caring, loving person), I have the joy back in my life and most of the pain is gone. I have gone through the fight/flight/freeze part of the therapy. It is a freeing experience. I am able to set goals for my life now. I have learned to love myself. I know that I'm a good person. You can see the light in my eyes now!

What does this mean to me? Even though I haven't had a treatment by John Barnes, I feel as though I have since my therapist was trained by him. Also, I think that my therapist has received the essence of what John is teaching, so I am very blessed to have him in my area. I am in the process of starting massage therapy school, then to take the John F. Barnes Myofascial Release Seminars. I want to be able to help others like me.

Now let me go into goal-setting more deeply. It is helpful for your patients to set goals. If we don't have goals we are aimless. We are squandering energy. We are all over the place. A lot of people are afraid to set goals because that means that they have to commit to something; they get real slippery about things. They don't want to do that. That's the way the human being tends to be. So, let the patient know that goals are not set in concrete. It's better to have a wrong goal than no goal. Because even if you set the wrong goal, you are going to be able to determine in a short period of time that it's not right for you, and you'll be able then to set a more appropriate goal. That wrong goal, then, actually helped you.

It's a known fact in the aeronautics industry that a missile is only on course about 2% of the time. We all have a negative feedback system that is similar to the negative feedback system of a missile. We have to stop being so concerned about making mistakes. That's how we learn. And that's one of the things that has destroyed a lot of your patients' images of themselves: they made mistakes in the past. You let them know that we all make mistakes. It's only a mistake when you don't learn from it, because you'll keep repeating it over and over again. Let them know that their mistakes are not really mistakes. Change their perspective of it, and tell them that mistakes are opportunities to learn. As you learn this, the zigzag in your life becomes less violent and you start to flow. Let them create short-term goals of a couple of days, or a couple of weeks; mid-range goals, which might be a couple of months to a year or two; and then long-term goals. In other words, what is their life purpose?

There is no pressure to come up with an answer right now, but I would like you to ask yourself this. You don't have to have the answer right away, but let's plant the seed. Relax your bellies. Take a nice deep breath in, and let your bellies puff out as you breathe in. Nice slow breath out. Each time you slowly breathe out, allow your bodies to soften. You want to be able to set some goals. I want you to consider stretching beyond your comfort zone. Remember that mediocre goals produce mediocre results. You don't have to come up with a goal right away. We're just going to plant the seed and we'll see what comes up for you.

Now I want to ask you a question. Again, there is no need for an answer right away. **What is the purpose of your life?** Very few of us really have gotten in touch with our purpose, and when we don't have a mission or a purpose, we are squandering our energy. We are wasting time. I want you to give yourself permission to get in touch with the purpose in your life. When you have a purpose, when you have a mission, you have incredible focus and power. Let your patients know that, too. Let them get in touch with their purpose or mission. We've all had problems. We've all been hurt. But sometimes we can look at that as a catalyst that made us stop and really look at who we are, what we're doing, what is meaningful to us. If we can give our past problems value, we can move on and grow. Once we have determined our purpose, all of our goals should be in alignment with that life purpose. So it's best first to get in touch with that purpose, and then set your goals after that. Give yourselves permission, and it will come to you. It might come as a picture, as a thought, an emotion, or an urge. Just say, "I give myself permission to get in touch with my true self, my essence, so I can align with the purpose of my essence." What I've seen with so many of us is that we've disconnected from our real self, our essence, and most of us are in more of a survival mode than really living. Just know that it's not selfish to take care of yourself, to get in touch with your real self. For as you do, it will give you the power to let other people, through your presence and your experiences, get in touch with their power, their true self. It's very profound. It's very necessary. Now, place the book down, close your eyes, slow your breathing, soften your body, and ask yourself, "What is my life's purpose?" Move into deep silence and ask for help.

Now I would like you to soften even more, and open your heart and read what has been paraphrased from a poem called *Invitation* by Oriah Mountain Dreamer:

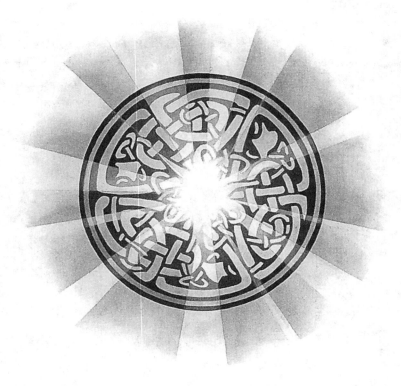

It doesn't interest me what you do for a living.
I want to know what you ache for,
And if you dare to dream of meeting your heart's longing.

I want to know if you have touched the center of your own sorrow,
If you have been opened by life's betrayals or
Have become shriveled and closed from fear of further pain!

I want to know if you can sit with pain, mine or your own,
Without moving to hide it or fade it or fix it.

I want to know if you can be faithful
And therefore be trustworthy.

I want to know if you can see beauty
Even when it is not pretty every day.

It doesn't interest me to know where you live
Or how much money you have.
I want to know if you get up after the night of grief and despair,
Weary and bruised to the bone, and do what needs to be done.

It doesn't interest me who you are, how you came to be here.
I want to know if you will stand in the center of the fire with me
And not shrink back.

It doesn't interest me where or what or with whom you
 have studied.
I want to know what sustains you from the inside
When all else fades away.

I want to know if you can be alone with yourself,
And if you truly like the company you keep in the empty moments.

I want to know if you can be with joy, mine or your own,
If you can dance with wildness and let the ecstasy fill you
To the tips of your fingers and toes without cautioning us to be
 careful, be realistic, or to remember the limitations of being human.

It doesn't interest me how old you are.
I want to know if you will risk
The adventure of being alive!

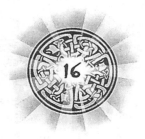

the recluse

My schedule in the spring of 1998 had gotten a little messed up. I am scheduled well over a year ahead with my seminar schedule. My treatment schedule at my Myofascial Release Treatment Centers in Paoli, Pennsylvania, and Sedona, Arizona, is then integrated into and around the seminars and other speaking engagements outside my regular schedule. Basically I work every day, with one long weekend off per month. This means I treat patients Monday, Tuesday, and Wednesday until nine or ten in the evening; Thursday is a travel day, and Friday, Saturday and Sunday are for my Myofascial Release Seminars. It's a difficult "juggling act" for my staff. To make a long story short, I was accidentally scheduled to work three months straight without a day off. This occurs every once in a while and I was prepared for it. I had purposely taken off a weekend in June, to rest, just before I was to give three advanced seminars in a row in Sedona.

The Friday night of that weekend, I woke up shaking violently at three in the morning. I was cold and very weak; I could barely get out of bed. This went on all weekend, and I don't remember too much. I found a bite mark on my left thigh in the vastus medialis area, in the form of a painful, inflamed "bullseye" with a red center, surrounded by numerous purple circles. The poison control center said that I had been bitten by a brown recluse spider. They said it is one of the worst and most dangerous of spider bites, close to the impact of a rattlesnake! They said people could die from the recluse bite; there is no antidote. If I got worse, I was told to go to the emergency room and there I would be put on intravenous medication to try to save my life!

I decided to tough it out. There really was no alternative anyway. It felt like all my strength had been drained out of me. I was so weak and shaky. My heart hurt, and felt like it was being crushed by a gorilla's hand. My left lower leg and foot were swollen, and my left foot dragged when I attempted to walk. My left tibialis anterior was weak, and very hard and leathery to the touch. I had fever and chills all weekend long, barely sleeping. Monday morning arrived, and still no improvement. I didn't know what to do. I was weak and shaking, and I had a full schedule of patients arriving from all over the country. I didn't want to let them down, but I could barely move. I followed my habit, when uncertain, of quieting down and asking The Ancient Warrior what to do.

Stay in the moment. You are thinking too much and trying too hard. This important test will be a time of deepening for you.

I don't have time for lessons right now; I have patients that I am responsible for.

Renegade, stop it. You are crying over spilled milk. Accept what has happened and make the best of it! This is your time to deepen. It is time to relearn your lessons on a deeper level, to their core, so that the concepts you teach go beyond intellectualization into true knowing!

But I thought that I had done that.

Just like fascial restrictions, there is another layer to the onion to reach the core. There is no end to learning.

I attempted to stand next to the bed and now noticed that my right quadricep was barely working. I thought, my God, I can't extend my leg, I can't stand!

Be quiet, center yourself....Now send your energy into the core of the earth...pull the earth energy up through you.

I very slowly stood up and was teetering.

Don't try to move the way you normally do. Change your pattern. Wait for the earth's core energy to meld with your core energy, your essence, and allow it to move you.

I slowly and laboriously showered, got dressed, and drove to my Myofascial Release Treatment Center, "Therapy on the Rocks." I started to treat my first patient and was shocked at how cold my hands were. They felt like ice-cube trays. My hands are normally quite warm and become warmer by the moment as I treat. I was so weak; I could hardly support myself as I sat on the stool to cradle my patient's head in my hands. I heard myself mentally saying, "What do I do? I have nothing to give this lady."

Renegade, get out of your way.

But I have been doing that for years.

Renegade, a master is always a beginner! Go deeper! Pull your energy back to your spine....Good, now pull your energy to the very back of your spinal canal and allow your essence to flow through you. Feel the flow of energy as it permeates your being and then open your heart and intend your energy to flow through this other being that you are touching. Never forget the sacred being that you are touching, touch her essence with your essence, feel the sacredness of the moment.

I could feel this warm tingle flowing through me, warming me and my hands, and then the patient jerked and started to release and unwind. I did this with each patient. It was more powerful than I can ever remember. I felt like and imagined that I was transparent, with light pouring through me and into my patients. Finally, I was done for the day and went home and collapsed in bed, exhausted. But with my left foot dragging and right thigh barely functioning, my old back problems were flaring up. My back was in such spasm and pain that though exhausted, I could not sleep.

The next day just before I started my first patient, one of my therapists walked up to me and said, "You look horrible, I know you don't feel well, but whatever you are doing, keep doing it. People always rave about your treatments, but they all described their sessions with you yesterday as profound. Each one felt they had a significant 'breakthrough' from it." I allowed myself to be a beginner. I got out of my own way more than I had ever done before. I could feel myself reaching deeper and accessing more power, despite my pain and fatigue. That Wednesday night I still could not sleep and was concerned about the next task that lay ahead, three advanced seminars in a row—twelve days of deep interaction with three hundred different people, and leading the class on a hike into the red rock canyons.

At three o'clock Thursday morning my body started to shake again. Then, all of a sudden, my body was being thrown into the air, as if I was being hit by a lightning bolt. I tried to resist, but the power was too strong and violent.

Renegade, give into it. You cannot fight it.

I gave into it and it began to take on the flavor of a past-life experience. My head whipped around and then it felt like I was punched in the stomach. I was all over the place and up in the air, then crashing down on the bed. What a trip! I felt like a gang of thugs was beating me up. This went on for over two hours! Finally, in exhaustion, I drifted off to sleep. The Ancient Warrior came to me in a dream.

Renegade, you have a long, arduous, ordeal ahead of you....Do not give up! Keep a proper attitude. Stay centered and grounded in your power. The poison of the spider has ripped the fabric of your electro-magnetic field. The energy of the vortex you are sleeping over is forcing open spaces that have not been open for eons. This increased energy and space in your being will throw you into chaos, and it will take you time to reorganize and adjust to your increased power and enhanced awareness. Don't fight the change! Flow where it takes you...and be aware, you are not done. This is just the beginning. Stay in the present moment; be in the center of the cyclone.

The alarm rang at seven—less than two hours of sleep. Time to get ready for the seminar. Many people are afraid of spiders and although I didn't get bitten in Arizona, I decided not to tell anyone, so that they wouldn't be concerned about being bitten. The energy in the advanced seminars is enormous, and the love from all of the therapists was very helpful. The seminars went very well, and no one noticed that I was having problems. By disciplining myself and staying in my center of power, we all benefited. Throughout the seminar, I kept treating myself at night, and every time I would get a new release, it seemed like I would release more trapped toxin into my system and I would go into a deep exhaustion. The exhaustion persisted. My right quadricep was barely

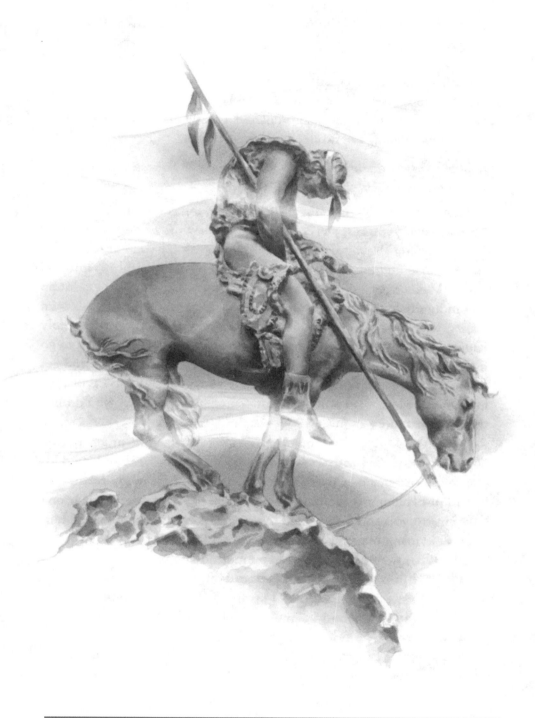

functioning. The weakness in my previously strong legs was flaring up my old back symptoms. On the way to a seminar series in Monterey, California, my lumbar discs above my fusion started to bulge and throw me into tremendous spasm and pain.

During the myofascial unwinding aspect of my seminar series, a few of the therapists saw that I was in pain and helped me unwind. It was very beneficial to have multiple hands unwinding me, which reduced the pressure on the bulging discs. I finally slept that night.

Question: What do you do when you feel yourself resisting the feelings that are emerging?

Feel the anxiety. When a sensation or emotion comes up, lean into it. Embrace what you resist! Feel the fear. Go into the anxiety. Give yourself permission to really tap into it. If you sense that you are resisting, catch yourself and say, "To hell with it," take a breath and tilt into the wind! Make it your clear goal, all of you, that every time you assist an unwinding or unwind yourself, that you're going to add to your own clarity, your own skill level, and your own awareness. It will definitely happen each time. The learning never ends. It's important for you to go into your anxiety through feeling. Let yourself scream or shake, and get to the very core of it. It will release its hold over you in all aspects of your life. On some level, you're probably anxious about everything you do, but that will pass more and more with each release.

After the Monterey seminars my back was feeling much better. However, I struggled with severe exhaustion for over a year, and my mid-back and ribs remained stuck, which made it hard for me to breathe or sleep. I just couldn't get to the mid-thoracic area. At another seminar, one of my instructors was a very good therapist and chiropractor. I asked him if he could manipulate my mid-thoracic area. That night I lay on my back on a treatment table and he lunged on me and attempted to manipulate me with all of his weight. He just bounced off my chest and said, "I can't do it. Boy, are you screwed up!" I said, "Let's try an arm-pull." So, he began to pull my arm and I centered myself deeply. After a little bit, I noticed through my proprioceptive awareness that his concentration was wavering. It felt like he was losing his connection. I looked at him and he said, "I feel funny. Are you unwinding me?" His eyes then rolled back and

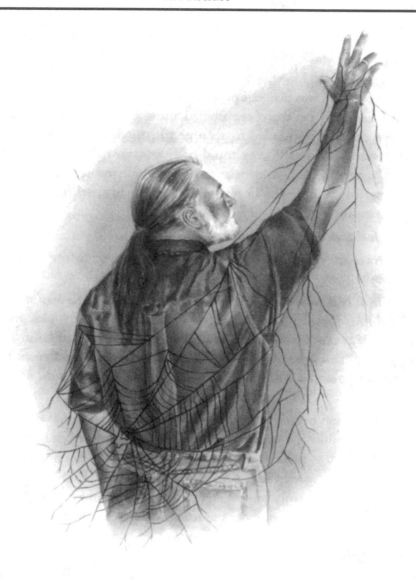

he collapsed on the floor. I got up and treated him. Oh well, so much for my back!

I felt trapped in the spider's web. The more I struggled to free myself, the tighter it became. My thoracic vertebrae and ribs remained restricted and painful for months. At night, I would wake up constantly. All positions were painful. I continued to struggle with immense exhaustion. It was hard to breathe, and my heart felt crushed. There were some nights that I felt that I was dying. I don't fear death, but I just felt that I wasn't ready to go because I have too much yet to do and I really love life.

I realized that I was biased. I purposely shifted my mindset to my preference of life. To be truly centered, I must be open to all options, including death. I responded to an urge to stretch, and then began to spontaneously unwind. As my mind-body continued to unwind, I felt myself slipping into a swirling darkness; I became aware of a deep fear emanating from a darkness in my heart. I began to swirl in a vortex of energy, into the crushing pain and into the fear.

Breathe, feel it deeply.

The Ancient Warrior came to me and whispered to me in a very gentle way.

Renegade, it is time to mend your broken heart. Your little boy still grieves for his father. Go back to the time when you were young and see yourself at the "father and son dinner" held annually at your grade school. You were the only boy there without a father. Remember and feel how crushed you were. You felt so alone. Feel the pain of your broken heart!

I started to sob from the depths of my being. My body was racked in pain, and it felt like my heart was going to burst. I was back in time as the little boy at the "father and son dinner." As I looked around at all the other boys with their fathers, I felt so alone, so hurt. I missed him so much; my heart was truly broken. The Ancient One took me, the adult, by the hand, and we put our arms around my little boy and encouraged him to feel and cry. We reassured him that he was loved and that my father was fine. We asked my little boy to open his heart and send my father and mother love and light; we sent love and light to let them go and be free. We reassured each other that we would always love each other and are together in our hearts.

My heart softened, and the pain left. I could feel my essence returning and filling my body. I felt present again.

They are very proud of you and the man that you have become. They love you and will love you forever. They ask you to keep your heart

open, to send them and the other beings that you are connected with
love and light.

I felt The Ancient One embrace me with a deep inner glow and warmth and fell into a deep sleep.

The next day, I felt like my power had returned; I felt present. I realized that I had been out of my body, which explained the exhaustion, prolonged pain, and why the treatments hadn't held.

I scheduled myself a Therapy for the Therapist Treatment Program at my Myofascial Release Treatment Center in Paoli, Pennsylvania, and received great myofascial release treatment three times per day. Now that I was back in my body, I made tremendous progress with the treatments. I then decided it was time to go off by myself and spend some time alone in the wilderness. The one-year anniversary of the encounter with the recluse spider was approaching, and it was time for me to go into solitude and to be open to any further lessons that I needed to evolve and heal deeply.

For years, I have been designing an advanced seminar, Myofascial Release IV, the "Path to Mastery." It will be held in the spring of 2001 and like Ernest Hemingway's book, *A Moveable Feast*, this unique adventure will be held in some of the most beautiful and powerful environments in the world: Zion National Park; Bryce Canyon, Utah; three to four days on houseboats up in the turquoise waters of spectacular Lake Powell; through the Grand Canyon; and finally into majestic Sedona, Arizona, one of the scenic wonders of the world. Although I had been in these areas before, I thought that it would be wise to travel through again from the perspective of leading a group of people. I would be able to check the timing from place to place and find beautiful private spots that would be appropriate to teach therapists the subtle intricacies of healing.

While out in these incredibly powerful areas, I also felt that this would be a ripe time to do a "vision quest." As I drove from Sedona, I felt very tired and sad, and headed towards the Grand Canyon. I had a room reserved in the lodge that had a balcony overlooking the abyss of this awesome area. A major myofascial/osseous restriction was still bothering me. Due to its location, I had not been able to resolve it. It was stuck just between my shoulder blades. The mid-thoracic vertabrae and a couple of ribs were severely restricted and radiating pain from my back around the ribs to the sternum in the front of my chest.

I walked up to the reception desk, which was about chest high. I gave the lady my name and she turned around to her computer to check my reservation. All of a sudden I heard The Ancient Warrior say to me,

Lean your chest into the registration desk and push.

I pushed into the desk with my chest and the pressure felt good. Then The Ancient Warrior said,

Put your hands on the desk and hold on tight!

I did that and kept pushing. I could feel a "good hurt" all the way around my ribs into the back of my mid-thoracic area. As the receptionist finished with her computer, she said, "Oh, Mr. Barnes, you have our best room, the 'El Tovar' room." At that moment it felt like a gunshot went off in my back. I felt a sharp pain and yelled! The pain was so intense and quick that if I hadn't been holding onto the desk, I would have fallen to my knees. As I yelled, the receptionist's eyes widened and she turned knowingly to her assistant, as if they were used to kooks and said, "Yes, Mr. Barnes, we are as excited as you about the 'El Tovar' room!"

As I moved away towards my room, they looked relieved that this nut had not hurt anyone. I was moving painlessly. My vision quest was off to a good start. The pain I experienced was a disc going back into place, and I was now breathing easier. The 'El Tovar' room had a wonderful view, and I thoroughly enjoyed my stay there.

The Grand Canyon is truly awesome. I drove for hours through this vast land, to where they dammed up the Colorado River to create Lake Powell, Arizona. The vibrant beauty of this inspiring area was ethereal. I climbed up onto a high ledge and I melded into the beautiful rocks. I enjoyed the beautiful view of the shimmering turquoise water and blue sky for hours. I sent my essence deep to the core of the earth and high into the sky, opening my focus to all the sounds, smells, and sensations that drifted through my awareness.

This image formed in my mind's eye:

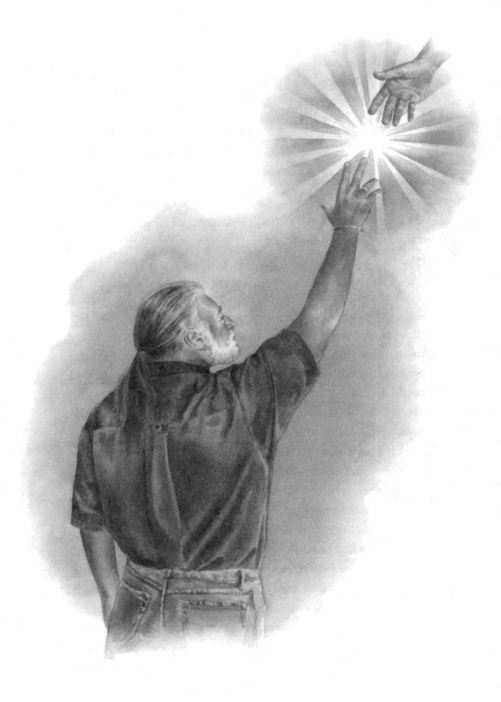

I heard, "I survived, I survived!" Tears streamed down my face and the image then transformed into my power animal, a cougar, that climbed up a rocky cliff to where I was lying. He lay down, exhausted and spent, with a paw hanging over the ledge. He was beat up, but alive; scarred, but victorious; enjoying the moment, the warmth of the sun and the breeze. I felt like I had left a cocoon of my old self, the remnants of my ego, behind; it was like the metamorphosis and transformation of the butterfly.

Renegade, you have done well. You have run the gauntlet; you have passed through the veil, through the gateway into higher consciousness. I love you. Always come from your heart with courage, wisdom, and kindness. Your example will inspire others. Tell those luminescent beings that you are connected with that they should respect and love themselves and embrace their struggle. They will find their inner light. Tell them the story of the butterfly.

The Butterfly

A monk found a cocoon of a butterfly. One day a small opening appeared, and the monk sat and watched the butterfly for several hours as it struggled to force its body through that little hole. Then it seemed to stop making progress. It appeared as if it had gotten as far as it could and it could go no farther. Then the monk decided to help the butterfly, so he took a pair of scissors and snipped off the remaining bit of the cocoon. The butterfly then emerged easily, but it had a swollen body and small, shriveled wings.

The monk continued to watch the butterfly because he expected that, at any moment, the wings would enlarge and expand to be able to support the body, which would contract in time.

Neither happened!

In fact, the butterfly spent the rest of its life crawling around with a swollen body and shriveled wings. Although the monk took very good care of the butterfly for all of its days, it was never able to fly.

The monk, in his kindness and haste, did not understand that the restricting cocoon and the struggle required for the butterfly to get through the tiny opening were God's way of forcing fluid from the body of the butterfly into its wings so that it would be ready for flight once it achieved its freedom from the cocoon. Freedom and flight could only come after a struggle.

Sometimes struggles are exactly what we need in life. If we were allowed to go through our whole life without any obstacles, it would cripple us. We would not be as strong as we could have been. We don't always need to be in a struggle and not every struggle has a positive outcome, but many are better for us than we realize. Often, it is in the struggle and the striving that we become truly alive and are able to recognize and appreciate the beauty of this world and all the wonder around us.

I feel that I was dragged back through every lesson I had ever learned in my life. I was to learn on an even deeper level, another layer of the fascial onion, so to speak. Having done that, I now feel great, with more energy, power, and awareness than I've ever had. It was tough, but worth it!

Embrace your essence and allow your essence to embrace you lovingly. Appreciate your beauty, step into your power; identify with your spirit and soar with the wind!

A Therapist's Perspective

John is the "Calm Before the Storm!"

There's something different about him. Something so sure. He has a sense of stillness within him. He looks so peaceful and calm. People study him day in and day out, but can't seem to figure John out. What is it about him? How is he so free when everyone else has turmoil within themselves? He speaks; you listen, wholeheartedly. You find your soul listening rather than your ears. What is he saying? For John is the Calm and we are our Storm.

The storm lives in us. John's spirit is strong; his energy purposeful; his essence, beautiful. This man has a beautiful soul. The clouds roll in; your sky turns gray, you fight bad thoughts. You lose your way, you're out of control, and your ship starts to twist. I don't understand what this is. You're frightened, you're scared, but in the air you feel John's presence. He'll guide you there, you'll hear a quiet whisper through this noise, "just let go and be there." Your innermost strength will get you through it. "Don't be afraid, just go with it." Trust yourself: it's John's gift to you. This new awareness, the power in you. I now feel strong, I'm not gonna quit. The storm picks up, there's crashing waves; you should be scared, but you feel safe.

That voice comes back. What message does it bring? "This is your journey, confront your storm, feel it, breathe it." You find what John has been saying is true. I follow the path, the storm is huge. My will is stronger. I ask it to leave. It doesn't belong here. I make it leave. The wind dies down, the clouds unfold. The storm fades into a gentle rain. I sigh, I smile. I feel so calm. It all makes sense. I thank you, John, for showing me this, for you were there beside me.

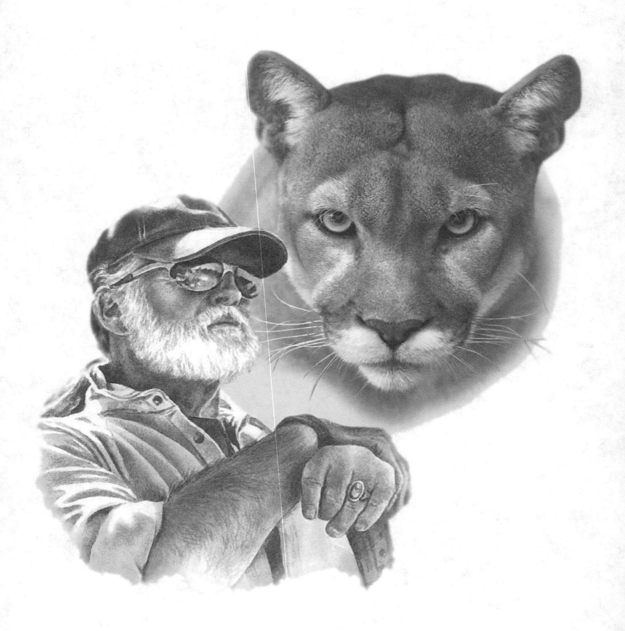

your power animal

Question: John, when I was last out in Sedona, Arizona, with you, you took me and a group of therapists and patients out into the Red Rock Canyons. Your "Therapy on the Rocks" adventure was wonderful, and the others and I had an invaluable experience as you guided us into the connections of our "Power Animal." Could you explain this concept and its therapeutic value for us?

Yes. As I have mentioned, health care has overly focused on the intellectual and symptomatic aspect of our problems. It has ignored the importance of emotional expression and tranquility and a deeper level of our mind-body's instinctive nature via myofascial release.

We are animals. Our instinctive side is the natural animalistic nature that has also been ignored in our society and health care. The Myofascial Release Approach addresses our intellectual side and symptoms, but we also go deeper and more comprehensively. We allow for natural emotional expression in healing, which also triggers our mind-body's instinctive response. In other words, we truly treat the whole person! As we clear our intellect (belief systems), our emotions, and our intuitive side, we open to the deeper dimensions of human experience, our internal guidance system, our instinct.

Myofascial release is, then, a left- and right-brained approach. The left brain communicates in thoughts and words, which are symbols for experience. The right brain's form of communication is visual/spatial relationships (pictures and feelings), which are another form of symbolism. So, it can be helpful and therapeutic to allow deep, meaningful cognition through symbolism to guide us, and use words, thoughts, pictures, and feelings as a way of accessing the deeper realms and dimensions of reality and healing.

I have chosen to symbolize my intuition as The Ancient One or The Ancient Warrior. I have found that it helps to use symbols to separate your normal consciousness from other forms of consciousness, i.e., intuition or instinct. This can help one's clarity, so that you don't confuse linear, intellectual thought with intuitive guidance or an instinctual response. Communication in book form is linear, and it serves in this medium to present my intuitive guidance as a separate form and voice. In reality, since intuition comes when one is silent and centered in the timeless-spaceless dimension, my communication with The Ancient One is instantaneous and part of me, or within me. It is another important dimension of me. The light energy flowing through our liquidity is a "hologram." We really think in pictures (holograms) and our brain converts these light pictures into symbols, i.e., words and thoughts.

So The Ancient Warrior expresses himself to me in the form of a hologram. I am centered most of the time. It is effortless and natural for me. My whole being feels energized and expansive. I am very aware and when I move, think or talk, my motion, energy, and information come from a very deep, silent, still place. This information is a "knowing"; it is very different than "to know." It is the "center of the cyclone." As the events and circumstances of life swirl around you, you remain in the center. This is where your source of power, awareness, and clarity come from.

This is the ultimate goal of this way of being and this form of therapy. The experience of your centered presence allows the patient to find their center. As these two centers of power merge, healing occurs.

Any talk about being quiet, tranquil, and powerful is just empty words or sounds until these concepts are coupled with the reality of the experience of one's personal power. One cannot appreciate or understand the experience of the center of the cyclone until one has been there! This is where the value of an experienced teacher or therapist comes into play, for she or he can guide you to this sacred space, and once you have "got it," you have "got it." It is very profound!

Your center has always been there. You were born with the potential to be centered and clear. Then through years of mass education and mass hypnosis, learning rigid and limiting belief systems thrust upon us by society, and limited by unexpressed emotion and physical trauma, our center—our source of power—became clouded and eventually inaccessible to us. Our role is to clear away the clutter of the past in ourselves. Then we will have the power and clarity to guide others into their own power and healing.

This same symbolic concept can then be applied to our instinctive side, our power animal, for it is through accessing our instinctual responses that deep growth and healing can occur. So, finally I can answer your question, "What is your power animal?" I wanted to develop a wider concept of the importance of symbolism to better understand the symbolizing of our instinctual side. Myofascial release safely and effectively triggers and deactivates the fight/flight/freeze response for instinctual deep healing.

I have always identified with, felt like, and been described by others as a big, calm, powerful cat; a panther or a cougar. This magnificent, luminescent, vibrant, shimmering panther with blue eyes slips into me during the seminars and while treating. It feels like a bristling form of power, light, and energy that permeates my being, heart, and the person that I am touching. When I go deep into this dimension of consciousness my energy fills the treatment room or even the entire seminar room, profoundly affecting all that are open and receptive to it. A quantum shift occurs as this catlike power penetrates the person. The feel and experience of that deep, still power empowers that person to connect with *their* power. This blending of energy is never forced upon anyone; it is simply available to those who sincerely wish to learn, grow, and heal. This is the power and clarity of being in the present moment, in the "now," as animals are. This is what it means to have a "presence." When a person is centered, they have a presence that can be felt by others when near them and at times even when they are far away.

The panther is also known as a cougar or mountain lion. In Native American mythology he is known as the "spirit of the mountains," symbolizing power, courage, grace, physical strength, intention, and balance. Panther or cougar energy involves lessons on the use of power in leadership. It is the ability to lead without insisting that others follow. It is the understanding that all beings are potential leaders in their own ways. By observing the graceful pounce of the panther you will learn to balance the body, mind, and spirit. The panther comes from his or her heart with courage! Courageously act and lead yourself where your heart takes you.

Animals are responsive, while humans tend to react, since their intellectual side has become overly dominant. Humans react from programmed filters, acting in habitual ways to stimuli. Over the years the reactions become more and more narrow, rigid, and automatic. Clearing the dysfunctional patterns of the past allows us to return to a responsive mode, opening our focus so that now we have a multitude of possible responses available to us.

Most people live in the world of "shoulds," and relying on our linear side has forced our ego into a very narrow viewpoint: tunnel vision. If you put a mouse in a maze, with a piece of cheese in one of the tunnels, the mouse will explore every tunnel until it finds the cheese. The human being will go down the same tunnel over and over and over, because the cheese "should" be there!

Just for a moment, stop and put the book down. Slow your breathing, soften your body and quiet your mind. Go back in time and remember….Which animals intrigued you as a child? What animals intrigue you now? What do you appreciate about their appearance? What can you learn from their characteristics and way of being? If you were an animal, what would you be? Allow yourself to play now, and become that animal. Without thought—simply sense. Perceive the world through the aminal's eyes and senses. Slip into a dreamlike state and ask your power animal to express itself and help you. Go ahead now, put the book down, and drift, and enjoy.

Practice that regularly, and you will discover a hidden part of your nature that will be invaluable to you. Your power animal can be any living being. In the mad rush of our society, we have stopped being "human beings" and have become "human doings," always doing something, always thinking or talking. So to return to a healthy balance we need to quiet ourselves and be in a sensing/feeling state; just be. Myofascial release treats the "being" of the human being. This is also how we can treat our animal friends without the need to talk. With myofascial release we are one being with another being, utilizing a very deep and fulfilling form of communication and therapy.

I received a letter from a therapist recently and I would like to share it with you.

> Dear John,
>
> I had a symbolic "power animal" experience that helped me quite a bit. I'd like to share my story of the "white buffalo-calf woman."
>
> The journey of the white buffalo-calf woman began when another therapist and I were helping at a myofascial unwinding class. It was during a time when I felt I had no right to be helping anyone, because I was an emotional train wreck. As it was, I arrived at the seminar and asked you if you thought I should stay. You held me, reminded me to breathe and said, "I think you're just where you should be." One by one the seminar participants revealed their personal and professional goals to the group. None cried—a little unusual. When it was my turn to reveal my goals I became very emotional. I cried, a lot—as did the rest of the instructors—also a little unusual.
>
> As the weekend progressed I began to experience "snapshots" of a beautiful Native American woman adorned in pure white buffalo robes. She was kneeling by the side of a river washing clothes on a rock. She was clearly expecting the arrival of someone and frequently raised her head to the right in hopes of catching a glimpse of this special person. I could feel her purity, naïveté and vulnerability. She was aware of her beauty but was not tarnished by that awareness. Suddenly there was a noise coming from the direction where she previously had been gazing. I could feel her excitement and anticipation. There was a glow of wonderment, and I could feel how full of hope she was. I had the sense that she was awaiting her "Prince Charming." Without warning an arrow flew through the air. I felt it strike her in the right side

of her neck just below the ear, and knew it sliced all the way through her neck to exit out the left side. I could feel her fall heavily to the ground, where she remained motionless.

My next encounter with the white buffalo woman was at Myofascial Release III. A friend and I were randomly paired for the "inner journey" unwinding. This is a special part of the seminar where two partners treat each other continuously for three hours. Initially we tried to avoid each other because we were acquainted, and thought we were supposed to be partnered with someone unknown. As fate would have it I was catapulted toward him precisely when everyone else was partnered up.

What continues to fascinate me to this day is that we didn't take turns during this unwinding. We were both in the same unwinding for three hours. Initially, it was supposed to be his turn as the patient. As the lights began to dim and the drums began to beat I could feel us spiraling backward. He appeared to be shape-shifting from a small four-legged animal into this massive beast. His back grew and grew and he began to look top-heavy. He became the white buffalo.

There was much chanting and primitive dancing. I could feel the earth vibrate under us in a common beat. There was intermittent firelight, and the room was spinning. The white buffalo began to take a defensive posture as if it was cornered and fighting for its life. It reared and snorted. There was massive power and strength. Intense vitality. And then a thunderous crash. As the white buffalo fell the earth shook with its weight. An arrow pierced the white buffalo, and blood spilled all around and into the earth. A torturous struggle ensued with this massive beast attempting to rise and falling, time and time again, in a thunderous heap.

After trying unsuccessfully to pull the arrow out of the buffalo, stillness was a part of us for a long time. I then found myself chanting and dancing around this still form. I felt my feet become a part of the blood-soaked earth, and my arms were rhythmically chopping the air as if rattling a rattle in time with the drums. Around and around the buffalo we danced and chanted, connecting with a deep central core. A universal heartbeat.

Then the buffalo once again began to struggle to its feet. This time, however, it was like watching Bambi take his first steps. Up the buffalo would go, only to wobble on its gangly legs and fall flat on its face. I giggled and laughed as I watched this clumsy youngster find its feet and run off. Swirling and firelight again, as the white buffalo woman lay motionless on the ground. I could see the firelight dancing on what looked like teepees, and Kachina-like figures were present in the fire spaces. There was chanting and dancing again. Around and around the body of the white buffalo woman, the tribe chanted and danced. Drumming to the universal heartbeat.

They were calling her back into existence but she was frightened of hearing them. She was confused by their betrayal. She wanted to share her beauty but was speared instead.

She then became a turtle. Carrying a shield on her back and the safety of the earth within her, so she could emerge a little at a time.

In a safe environment, in the presence of a virtuous man who could see her beauty and respect her being without expectation, she could emerge for short periods of time, growing and experiencing when it was safe, then hiding in the comforts of her shell when danger seemed eminent.

And so the white buffalo woman progressed through childhood and into womanhood. Experiencing the evolution of her sensuality and the depth of her beauty. Because she felt safe, loved, respected, and accepted, she did not feel the need to shrink from her power or beauty, internal or external, and was able to experience her whole being as an intact entity.

In the time that has passed since this experience, I have heard several versions of a Native American legend which involves the White Buffalo-Calf Woman. I'm not sure why it was our privilege to experience her presence or that of the white buffalo. I do know that this experience had a profound impact on my life. Not only did it shift my perception of the realm of possible experiences and realities available to us, it also gave me great clarity into who I am and how I have perceived my own life experiences on a subconscious level.

At the time I had this experience, my husband (now ex-husband) had left me and my two-year-old daughter. It was a complete shock to me and it came at a time when I thought things were finally going "according to the plan." I allowed myself to feel safe and was experiencing some of my own internal beauty for the first time. I was filled with hope and anticipation for the future. I felt literally slain by his decision. Not only was I devastated by my husband's rejection and the loss of my family network, I was totally uprooted by the loss of my community. I was forced to give up my private practice in order to be more available to my daughter and to provide consistency in my income. I was equally disappointed to realize that many of the people I considered my close family and friends were forced to "choose sides," and they were no longer a part of my life.

Like the White Buffalo-Calf Woman, I have also heard the call of what is left of my community drumming me back to life. Providing support, love, acceptance, and above all patience and trust that I will return to my fullest capacity as time moves forward. I find myself emerging in tiny increments, hiding under the turtle shell for long periods of time. Allowing myself to feel power and beauty in small increments when I am in situations when I feel totally safe and nurtured.

I am thankful for this experience. I am thankful to my friend for allowing me to feel safe at a time when I really needed a friend. And I am thankful to you John, for having the courage to follow your dream and provide us with the opportunity to broaden and deepen our life experiences.

Question: John, was the reality of her husband leaving too shocking, so she was allowed to look at it in a symbolic way?

Many times when something is too intense or painful, our mind presents a lesson to us in symbolic form. Her partner is here. Would you be interested in sharing your interpretation of your experience?

THE THERAPIST'S RESPONSE

I thought what was so unusual at the time was that I began the session in my own world, the world of being the white buffalo. I didn't verbally communicate any of this to her, yet she was completely participating, fully aware of what was happening. My senses were dulled throughout most of the session, as if I were thinking through the mind of the buffalo.

I remember the still point of anticipation while the arrow was approaching me. I'm not sure of its originator, but it seemed like it remained in the air for an eternity. Time truly stood still as that arrow arched through the sky. There wasn't a sense of dread, only amazement. When the arrow struck me, I dropped like a stone and the heaviness of my dead or near-dead white buffalo body was oppressive.

As I tried to regain my feet, I was aware of her physically in the seminar room, encouraging me, while at the same time aware of a presence in the buffalo vision. This presence followed the same sequence of actions that she just stated in her letter.

I can also remember when she emerged from her turtle shell, attempting to see if I, and the world, could be trusted. Although we spoke no words, I knew exactly what she was experiencing. Trust.

What did you learn from this experience?

THE THERAPIST RESPONDS

In the two years that have passed since this encounter, I have many times attempted to find meaning in it. My struggle for understanding seems to mirror my stance in life.

I am always looking out for myself. I am always wondering what is in it for me. It has taken me this long to see that my role in the white buffalo saga is one of a helper—it is not a story about me. It is, however, a lesson. Reflecting on it has shown me that I can contribute significantly to another's life if I only quiet myself and allow it to occur. The white buffalo, disguised as me, was there to support her in her journey. The reality of her life events were too shocking to face, so this experience allowed her to look at it in a symbolic way. I, as the buffalo, acted as a conduit to show her the struggle she was going through. The arrow hits in her most vulnerable spot. My buffalo's struggle ended with the arrow; a calf was born.

After my death, the buffalo calf struggled to stand. I see this as her emergence, as a new birth for her.

It is very freeing to finally see that this story is not centered around me. I see that I can give to others and help them with their struggle. I can actually feel a weight lifted from me by simply stating this out loud. Thank you.

It's fascinating that when entering an experience with another, we can both benefit.

A Therapist's Perspective

When you mentioned entering another person's experience, I remembered another episode during Myofascial Release III. The assignment was to treat a partner with the patient's and your eyes closed, in an effort to lessen your reliance on the visual so you could tune into your extraordinary senses. I was acting as the therapist and I thought things were going along pretty well. My patient/partner ended up in a position where she was sitting at the edge of the treatment table. My focus was nowhere in particular when all of a sudden I was heading over a waterfall, completely surrounded by lush green vegetation. We were both falling fast down this waterfall, and it was very real. It turned out that my partner was experiencing the same image at the same time, and she fell forward off the table with me following right behind. Luckily, neither one of us was injured. It was a lesson to me to remain grounded and aware, but it was also an incredible glimpse into how energies can converge.

⚡

Question: John, someone told me that you have a funny story about you and power animals on Bell Rock in Sedona. Would you tell us that story?

Sure...

As I was about to answer, I felt a sharp pain in my back and The Ancient Warrior transported me back in time. Back to a time when I had injured myself while weight lifting with over three hundred pounds. I fell, and a lightning bolt of pain ripped through my body.

Ride the pain further back in time!

All of a sudden I was transported back to when I was fifteen years old. I was viewing and feeling an incident that happened when I was working out with weights in my backyard in Pennsylvania. It was a hot, humid August afternoon. I was working out hard. I was hot and sweating profusely. I was doing overhead presses with heavy weights and as I completed the last repetition, I started to feel dizzy. I threw the barbell down as I passed out. All of a sudden, I was having an out-of-body experience and was looking down on my crumpled body with barbells strewn around. Then I was caught up in this vortex of swirling energy. To my surprise and shock, I had become an animal. I wasn't *thinking* about an animal. I *was* the animal, looking out through its eyes! My sense of self and body had expanded tremendously. I was perceiving with all of its senses.

I had long powerful tusks and I was ramming my tusks into a wall of ice. I was trying to get to some plants that were embedded in the ice wall. I was furious! The sound of me ramming into the ice was deafeningly loud, and I felt a sense of bristling power that was beyond my wildest imagination! Then all of a sudden I was aware of being back in 1954 and waking up and looking around. I was in shock! What had just happened to me? I was so confused. Back in the mid 1950s I had never

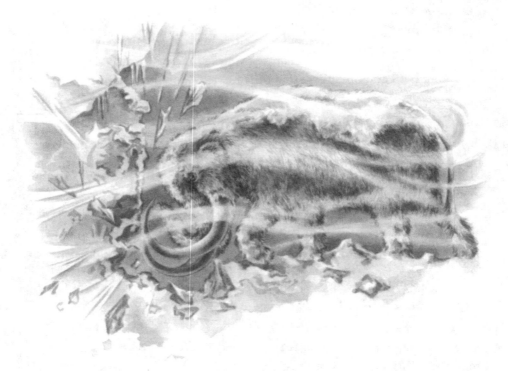

heard of out-of-body experiences, past lives, or anything like what had just happened to me. Was I crazy? I felt so sane, but it was so real, so vivid. Even today as I relate this story, I am right there as if it is happening now. I can feel the same power, vividness, and intensity. Interestingly, about two weeks after my experience with the power animal, I picked up a *National Geographic* magazine. As I thumbed through it, I came to a dead halt when I saw for the first time in my life a drawing of a Mastodon with huge tusks ramming into an ice wall. There I was. I was that animal. I had never seen nor heard of such an animal before.

I once asked The Ancient Warrior what this experience was all about.

That awareness and the pain of your weight lifting injury has helped you break out of your conditioning. These experiences have helped you to see there really is not one, concrete reality, but a multitude of realities accessed through an open mind via different levels of vibration and consciousness.

Do other people have these experiences?

Yes, all of the time. But the fear of them leaving their habitual mode of reality blocks or discounts the experience. Their present, limited reality is an illusion. It may not be working for them, but it is familiar and they cling to it desperately. This is why it is necessary for a true healer to straddle realities and be the safety net for the injured individual to take the risk to leap into the unknown; that leap takes courage! As they leap into the unknown—the void, the chaos—nature will help them reorganize into a higher level of reality that is more comfortable, effective, and healthy for them.

You are the catalyst! You leap with them. Your energy guides and provides safety, so that nature can help them. Nature loves you. All of you now hearing John's words hear this clearly. Get out of your own way and allow nature to nurture and heal you. Nature loves you!! Your essence is beautiful, powerful, and loving. Your essence is impeccable and wants to love and heal you. Give yourself the opportunity to connect with your true essence.

I became aware that I had been transported back to another time, another reality, and heard myself speaking to the group, answering their question. This happens to me quite often. I seem to be able to straddle and function in multiple realities at once. So, when you are with me, I will be immersed in and totally aware of you and our interactions, but I may also be somewhere else. I heard myself continuing on with the seminar, answering their question about power animals.

⟋

A number of years ago, in one of my advanced classes, Myofascial Release III, we were involved in what I call the "Fantastic Voyage." It was the second night of the seminar. We were all in a candlelit room with loud drumming music playing, and the therapists were paired up unwinding each other for one and a half hours each. During this time they were also breathing deeper and faster than normal. The breathing, the music, the touch, the unwinding, the atmosphere, and the fact that this was all occurring in the middle of a powerful "vortex" in Sedona create a substantial life-enhancing experience.

⟋

Prior to this Myofascial III experience I had gone over the concept of power animals and encouraged the group to allow their instinctual side to emerge and get in touch with their individual power animal. I assured them that I would keep them safe. About two hours into the experience, I heard a whinnying sound. It sounded just like a young horse whinnying. I looked around and saw a seven-month-pregnant therapist up on a table, both hands in the air, pawing the air, whinnying! Her power animal was fully expressing herself through the totality of her body-mind. After class that night I asked them to stay with their feelings and energetic levels in silence, so that they could integrate their experiences to their core. Thinking or talking about it too soon would diminish their experience. I then asked that they remain in silence until we went out on the rocks the next day, into the canyons, and we would then have time to share.

About forty of us climbed high up Bell Rock in silence, until we reached a flat ledge. One of my instructors turned on some music, and I told them to pair up and dance as long as it felt right. Then they were to split up into different pairs, taking turns treating and unwinding each other in silence with their eyes closed. This would encourage their extra-ordinary senses and skills to emerge. They began dancing and soon became aware that there was someone among us that was not part of our group. He wore a green forest ranger uniform and a large-brimmed, green hat that looked too big for him. He looked very ticked off, so I went over to him and asked if I could help him. He angrily shouted at me, "What the hell is going on here?" I said, "We are just dancing and enjoying ourselves." He snapped back, "Do you realize that you are breaking Federal law? You are not allowed to use motorized equipment on Federal land!" I said, "We don't have any motorcycles here." He pointed to the stereo and said that was motorized equipment and I was to take it down the mountain now!

In the meantime, the therapists were beginning to treat each other, oblivious to my confrontation with the ranger. Now, this twerp was beginning to annoy me. He was about 140 pounds soaking wet, and I was a solid 220 pounds. My panther was beginning to stir inside of me, and I wanted to pounce on this annoyance. We both had our hands on our hips, glaring at each other very aggressively and I said, "NO! I will not take that stereo down the mountain now. I will turn it off and take it down later. I am responsible for these people." His eyes were bulging out of his head in fury. Now, you know that when you are in a confrontation with someone, you don't take your eyes off of each other. I was becoming more menacing by the moment, when I noticed that his eyes kept shifting to my left. Something was beginning to distract him.

Then all of a sudden I heard whinnying. We turned around to see this seven-months-pregnant woman prancing around like a horse, whinnying at the top of her lungs. It was a funny sight to me; quite strange to him. He was now panicking, totally out of his element. His reality was broken. He stammered, "Okay, I'll let you off this time with just a ticket." He shoved a ticket in my hand, and ran off stumbling down the cliff. While I had no intention of hurting him, he didn't know that. From his perspective, he was looking up at this man, much bigger and stronger than he, glaring at him with the ferocity of a wild animal. He was prepared to stand his ground, until he was challenged by the unfamiliar. What he saw and heard broke his reality, and he became terrified and fled. This is just another example of how we cling to the familiar. We may hate the fact that we hurt, or can't work or play, but what scares us the most is the unfamiliar, the unknown.

So, for healing and growth to occur we must be willing to leap into the unknown. We, the therapist, acting as the catalyst for change, create the safety for our patients to move into chaos, into the darkness, to reach the light.

Long ago, the famous psychiatrist, Dr. Carl Jung stated, "…we must go into our shadow side to find the light." He went on to say, "…if we don't express all aspects of our being, the darkness, or the shadow will express itself in some form of abnormal behavior or symptomatic complex." Traditional medicine and therapy is about treating or masking the symptoms, or just teaching us to cope with our problems. We were told not to go into the darkness, and even if we did the traditional methods didn't provide us with a safe or effective way to deal with it! Myofascial release allows us to go into our shadow side and find the light safely, efficiently, and effectively.

A person who is always nice and smiling or always mean and nasty is not real. They are living in fear, controlled by the filters of the past. The

Ancient Warrior has shown me over and over, that there are times to bend and turn the other cheek, and there are times to stand your ground, be strong, and fight for your or others' protection and beliefs. Remember the fortune cookie: "Be as soft as you can be, yet as hard as you have to be."

A Therapist's Perspective

I attended the Myofascial Release I, Unwinding, and Myofascial Release II seminars a year and a half ago with the goal of finding a new direction professionally. I had found myself in management positions and feeling very disconnected with the reason I had become an occupational therapist in the first place. I expected to gain some information to help me find this new direction. I did not expect those courses to help me personally as much as they did. I have been amazed and grateful that they did!

The first day of Unwinding, I went to John and asked him if he had any suggestions to help me with recurring shoulder and sinus problems. I told John that my shoulder will "act up," and then within two or three days I will have a sinus infection. I would cycle through these about every four or five weeks. I told John that I have never felt like my pain fit into the normal descriptions of pain, i.e., sharp, dull. It has always felt like a snake that stays curled up under my left scapula (a constant presence) and will occasionally "act up" and coil around muscles and bones in my left arm, shoulder, and neck. I can feel it moving slowly, smoothly, and strongly around in that area. Needless to say, my doctor has always looked at me strangely when I have described the pain to him, and I therefore expected John to do the same.

Much to my surprise, he did not. Instead he suggested that my goal for unwinding be to "ask the snake to complete his journey." I walked away with the feeling that someone had actually listened to me and that I was not as crazy as I thought I had been.

During the first two days of the Unwinding Seminar I was pretty scared. During the last activity on the last day of unwinding, I finally decided that it was now or never. I asked my snake to complete his journey. I was lying on the floor with my arm writhing around like a snake; there was some drumming music playing, which I think of fondly as my "jungle music." I remember asking my snake to quit playing around and get on with it. My left hand began to flop around. I asked the snake to quit flicking his tail. My hand then got very still. I remember laughing and asking the snake, "If that's not your tail, then where is it?" At which point my head snapped hard. That scared me, so I asked the snake where his damn head was, and my left hand lifted up and turned toward me, and all I could see was a snake's head and he was laughing at me! As I went to stand up I found that my left hand was stuck to the floor and I could not lift it, so I yanked it real hard, just as John walked near me. I started crying and stopped John and told him that I couldn't find my hand. He very calmly took me over to a table and helped me.

He asked me what had happened, and boy, was I surprised when I told him that I had cut my hand off using a kitchen knife. He did something with my neck and head and I felt much calmer, but still lost. He then talked me through seeing my hand reconnect. I remember telling him that I couldn't, and that it was stupid. He asked me to forgive myself, that everyone makes mistakes. I remember repeating over and over that I couldn't because it was "really stupid." John told me to give myself permission to feel stupid.

I went home that night with the sense that my hand was connected on one side and gaping open on the scar side, all bloody and cold. I tried some of the energy techniques he had told us about in class, and found that my energy hand was about three feet from my physical hand. I then "saw" my hand reconnecting. It took about two weeks before I felt like my hand was "healed."

What I had done as a five-year-old child was cut my hand while cutting a hole in a box, and I must have been afraid that I had almost cut it off and my body believed I had! It probably didn't help that I also ran my arm under cold water trying to get the bleeding to stop, which explains the sensation of coldness during the unwinding.

How was I before unwinding? My answer is: I was very confused and felt disconnected sometimes from events around me. I felt like I should have been left-handed and couldn't be, without knowing why. I found that I had gone through almost thirty years using my right hand but wanting to use my left, but I couldn't. I would start to do something left-handed and then pull back in confusion before going ahead and using my right hand. I write with my right hand, but as a left-handed person does with my wrist flexed and twisted away from my body. I also used to sleep with my hands curled up under my chin to the point where they were numb in the morning. As an occupational thera-pist I tried splinting them, but it didn't work. I would just take the splints off in the night.

How am I different now? I now find myself using my left hand spontaneously for things like brushing my teeth, playing Frisbee, etc. I feel more connected and whole. I no longer sleep with my hands curled protectively under me, and have the sense that my hands are safe now that I have found my left hand and know what the cause was. I am less angry with myself, especially when I make mistakes. I have more patience with my kids and their mistakes and accidents. I also find myself excited to be on a journey, but not impa-tient to complete it. I'm willing to go at the pace that my body sets.

John's touch was powerful yet calming, a strong sense of safety and of being able to relax.

I guess my power animal is the snake (smile). I have always been afraid of snakes and have had nightmares of snakes around me; socks on the floor and stripes in bed sheets would become snakes. They never bit me, but would just surround me. I had two incidences with snakes around the same time that I cut my arm, where the snakes were killed by someone chopping their heads off. Somehow I believe I must have absorbed/related those incidents and connected them to my experience. I find I am no longer afraid of snakes. I spent almost thirty years being frightened by snakes instead of realizing that it was only trying to guide me. Power animals are useful to us consciously, as a symbolism of our instinctual side. They can help us access within us the lessons their essence represents.

The vision and experience I had as a teenager, of the mastodon ramming into the ice wall, has returned to me a number of times. Over time, as I was initially developing my Approach to Myofascial Release, I realized that I was using too much force in attempting to release the fascial system.

One day while pushing into a myofascial restriction, the picture of the mastodon came into my mind's eye. I saw and felt this powerful beast ramming into the ice wall for food. I felt its frustration. The message from this experience was, "ease up." Be and meld with them with finesse and awareness. It reminded me to be patient, and to use my strength intelligently by following the laws of nature. "Go with the flow!"

our luminous essence

I would like to tell a story that illustrates a lot of the principles that we have experienced up to this point, and hopefully deepen your understanding of them. It also will show you the depth of the possibilities of myofascial release. I have had many similar situations like it and I think you will, too, so I want to prepare you for it. I was in Kauai, Hawaii, a number of years ago, and I was doing a Myofascial Release Seminar series there, and a physician showed up. He was a local doctor, an emergency room and family physician. He had some friends who were therapists, and they had told him about the course, so he decided to take it. The first morning at the Myofascial Release Unwinding Seminar I asked for a volunteer, and he came up on the stage. He turned to the audience and said, "Well, I'm a total skeptic." I put my hands on his back and head and in about thirty seconds he's upside down with his butt in the air, shaking violently and screaming his head off. Finally, he collapsed in a sweaty heap and he said,"Wow! You know what that reproduced for me? I hit a high-voltage line on a surfboard and was almost electrocuted eight months ago. I've had horrible shoulder pain and I haven't been able to raise my arm since then." He then raised his arm through a full range of motion and said, "The pain is gone! Well, I guess I'm not a skeptic anymore!"

We've become friends since then, and he's really a great guy. The next time I was back in Hawaii, he called to go out to dinner. His wife had been in a bad Jeep accident on the beach, where the Jeep had turned over and she had broken her back. He asked if I could come up and meet him at the hospital to show him some myofascial release techniques to do for his wife. I met them at the hospital, and in the process of treating her, he was called to the emergency room. There had been a bad car accident. He left for a while, and eventually he came back, looking rather bemused. He said, "Boy, I had an interesting experience. I went to the emergency room, and a lady had a very severe fracture of her pelvis. The x-ray showed that there were multiple pieces. The lady said, 'Doctor, I'm in agony. Is there something you can do for me?' And he said, "I was about to do my normal thing and give her some medication, when I remembered the myofascial release energy work that you had taught me. All I did was put my hands an inch or two off her body, above her hips, and in about three or four minutes, we both felt this tremendous heat build up and we heard, click click, click, click, and she said, 'Doctor, my pain just went away.' I x-rayed her again, and all the fragments had reoriented."

So, energy work, combined with myofascial release, is very potent. It's very important, because it's charging the electromagnetic field.

The next time I was in Hawaii, I was doing some treatments and a Skill Enhancement Seminar over there. When I treat away from the treatment centers I always want to treat people at least three times, because just once isn't enough. It might stir them up and I have no way to follow up with them, and I don't think that it is fair. My schedule had been booked well in advance, and when I came back my friend called again and wanted to get together. He said a friend of his had just had a very severe accident; a runaway truck had hit his car. He wanted to know if I could help him and I said, "I'm really sorry, but I'm totally booked right now." So he called me every day, he was very persistent, and eventually he found out that I was going to Waimea Canyon. He said, "Hey, my office is right at the bottom of the canyon." I said, "I can't imagine what you are going to ask," and he replied, "Could you just stop by and see my friend for a little bit?" I said, "Okay, but I can only treat for a half hour, because I have to get back to the seminar."

This proved to be a good lesson for me in expectations and assumptions. I would have thought if someone had been in a severe accident and I was going to have someone else treat my patient, I would have told him or her about it. I think I would have told them about the person and what they were going to do, and get their permission. That was my assumption. I walked into his office, and he brought me into this small treatment room. The man was lying on the table with his head facing away from me. There was so much stuff around the table; I couldn't even get around the table to introduce myself.

The physician walked in and said, "This is John," and walked out! The patient said, "What are you doing here?" I got really ticked off , but then I realized it wasn't this guy's fault, so I centered myself and figured I would deal with my friend later. I sat down at the head of the table and I just started to touch his head when he agitatedly asks, "What are you doing?" I said, "Well, your doctor wanted me to treat you." He said, "You're not going to manipulate me, are you?" I said, "No, I won't do that." "Well, don't manipulate me!" "I won't do that; I promise you. I will just touch you lightly, and if anything bothers you too much, I will take my hands off you right away. I will not injure you. Is that okay?" He said, "Well, alright."

What had happened in his accident was that he was sitting at a stoplight in a convertible, with his two children in the back seat. There was a sugarcane truck up on the hill. In Hawaii, they have these double trucks with tons of sugarcane in them. Evidently, the driver of the truck had fallen asleep, so it was a runaway truck that came down the hill at about sixty miles per hour and hit the front of the car. The man was trapped behind the steering wheel and was knocked unconscious. When he woke up, he was in severe pain, his ribs were broken, he had a concussion, etc., and he was in a state of panic because he was trapped behind the steering wheel and he didn't know what happened to his children. He didn't know if they had been thrown out of the car, or killed. Since the accident, which was about two weeks before I treated him, he had a lot of head pain, neck pain, and severe rib pain because of the fractures. He also had severe vertigo. He was so dizzy he could not even stand up.

Anyway, as I sat down, I started to touch his head very, very lightly, and within thirty seconds, he said, "What's happening? I'm back in the accident again! What the hell is going on?" And BOOM! I could feel a tremendous impact go through his body. I felt him get hit by the truck and then he became very quiet, and everything stopped; his body started to cool off, no breathing, no energy, no sound. It was very quiet for a while and then I heard him say, "Where am I? What's happening? I'm spiraling up a shaft of light. This is the most beautiful, incredible light I have ever seen!" He kept going up this vortex of light and eventually he became emotional. He was having a reunion with his dead grandmother, and then he became emotional again and he was having a reunion with his dead father; and then he saw Jesus. After a while, his voice really changed and he started to describe a beautiful woman. He described her as having black hair, black eyes, and he really seemed to love this woman. He cried, "Who are you, who are you?" Then he started getting agitated again, and I said, "What's the matter?" He said, "They want me to go back. I don't want to go back. They said it's not my time, but I don't want to go back! I've never had an experience like this in my life; this is so wonderful."

I said, "Well, what about your children? Do they need you?" "Yes, yes," he said, "I have to go back and help them, but I don't know what to do." I said, "Why don't you ask these people if maybe they can give you advice; maybe they can be your guides." He became very quiet and he said, "They told me that they have always been my guides, that they will always be there for me and all I need to do is ask. It's not my time and I need to go back." So, he started coming down the brilliant vortex of light again.

Then he became the most agitated of the whole experience. He was now having an out-of-body experience in the emergency room, hovering over his body, watching the doctors work on him. He started yelling, "Get your hands off me! You don't know what you're doing! I just need to rest, leave me alone." Then slowly he started to come down towards his body and then all of a sudden, I felt this weight and energy enter his body and I felt this buzzzzz; his body warmed, he came back in, and opened his eyes. Time was up, and I needed to get back to the seminar site, so I told him to rest and his physician would be in shortly to check on him. I told his physician he did fine, and left. His physician called the next day to tell me the patient said all his headaches and vertigo were gone! All that was left was some pain in his chest where his ribs had been broken, but he was feeling much better and was able to play with his children on the beach. He wanted to thank me.

I've had many experiences like this, both myself and with my patients. This is why I really feel that the still point is what you might consider "the death experience." It's really a wonderful space; this is where we go out into some other dimension, whatever you want to call it; we reorganize, then we come back in and something has significantly shifted. You will feel them get lighter during the still point. They'll become quiet and then when they come back in, you feel this weight, this energy, this motion comes back in again. Then they move into the next significant position.

Now before I go on let me explain something. He saw Jesus. A lot of our patients have seen angels, celestial light, Buddha, whatever their belief system is, whatever the context, they perceive this energy. The point is this energy is out there, it's therapeutic, and I've found it to be very loving, helpful, and healing. So, it doesn't matter what context or label they put on it, it's what is important to them. It's important, I believe, to speak their language. So allow them to be able to describe it in whatever language they want to use. I don't think it's up to us to be judgemental in any way. You'll find you get much better results that way.

Question: Is there always motion?

Some unwindings will be profound, and there's no motion. During this experience I just related to you, the patient didn't move at all.

Now there's another piece to this story. A year or two later, I went back to Hawaii for more seminars and another treatment clinic. My friend called wanting me to see his patient again, but I was already booked up. His patient was still having some problems that weren't resolving. I said, "You always call me so late. I'm filled up again." Eventually, he found out that some appointments became available; someone had gotten ill and cancelled. We slipped his patient into the three treatment slots. When his patient arrived for his appointment, he hugged me and thanked me for what I had done for him before. We laid him on the table and within thirty seconds, he was becoming very upset again. He said, "What's going on? I'm back in the accident again! I don't want to go through this again, I thought I did that." I said, "You did, but you know, we only had a half hour together, and you pretty much became involved in the spiritual component of it. You have yet to really tap into the emotional or some of the physical aspects that were traumatized at the time." I added, "If you can trust me, I encourage you to let yourself go into it. It wouldn't be coming up unless you needed to go there again. Are you okay with that?" He said yes, and a lot of emotion came out this time. Deep sobs. It was really good for him. The next visit he came back and this time he was really afraid of the whole process. As I touched him, I could just sense he was really shut down and wasn't going to move. It just wasn't going to happen. I wasn't going to force him, I didn't want to, nor should I, nor could I. So, this was the day to focus on structural work. We balanced his pelvis and released many of his physical restrictions.

The last day when he came in, he was still shut down. I sensed he still needed some type of myofascial unwinding, but he was still scared. I wasn't sure what to do, so I quieted down and listened for my intuition, The Ancient Warrior.

Go off the body and unwind his energy field.

There were a couple of therapists participating in a Skill Enhancement Seminar with me, where they assist me in treating the patients to deepen their skill level. One of the therapists who was part of the skill enhancement team was very good at energy work, so I had her stand at the feet, maybe six inches or so off the body. I stood above his head and we contacted his energy field. It was unbelievable, it was so magnetic and strong. I felt his energy field start to float. It was very interesting. A couple of other therapists were watching this from the side. One of the therapists watching describes her perspective of it. "They both would approach the body from opposite ends. When their hands were about two feet above his body, they would spin and then take a side step while they were holding what looked like a big, invisible beach ball up in the air. Then all of a sudden you'd see them do this little spin again, step back in toward the patient's body. They were both in sync with each other as if it was a choreographed dance. It was like they were watching each other, but their eyes were closed. The patient's eyes were also closed. When their hands got close to his body, they would whip over his body, and it would shake violently. It was like the patient was plugged into an electrical outlet. Then their hands would whip away to the other side, do the spin thing, and then come back toward his body again. His whole body would shake, and they would be whipped away to the other side. This went on for three or four repetitions."

If you go back for a moment to the image of the luminous essence connected by a silver cord, my sense is that his luminous essence had been knocked out of his body with the impact of the car accident. His whole body was like a high-voltage line; it was so charged, as it was still full of memories, fears, and pain. As it would attempt to pass through his physical body, he would almost levitate off the table. When we attempted to connect his energy body through his physical body, it was just too powerful, and it would just whip me right out. Back and forth, back and forth, we had no control over it whatsoever. He obviously was not ready to accept this charge. So eventually, we stopped for a minute and he said, "That's just too much energy, I just can't take it." I said, "I can see that. Do you remember when I saw you last time and you said you had met your father, your grandmother, and Jesus, and that lady, and I suggested that maybe they would be your guides? Have you ever used them as your guides?" He exclaimed, "Oh yes. It has changed my life!" He continued, "We communicate every day, it's been wonderful! They've helped me significantly." I asked, "Do you trust them?" and he replied, "Absolutely." So I suggested, "How about if you quiet down now, and why don't you ask them what would be best for you." He became very quiet, and eventually he said, "Yes, they said you are to be totally trusted, and it's time. I will go for it."

So I said, "Okay, it's going to be strong, but you will not be injured. I will stop anytime you need me to. I will be right here with you."

We probably worked with him another fifteen or twenty minutes. Every time the charge went through him, it would get a little less, and a little less, a little less, until eventually, it just settled into his body, and you could see color come back into his face. He was totally exhausted, and my schedule was shot at this point. I turned to the therapist who was helping me and suggested we help him sit up. I asked her, "Will you stay with him for a little bit and make sure he is okay? I'll go start the next patient and you join me when you can."

We sat him up. We were standing in front of him, but his head was down. Eventually he lifted his head up and looked at her. Big tears ran down his face as he said, "Oh my God, you're the woman!" She had black hair, black eyes.

How these things happen, I don't know, but somehow, she had come back to help him again! After this series of treatments, he made remarkable turnarounds, reporting that he felt more fully alive than ever and was leading a pain-free, active life once again.

There does seem to be this luminous energy body, our mind. It is the part that heals us. It can become disassociated from us in fragments, or sometimes almost as a totality. Myofascial release seems to bring our essence back in. I think this is the essence of healing. We need that energy and that awareness to heal. You can keep it in a language that's not offensive to anybody so they don't have to resist. We don't have to thrust our belief system on anybody. We just go with their belief system and work with that. Be gentle and create an environment of acceptance and love.

Question: Wow, what an experience! Do we really have the potential to do that? You mentioned that you have had a number of similar experiences like that yourself. Could you relate another one to us?

You do have the potential! We all have latent untapped talents and powers that we can learn to use to help others. We need to learn the principles and do our own personal growth work so that we can open our heart and have the wisdom, courage, and loving power to use these refined principles with integrity, clarity, and awareness.

To answer your question about the death experience, I have had a number of fascinating experiences where I have flowed into the death space. To reassure you, it is a very nice feeling and extremely therapeutic. I believe the still points are the death space or a higher dimension full of love. I believe that it is in this loving dimension of expanded awareness where we receive information, reorganize, and come back more fully into our physicality, so we can release, improve, and grow.

So maybe moving into still points is a form of training, clearing, and growth, preparing us to evolve and get ready for that transition we have labeled death. Our physicality may eventually cease to exist, but our essence may live for an eternity.

In a Myofascial Release III Seminar in the 1980s, I had been injured and the therapists at the seminar offered to treat me. We decided to unwind in a pool. About six therapists supported me as I floated on my back. I started to unwind and eventually my head went under the water and my whole body sank to the bottom. I stayed on the bottom of the pool for a long period of time with no urge to breathe. I was having a past-life experience, where I had drowned. A number of other therapists who were standing by the side of the pool watching began to time the amount of time I was under the water. I was now having an out-of-body experience; my awareness was above the pool looking down at the therapists treating me. I could see their heads and shoulders and all the people watching, surrounding the pool. After about three minutes my body started to float to the surface. Now, I wasn't capable then or now of holding my breath for over three minutes and I was under the water, so I couldn't cheat. Try it yourself now. Take a few deep breaths and see how long you can hold your breath. Most people don't last longer than thirty seconds to a minute. Try it!

Amazingly, when I reached the surface, instead of gasping for air, I just took a normal breath and felt very calm and peaceful. These types of experiences break our reality, but as I have said before, "reality is just a figment of our imagination!"

Whatever the explanation, my pain was gone and my range of motion returned to normal. I felt great!

Myofascial release and myofascial unwinding can be utilized successfully and safely with any or no belief system. What I've tried to do over the years is to construct a model of healing from my experience that is intelligent, compassionate, safe, and highly effective. The bottom line is that it works!

A Therapist's Perspective

I was contacted by a private practice across town "on a whim" to help with a Pediatric Myofascial Release course by recommending a child for demonstration. "MFR what?" I asked. Without a clue that my life was about to change, I went to the course. By the end of the two days, my body had shifted so much that I was totally disorganized and very aware that my body was way out of balance.

I proceeded out of pure curiosity to Myofascial Release I, taking a trusted friend who thought like I did: "Prove that this stuff is real and valuable." We sat in the back skeptical, despite my previous experience. By the end of the third day my body was a vibrating mass of Jello, and I could hardly pull myself loose from the table! My friend and I left, scratching our heads, but fully aware something "real" had happened, because we trusted each other's experience. It was also during Myofascial Release I that I became aware of presence, thanks to John. While we learned techniques, I noticed/felt something I had not felt before, and when I opened my eyes, it was John who was walking by every time! By the end of day three I "noticed" where he was from across the room!!!!!! I left unwinding to the last of the series because I wanted to be "prepared." This is the story of my life!!!!! Needless to say I had a lot to learn about trust and process. I did know that I hated the drum music (which I grew to love in Myofascial Release III) but I wanted to keep learning.

When I went to Paoli to complete the Skill Enhancement Seminar, I had completed four courses in less than a year, and knew for a fact that myofascial release was "real and valuable." I had only one dilemma...I was terrified of John! This made no logical sense to me. He was warm, kind, obviously compassionate, and a great teacher, so what was the story? I had a sense that he would know more about me than I knew myself. I knew I was standing in my own way. Before I began this journey, I felt I knew myself very well. By the end of that first year, I realized I had found something that fit my professional hands like a glove, and I could no longer hide from myself.

Fast-forward seven years to now....How am I different? First off, I am no longer afraid of John, and can embrace his presence with all of the loving support I have come to know is "real and valuable," and is a huge part of my growth. I am now less "prepared" and have had some great experiences because of it. I am allowing the layers to peel away in order to get out of the way of my own progress toward becoming the person I was born to be. Most of all, I have discovered how deeply I am capable of feeling, and this used to scare me too. Thanks to advanced unwinding this past June, the barriers of embarrassing myself in public are being broken. Oh, by the way, the other benefits are that I've regained much of my physical structure, restoring an upright posture lost to three spinal surgeries and nine months of a body cast. I now have mostly pain-free days following fifteen years of constant back pain that threatened my career as an occupational therapist.

A THERAPIST'S PERSPECTIVE

I have spent a lifetime trying to stuff my emotions down to be "stronger." Since attending the Myofascial Release Series, I now let myself cry when I need to, and as a result, I cry less often. I was considering taking antidepressant medication and I was trying herbs first, but I didn't need either after the course. Interesting. I now feel I have more tools to deal with my emotions. I have a greater understanding of their purpose in my life and how they can serve me.

Through John's teachings I came to a large awakening. Things I viewed as religious are actually natural phenomena. They can be accessed by anyone, regardless of religious persuasion. It is a skill that can be developed, with proper training and practice. The MFR training is demystifying the mind-body-spirit connection for me. It explains it, in part, in scientific terms. I love this combination of scientific theory and emotional/mental awareness.

I look forward to more learning and further "ah-ha" experiences ahead of me. Thank you to everyone for sharing. It helps me to understand the process and be more comfortable with my own journey.

ancient wisdom

I believe that myofascial release is an evolution and blending of ancient wisdom and recently discovered therapeutic principles. This information is for those interested in the more esoteric aspects of therapy and life. In all of my seminars, I encourage people not to believe a word that I say. I do not believe in forcing any belief system on anyone, ever. Words and explanations can never replace the actual experience of receiving the treatments yourself. It is only through your own personal experience that you will be able to understand the importance of myofascial release. You can then describe myofascial release in words and concepts with which you are comfortable.

Myofascial release is not a religion or a cult. I believe that the myofascial release experience can be used as the action component of any religion or philosophy that expresses love, respect, and helping oneself and others. A cult is where someone tells you what to think and what to feel. Your power is taken away. Instead, I believe in helping others tune into and develop their own personal power and awareness. This is true and authentic empowerment.

A THERAPIST'S PERSPECTIVE

When my parents found out that I was going to leave my profession in traditional physical therapy to do the John F. Barnes Myofascial Release Approach, they became very concerned. They became even more concerned when I used words like energy and transference. They thought for sure I had joined a cult in Sedona that worshipped the vortices, and had turned my back on my Christian upbringing. I gave them this answer:

When God created us, he created a marvelous human being. One that knows what it needs and one that can heal itself in many instances. We are electromagnetic beings and because of the electromagnetic fields found in mountainous regions or at the ocean, our bodies recharge and reorganize. The same is true with the piezoelectric effect that John speaks of. We are merely the facilitators. One electromagnetic being to the other. I believe that some of the perceptive or intuitive capabilities that I have are a gift from God. I assured them, I cannot speak for others but as for me, I will always worship the Creator and not what was created.

Because of scientific advances, we can now measure the electromagnetic energy. I have found it to be true, especially of very religious people, that grasping new facts is difficult. If it's not understood, or it doesn't say so in the Bible somewhere, it must be of Satan. Nothing could be farther from the truth. Know yourself and your beliefs and know that you have been given the wonderful opportunity to help others heal themselves. Don't be afraid. Trust yourself.

The Myofascial Release Approach is simply a loving, compassionate, and effective way of taking care of yourself and others. The inner growth potential is also enormous and fulfilling, if one chooses to engage in that journey.

Before reading the description of this picture, please quiet your mind, slow your breathing, soften your body and visual focus, and softly look at this picture. Take notice of emotions, sensations, or images that may emerge. Then dissolve into the visuals, sensations and/or emotions that may arise for you, and let them take you away. Flow with the experience and see and feel where it takes you. Ask for help. Ask, "What can I learn from this?" Soften your visual focus until your vision is blurry, slow your breathing, soften your body, and "be" with your feelings...

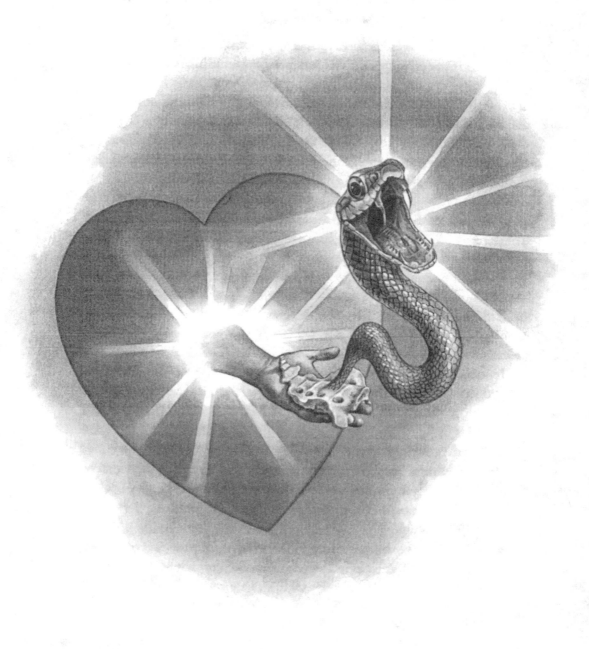

This picture appeared in my mind's eye one day from my intuition, The Ancient Warrior, while I was treating a patient's sacrum. My description of this vision is that other therapies are intellectually and ego based. Myofascial release is from the heart, where our compassion and wisdom lie. Important acupuncture meridians run from our heart down and out through chakras, spinning vortexes of energy, through our hands.

The therapist's hand is holding the sacrum, the keystone of the spine, considered to be the "seat of the soul." The Kundalini energy arises from the second sacral segment, where the sympathetic and parasympathetic nervous systems join at the ganglion of "Implar." The Kundalini energy is symbolized as serpentine energy; our life force.

The medical symbol is the caduceus, which is two intertwined snakes with a shaft of light flowing down the center between the snakes. The two snakes represent the balance of the male and female energy emanating from the light or the life force.

This vision symbolizes how myofascial release allows us to become aware of and face our fears. If we don't, we are imbalanced and our primal energy is stifled, leading to symptoms, chaos, and dis-ease. Myofascial release safely and effectively allows us to face our fears to be able to heal. Otherwise, we are living in a flight-or-fight response, and healing and living life fully is not possible. We were not meant to function in a fight/flight/freeze response, with our internal alarms ringing for more than a short period of time. Unresolved anger and/or fear disconnects us from our essence or life force. This can, over time, undermine the integrity of human physiology and the proper protection and functioning of our immune system. Neither fear nor anger is negative; they are considered vital to our survival. But these lifesaving emotions were never meant to last more than a short period, just long enough to move us out of danger.

This mysterious energy is actually the flow of information carried by the biochemicals of emotion, the neuropeptides, which is a vast superhighway of information exchange taking place on the molecular level. Dr. Candace Pert in her book, *The Molecules of Emotion*, states that this flow of information is bi-directional. While the release of endorphins and other peptides brings about changes in our emotions, our emotions can also bring about the release of these same neuropeptides. Dr. Pert suggests that, while some have called this innate intelligence, the wisdom of the body, still others have called it God. Whatever word you are most comfortable calling this power and wisdom, the bottom line is that this energy/information flows through the ground substance and microtubules of the fascial system, and myofascial release opens up our mind-body systems to allow for proper functioning and awareness.

Another word for this energy or information is love, the most potent healing force in the universe! Our emotional reactions have a tremendous impact upon our physical bodies. A twenty-year study from the University of London revealed that neither smoking nor eating high-cholesterol foods was the best predictor of heart disease and cancer. The best predictor was unresolved emotions. Love brings a powerful transformative influence upon our physical and emotional well-being. Love has power. We need a compassionate relationship with our shadow side in order to be compassionate and loving with someone else. Love provides the compassion needed to face and embrace our shadow side. As long as we are afraid of some aspect of ourselves, we will not be whole and balanced. The famous psychiatrist Dr. Carl Jung said that if we don't acknowledge and learn from our shadow side there will always be an imbalance, producing a symptomatic complex or aberrant behavior. Society teaches us to be afraid or ashamed of our shadow side and to mask it. Traditional medicine has focused on medicating people so they don't feel their shadows. Unfortunately, it just treats the symptoms and just barely enables us to cope. While this is fine for the short term, if that is all we are doing, it is disastrous for the long term.

We must go into our shadow to find the light. The myofascial therapist gently guides the patient into their shadow (chaos and fear) so that they can learn, heal, and find the light. Darkness is a choice. There is not an absence of light; there is a denial of light.

Going back to the image of the caduceus: intertwined snakes wrapped around flowing light. DNA has the shape of a double helix, often described as a twisted rope ladder or spiral staircase. The double helix of the DNA resembles two entwined serpents.

Shamanism talks of two serpents symbolizing the male and female energy, water and land, spiraling rhythmically in a swaying motion from one side to the other. This represents the concept of the oriental yin and yang, or binary opposition, which has to be overcome to achieve individual awareness and integration.

The serpent symbolizes the sacred energy of life, which creates life by transformation. Western culture has cut itself off from the serpent/life principle—in other words, DNA—since it adopted an exclusively rational point of view. DNA transmits visual information by emitting photons, which are electromagnetic waves. Scientists have discovered that

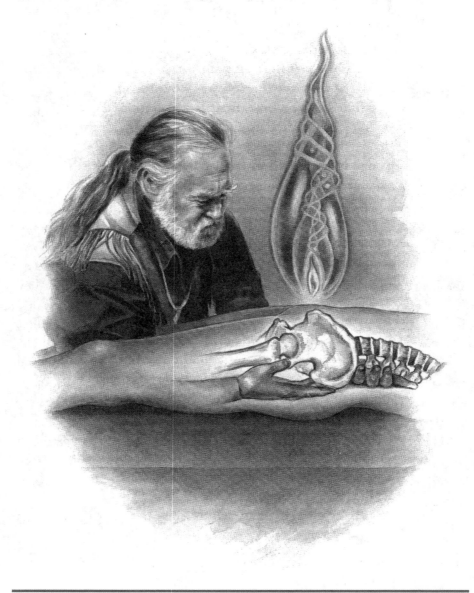

all living cells emit photons, producing a luminescence. For centuries we have been called "light beings," and our energy body has been described as looking like a "luminescent mist." Could this be what has been described as a halo or aura?

I believe that we are liquid light flowing through the microtubules and ground substance of the fascial system throughout our bodies. This liquid light flows in the micro-fascial system of our cells and beyond our bodies into the universal web of life, and back into our being as a loving wave of light energy. We are mostly fluid beings with light energy flowing through us; DNA living in water and emitting photons. To transform, a person must face his or her fears, or serpent, with another serpent, the life energy of our spirit. As we face our fears, love emerges and transforms us, as depicted in the picture on facing page.

A THERAPIST'S PERSPECTIVE

When I took my first Myofascial Release Seminar with John, I thought I was going to learn just another tool for my bag of tricks. Boy, was I wrong! After the first half of day one, I felt I had found what I had been waiting for my whole life. I felt I had known John forever.

Every time John touched me during the seminar, I went into a state of deep trance, even if it was just a passing touch with my partner working on me. I couldn't believe what I felt when I went on to the stage and he treated me. I immediately went into an emotional response. He is the most balanced of left and right brain of anyone I have ever met. His powerful energy field fills an entire room. He is extremely humble and is also the most patient listener of anyone I have ever met. He treats everyone with the utmost respect and love.

We were trained traditionally to view the body as a solid mass and treat it with mechanical principles. I treat the body mechanically with joint mobilization, muscle energy, exercise, and massage techniques. However, I also realize that the instant the person moves out of a slackened environment on the table and stands on the floor, gravity exerts its influence and fluid dynamics are in play. Myofascial release employs both biomechanical principles and the principles of fluid dynamics, since the body and myofascial system are mostly fluid.

The implied message in school was that the patient never gets off the treatment table, so the influence of gravity, the fascial system, the body's liquidity, and the mind were not considered relevant. The fragmented myth that is called traditional health care only provided physicians and therapists with an incomplete set of rules. I believe the Myofascial Release Model of healing provides an encompassing, comprehensive view and method of treating all aspects of the physiology, mind, emotions, and spirit of the whole person.

A THERAPIST'S PERSPECTIVE

Before myofascial release I was becoming dissatisfied with mundane, conventional physical therapy treatments. I had nothing to offer the chronic neck and back patients. I was beginning to wonder if I wanted to continue doing physical therapy.

I first heard of myofascial release in 1987 when John was in Bermuda lecturing at a dental seminar for TMJ. What he said made so much sense, I was excited by what I had learned.

I can now treat anything you throw at me, and I enjoy doing it. In fact, a large part of my caseload are the very problems that I couldn't treat before.

John's presence is powerful, you can feel him even with your eyes closed when he's in the room. His touch is strong and firm but gentle, very reassuring and calming. I can relate to the comments made about John's presence transcending space. I have, at times when I needed something extra, called on his magnificent energy and have felt his presence. At times I need to remind myself to slow down and treat as if I really am a beginner especially when I am very busy and just trying to get things done. "Stay in the moment."

*

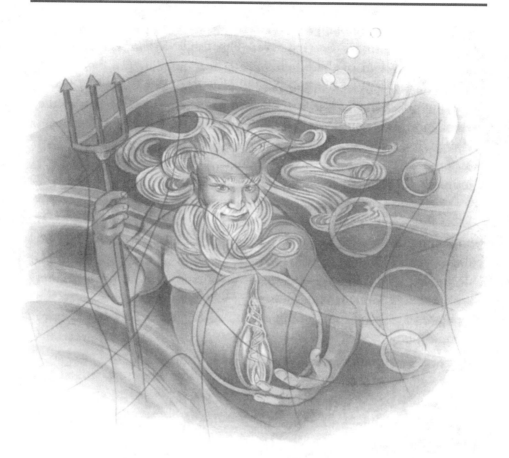

We are liquid light, a "luminescent mist." We are a fluid intelligence system. Instead of the mechanical traditional view that we are solid mass, we are a liquid vessel, a gelatinous being with fluid conduits (fascial microtubules) for the flow of energy/information, a liquid nervous system.

The picture above is Neptune, the mythical God of the sea and earthquakes. Neptune is depicted holding his trident, the symbol of power. This picture appeared in my mind's eye while treating. I felt as if I was transported down into the cellular level. The net is the fascial web filled with fluid. Neptune symbolizes the intelligence and power within this liquid light, holding a bubble with the spark of life within: love! We were conceived in fluid, developed in amniotic fluid, became fluid beings (the human body is approximately 70% fluid!), we live on the water planet (the earth is 70% water).

We are incredible beings, always vibrating within a liquid medium. Our bodies are like a flowing river. The fluids of our body are the transporting system of the biochemicals, nutrients, oxygen, hormones, neuropeptides, and antibodies, and they eventually flush out waste products and toxins for purification. *Drink a lot of water!* It hydrates the system and flushes out the toxins. Most of us, on a nutritional level, are walking around totally poisoned. We are in a toxic state because the restricted fascial system, on the cellular level, is not allowing us to eliminate all those toxins. The cells are not assimilating food well and are not getting proper oxygenation. This affects us on all levels.

The fluids of our body enhance the energetic movement of information, thought, and emotions. Unexpressed emotion and/or outdated beliefs create a holding pattern of stuck vibration that becomes unavailable to the whole. These imprisoned fragments build up pressure and become dense and stagnant, causing blockages and restrictions to the proper physiological functioning and sense of peace and tranquility to the mind/body.

Love is a vibration. So to lead a quality life and be healthy;
Love who you are.
Love what you do.
Love each moment, by being in the moment.

This allows you to move out of judgement and make the best of the situation. It's like mental ju jitsu—simply ask yourself, how can I make the best of this situation? How can I turn this supposed negative into a positive? This is truly going with the flow. You have a choice in each situation. Crying over spilled milk, being a victim, blaming others or bad luck, basically being a victim of circumstance, is a powerless reaction. In other words, you are either "re-*acting*" an old pattern or making a choice to respond to the situation in the moment. Accept what is! Learn from what is and create another choice: what is my best response? This is responsible action. Your power is in the present moment. Be here now!

If you are more comfortable with scientific jargon, allow me to convert these symbols that we call words into more scientific terminology. I am on the editorial advisory board of the *Journal of Bodywork and Movement Therapies*, edited by Dr. Leon Chaitow. The following information may be of interest to you, and has been paraphrased from a series in the *Journal* called "Healing Energy" by James Oschaman, Ph.D. He explains that not all bodywork effects can be explained in mechanistic terms. When dense tissue melts and softens, this release is not just because of neurological influences. Collagen fibers are embedded in a gel-like ground substance. Fascia is a piezoelectric tissue generating electrical fields when compressed or stretched. Since collagen is a semiconductor, the fascia is an integrated electronic network that allows all parts of the organism to communicate with each other. The new way of observing living tissue is as an interconnected molecular continuum referred to as "the living matrix." The matrix inside cells is known as the cytoskeleton, which is connected to the matrix outside of cells, classically known as connective tissue or fascia. In other words, there is a micro-fascial system within every cell of the body, a fluid nervous system, capable of generating vibrations throughout the entirety of the living matrix. Every conceivable kind of vibratory information is transmitted through this fascial web.

As the ground substance of the fascial system loses its fluid content and begins to become more viscous, this vibratory light energy is blocked. This interruption of the flow of this vital energy, or life force, causes many of our symptoms or dis-ease. The myofascial therapist touches the patient's body to sense structural myofascial restrictions and the vibratory flow of energy through the microtubules of the fascial system. Upon discovery of these structural, fluid, and vibratory blockages, the therapist quiets and allows for a flow of energy between the two beings. The therapist centers themself and moves into the timeless/spaceless dimension where healing occurs. The therapist applies light, gentle, and sustained pressure into the myofascial restriction or allows the body to move into significant positions of past physical or emotional injury through the phenomenon of myofascial unwinding.

The therapist's charge of energy raises the patient's energy level until their vibratory level is similar. This is called a state of attunement. Eventually there is a point where their energetic vibratory levels match identically; this is called "resonance." It is the therapist's sustained physical pressure into the restriction and their ability to achieve "resonance," that allows for a release. In other words, the dam is broken and the blocked energy begins to flow through the fluidity of the mind-body. As enough releases occur, the body's self-correcting mechanisms begin to function harmoniously. Eventually the patient is filled with a vibrant luminosity; this is authentic healing.

Where does the energy come from? My experience has led me to believe that we are like beautiful, luminescent dewdrops in the sea. As our awareness increases we see that we are not only a dewdrop, but also the sea. I perceive the sea as God. You may be more comfortable labeling the sea with another name. Whatever label you believe in; there is an infinite, vast sea of vibrations (love and light), a loving force that helps, guides, and gives us life and healing energy.

A THERAPIST'S PERSPECTIVE

Mastery is a process. There is a suspension of prior models of knowing. This may be the result of pain or inspiration. Frequently, current models just don't work. Recall John's injuries and his search for relief, the serendipity of some of his explorations.

Observation. Take an action and pay attention to the feedback. What did I do and how did that action affect me (or someone else?). John started as his own best guinea pig. If something felt helpful he did it again, and a little more consciously. Hmmm…what if I do it this way?

Suspend judgement. Accept the unacceptable, unconventional, unpopular. Current vogue thinking juxtaposes nature and nurture. Man over nature. We have antibiotics, antibacterial, weed and pest control, the war on poverty, the war on drugs and countless other battles. John went outside these boxes to man working with nature. Flow with the forces of life. Go in the direction of ease. By beginning to understand the nature of fascia, he found the way to nurture it.

Observe with heightened senses. Process experiences through the regular five senses in expanded ways. A wine taster or perfume maker trains their senses of taste and smell as John trained his sense of touch. This process demands attention to nuances. How does it feel if I stretch? Pull? Push? Sustain? Rebound? How does the tissue respond? What happens to the pain? Function?

Make associations. Connect the dots in a variety of ways. Like an infant—everything is new and explorable. No expectations. This looks at the "why" of what is being observed without attachment to explanations. Who knew John could treat the electrical system in the body through the connective tissue? Who thought the piezoelectric effect would stimulate unwinding and could affect pain and functioning so dramatically? And what about the body-mind-spirit interconnections that are all treated through bodywork? And of the body as the filing cabinet for traumatic emotions and memories?

Observe, associate, observe, associate, and observe. I am sure many dot-to-dot pictures got thrown out. Some led to new associations. Others may be sitting, gestating, and emerging in this new text of his. Everything has its own time.

Translate observations of what's happening to others with clarity and integrity. This is the mastery of educating. It involves the pacing of what is taught, when and how, so the students get both the art and the skill. How does John convey the balance, rhythm, timing, and coordination of the touch? How does he teach us to observe and follow our intuitions? How does he shape our growing skills in connecting, detaching from the outcome or becoming centered?

Hold the space for change. John does more than teach; he inspires the will to change and grow. He holds a bigger vision or space for us than we hold for ourselves. It is not limited by our self-concept or beliefs of what we can or can't do. He demonstrates principles of excellence every time he demonstrates a technique or leads a meditation. Who knew how profound or quickly an improvement in condition could take place? I never saw it demonstrated in college. His power of attraction conveys the confidence for us to "get it." And more... he builds our ability to hold an expanded space for others by promoting our continued work on ourselves.

The KEY: Total presence. Be here now! Harmonic resonance. The great gift of being totally with someone provides the space to confront the demons and to make happiness something that we bring to life. The focused attention in the moment lets us feel loved, important and valuable. It allows our own depth and courage to resonate with his, so that we too go to the top of the mountain for a moment. Having been to the top and seen the view, we better know how to go again. "Presence" teaches us that the quality of our lives is on the line every moment. This, then, is the mastery John shares with us all.

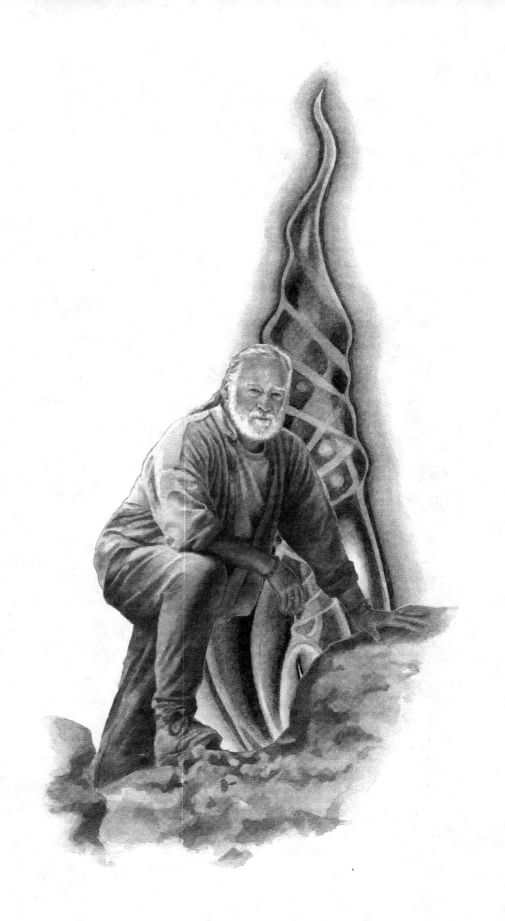

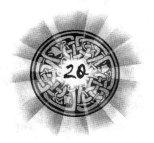

the path to mastery

I had just finished one of my advanced seminars, Myofascial Release III, "Beyond Technique," in Sedona, Arizona. I finally had a few days off to allow myself to rest and immerse myself in refining my book and writing this last chapter, "The Path to Mastery."

Sedona is one of the most exquisitely and uniquely magnificent places on earth. It was a beautiful fall day in late October, with cool and crisp air and a brilliant blue sky. Although I had a lot of writing to do, I had a strong urge to be outside and take a hike into the red rock canyons. Sedona is truly the "Wild West," still very pristine with incredible red rock mountains and abundant wildlife—deer, elk, cougars, coyotes, eagles, ravens, javelinas (wild boars), jackrabbits, chipmunks—I could go on and on. One never tires of the natural beauty there. I acted on my urge to explore when The Ancient Warrior said, "Go, you deserve a rest, the beauty will stimulate your creativity." My home, "Windswept," is situated high on a red rock pinnacle with a 360-degree view of Sedona's rugged mountains. My land abuts national forest land, drops sharply into the ravine, and then dramatically raises to the 7,000–8,000-foot level of the imposing Crimson Mountains.

As I climbed up a mountain ledge The Ancient Warrior said, "I will give you a 'sign' tonight. Be alert and centered, and the moment it happens tune into your feelings, then open up to the symbolism." At sunset I returned to Windswept feeling exhilarated from my day. I had seen coyotes, and deer, and ravens swooping and playing in the sky.

That night I was leaning on a desk which overlooks my deck and has a large plateglass window in front of it. Suddenly, the outdoor floodlights, which are motion sensitive, went on. Standing there looking at me was a huge cougar, only five feet away from me! Our eyes met and time stopped. We somehow "connected" in that timeless/spaceless eternal moment. His beautiful eyes and powerful, muscular shoulders and chest transfixed me. He was identical to the panther on the front cover of this book, my power animal. After a moment that seemed like an eternity, this "mountain spirit" gracefully disappeared into the shadows.

As The Ancient Warrior had predicted, I had a powerful visceral reaction in my solar plexus. There was a felt-sense of falling into space, expanding and going deeper, while at the same moment I experienced a profound level of consciousness that was deeper than I could ever imagine. I felt exhilarated afterwards. That sacred experience had a dreamlike quality to it.

Later that night, I slept soundly and had a very vivid dream. My power animal, the cougar, came to me. Now he was in my house! He appeared in every room. He wasn't menacing. I wasn't afraid. We were curious and communicating on some non-verbal level with mutual respect. He then leaped up onto a high ledge and looked at me intently! I felt my heart opening and he was saying, "free me!" I opened the door and he pounced down and out the door. He was free!

The timing of this exciting episode was certainly a synchronicity, a meaningful coincidence. This represented for me that the timing and thrust of this book was right on, and could be a meaningful experience for me and others who are open to grow and connect with their true self. I believe in learning from the emotions and feelings in dreams and not overanalyzing them. What this dream symbolized for me was that my "power animal," my instinctive side, was in all of my rooms (in every aspect of my being), and that I should further encourage my curiosity and full expression of my power to be free. By fully allowing the power of our instinctive side to express itself, interconnecting with all aspects of our being, we open to become fully human, creating the possibility of living life with vitality. We are free!

Unfortunately, most live worried about the past or fretting about the future. This is a state of disempowerment and distraction. We are always one thought away from the action, from true experience, from power and clarity. Our power, clarity, and awareness come from the silence of the present moment. The "now" is eternal! Love is eternal. Fear blocks love and our ability to be in the "center of the cyclone." Because of our cultural training, our emotional distress, our painful traumas, we live in an envelope of fear! To avoid the turmoil, pain, and fear, many are always thinking, talking, or doing something, instead of being. For too many, this way of thinking about their world has become a dysfunctional habit, an intellectual prison. We need to break down the illusions that restrict our actions, ideas, growth, and healing.

A person's depression, fear, and pain is a reflection that they lost their will and personal power by identifying into somebody else's concept of who or what they should be. The winds of change are upon us, and it is time to reclaim the power of your essence. Look through this illusionary facade that society taught us was physical reality. Your essence will guide you through the mists of illusion to the pathway of transformation!

One day I had taken a group of patients and therapists up into the red rock canyons of Sedona on what we call "Therapy on the Rocks" day. We go into the spectacularly beautiful red rock canyons of Sedona and treat each other and learn how to be in our power center. For as the therapist centers, they then can guide the patient into their own power center to allow for healing to occur. We all sat on the edge of a large waterfall and were discussing our experiences. We had been discussing the role of fear in our lives, and how it prevented healing. One of the therapists was visiting us from Germany and was telling us how he didn't have any problems, was very healthy, and would arise every morning around five to run for a couple of hours.

I sensed that he was talking from his head (intellect), not from his heart. I centered myself and observed his body language. He went on to say that he used his fear to drive him in his running and life. He said he thought that fear was a good thing. He was lost in an all too common and stifling illusion. He was identifying with fear. I turned to the group, knowing that he was watching me. I use words sparingly. I don't believe in telling people what to do. I teach lessons in story form. I never explain the story. It is up to the individual to ascertain what that story symbolizes for them. I don't believe in slapping people to death with words.

I use words like a karate strike. A well-timed word or phrase coming from the center of my being can go right to the heart of the problem.

I explained my belief to the group that fear is either driving you, and you are running from it, or it cripples and paralyzes you. I turned to him and looked at him in the eyes and asked, "have you ever considered just *being with your fear?*" It was like a bolt of lightning hit him. His eyes rolled back and his eyelids began to flutter, his breathing increased, his belly was quivering, and he spontaneously began to unwind. I reached over and held him behind his neck, and his back arched and his arms began to flail around wildly. He then began to choke and spit up fluid. This flailing and choking went on for a few minutes and then he moved into a still point, becoming very quiet and motionless. He stopped breathing for a short period. His eyes began to flutter again; he opened them and looked around in a state of shock. He said, "My God! I just went back in time to when I was six years old and almost drowned and had a near-death experience!" Tears welled up and he started to cry; deep, deep sobs. When he quieted, I suggested that he mentally tell that little boy that he survived…that he was safe now…that he could let go of the fear now. I suggested that he go off by himself for a while and "be" with himself. Later, he came over to me to thank me and said he was aware that something very significant had shifted in him, and he felt an inner peace that he had never had before.

My interpretation is that he had left his body when he almost died, and fear had driven him since. Most of us have had some incident where fear enveloped and overwhelmed us, and it was too scary to quiet down, because that horrible, deep fear at our core would emerge again. The fear either drives our behavior and we run from it, or we contract and collapse and it cripples us, it paralyzes us. When we have unresolved emotions and/or fearful beliefs, we are stuck on the subconscious level in a fight/flight/freeze response with our subconscious "alarms" activated. In this state no healing is possible! These primitive responses cannot be deactivated on the conscious level through willpower alone. They reside in our subconscious. Remember, "We don't know what we don't know, until we know what we don't know."

This is when the healing power of myofascial release, myofascial unwinding, and myofascial rebounding can create the safe environment for the patient to leap into the unknown. As we enter the chaos, the shadow, the fearful unknown, we find the light. The compulsive, driving, or crippling fear is converted into excitement, and we discover our inner light, our power, that still, quiet, tranquil space that lies within all of us: the center of the cyclone! So the hurt or fear that we embrace is the path to our inner peace and becomes our joy!

The German therapist came up to me a couple of days after his un-winding and thanked me again. He said, "What a massive internal shift. I don't *have* to run anymore. I now love to run!" Everything is mind at various levels of vibration. Humanity, in its unwillingness to face its fears, has put too many into a trance, locked up within a cocoon of limited awareness and self-induced amnesia. This unfelt fear is a state of shock, a frozen moment in time. The skilled therapist "shocks the shock" with their energy, which emanates from the center of their essence. When a significant position in space is achieved through unwinding, that frozen energy (emotion or belief) changes its vibration and begins to flow. The therapist helps the patient to move and enhance their vibrational level into a vibrant luminosity—their essence. This is awareness; this is healing.

One day in Paoli, back in 1987, I met a new patient referred to me from Hong Kong. She was a beautiful Asian woman about fifty years of age. She was very wealthy and had been all over the world to see some of the leading physicians for her problems over the past ten years. She had been suffering with crushing headaches, neck and back pain, and tightness. She had large cysts or growths all over her body, head, and face. Her most recent diagnosis was fibromyalgia. Nothing had given her more than temporary relief, and her situation was worsening.

Our first treatment consisted of getting to know each other and was mostly evaluation and structural myofascial release. She expressed how angry and disappointed she was at how she had been treated by the other therapists and physicians that she had seen. The second day, as I started to treat her, she quieted down fairly quickly! With her permission, I had three other therapists in the room. The therapists were participating in our Skill Enhancement Program. During this program they treat along-side me and my team of therapists to increase their skills and sensitivity, while also enhancing the patient's response to treatment.

I started with structural myofascial release and as she quieted down, she started to slowly move spontaneously and unwind. I could sense that her belly was quivering, and her emotions beginning to emerge. A rumble emerged from her throat as her body arched, and she let out a sound of fury that had been buried deep inside of her for so long. Then she became incredibly quiet, and without opening her eyes, she said, "It felt so good and freeing to let go of that anger and fear." She lay there peacefully for awhile, and then began to cry. She shared a vision which emerged during this experience. "I saw my rage as a molten volcano spewing from my depths, and from the torment of my volcano flew a baby eagle! I feel that by releasing my fear and anger, I am now renewed and free again! Thank you, thank you."

Then she became very quiet again and began to move gently and unwind again. Her eyes rolled back in her head and all we could see was the white of her large eyes. The atmosphere in the room shifted, the tone of her voice changed and she boomed from the depths of the universe, "John, you are an ancient healer, and those that are learning from you are ancient healers. They are all coming together at this time of evolving awareness. You will endure much criticism, you will be vehemently attacked, and you will suffer many hardships. You must endure! Let no one stop you! What you are all doing is too important to be stifled. There will be an awareness shift in 1993. Then there will be a cascade of massive shifts in global awareness, and you and your fellow healers will be the leaders. Develop your power and awareness and deepen your courage and integrity now, to be ready for these important responsibilities. All of your thoughts and actions must come from your heart. Touch only with compassion and love!" She then became very, very quiet....The next day all of the growths on her body and face had disappeared. Within two weeks her pain and headaches were gone, and her range of motion had returned.

It is important for your patient to understand that healing is not an event, it is a process! As a therapist, our role is to kick the pebble that starts the avalanche. In order for the therapist to be clear and powerfully effective they must detach from the outcome. On the surface that may sound cruel; however, it is the most loving thing you can do for another.

I once heard the inventor of the Bell helicopter, Authur Young, speak about the trials and tribulations he went through in his attempt to develop the principles of helicopter flight. He is a true genius. He stated that a helicopter must achieve a centered balance. Once it tilts in a particular direction, it has a bias. It must fly in that direction; all other directions are no longer available to it.

So as a therapist, if we are attached to an outcome, we are biased. In other words, no other options are available to us; we have lost our power. When we rebalance and move back into our center, we regain our power, for 360 degrees of options are now available. As we move into the center of our power we allow the patient to engage their internal power. Their inner wisdom can now move into the direction that is in their best interest. I love my patients enough to detach from the outcome. This is the healing power of the present moment.

A THERAPIST'S PERSPECTIVE

My college roommate and best friend had this vision prior to my going to my first MFR III class. Mind you, she has never had any contact with John or any other myofascial release therapist beside myself. What she said to me was, "I see you all on top of the red rocks. John is the eagle. You each are his babies. One by one he ever so gently nudges you off the cliff. He watches with pride as you fly off, each in your own direction. He doesn't need to follow you. He knows you're on the right path."

The first day I attended Myofascial Release III, John took the whole group outside high up on a ledge. He shared this poem with us…

He said, "Come to the edge."
They said, "We are afraid!"
He said again, "Come to the edge."
They did.
He pushed them and they soared!

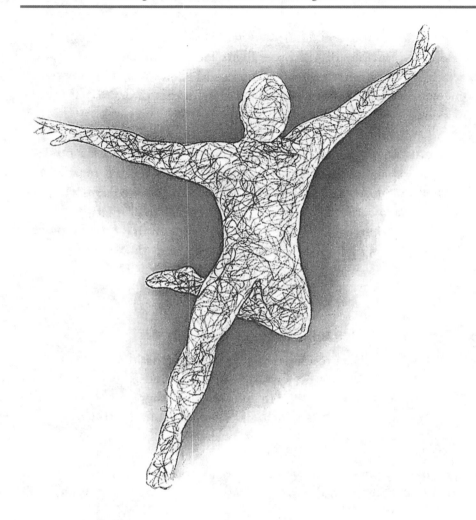

This important shift in awareness—from being locked into our fearful egos to evolving into our powerfully, aware essence—has already begun, and will be massive in the next few years. We need to "lean into the winds of change" and soar!

Myofascial release is the ultimate mind-body therapeutic art and mastery of life. My goal, my mission, is to help you achieve mastery as a therapist and in life's adventures.

Most people's conditioning has forced them into believing that physical reality is all that there is. All beings have the potential to experience a much vaster reality. Most have become stuck within a very small reality that is limited and distorted. As a result, they do not access their full potential for perception, experience and action. They are not being fully human.

Most are stuck in linear time or clock time, fretting about the past or worried about what will happen in the future. A being accesses their full potential and awareness in the present moment, in the flow of the "now."

A being is a presence in the now, a succession of moments of presence in the present. One is only truly living and growing when they are being present in the now, as opposed to linear, clock time. The present moment is real time.

Renegade, it is vitally important for you and others to understand that all other time, when one is not present, is a waste in terms of life, for there is no presence in it. Wasted time is when one is smothered in a cocoon of fear, fixated and stuck, existing only in linear time; basically, just walking in place, getting nowhere in terms of develop-ment of one's essence. How much one has been in real time, in the now, indicates one's true age, since this determines the development and maturity of the essence. Unfortunately, most people have spent only a year or two of their entire lives being truly present, so that is how old they really are from a perspective of the essence.

The key to a quality life and effectiveness in treatment is to be present, to be aware in the now. This is authentic power!

I request that you reread the wisdom of The Ancient Warrior's last statements and consider their importance and potential impact upon your life.

In other words, most are spending the majority of their life in a stupor, the trance of consensus consciousness. They are in a daze, just going through the motions. When one is lost in their linear trance in linear or clock time, they are on a meaningless treadmill. They are squan-dering their precious life! We are only truly alive and aware when we are immersed in the present moment.

When we are lost in clock time we are living in an envelope of fear. We all need to face our demons. We need to embrace our fear. As we summon our courage and move into the chaos, we will learn and grow from our fear. Accept what is; make the best of it and flow with the energy!

We then can embrace the present moment, where love exists. And in the most practical terms, flowing within the present moment is the most healthy way to be. Being in the "now" is when we are our most mentally clear, emotionally tranquil, and physically comfortable and capable. Mastery has to do with stillness…being calm, nonjudgemental, real, intelligent, sensitive, strong yet flexible, compassionate, empathetic and joyful! A master lives in the eternal moment. It is in the now, the present moment, where our power lies to transform, grow, heal, and live life fully and joyfully.

Wisdom means understanding that we do not know what is going to happen next. So, the only thing we can do is soften and relax. As we relax we slide out of the swirl of the cyclone and into our power center. Realize that as we soften and relax, we are in the present moment, going with the flow! Be here now!

There is a wonderful book I recommend to all therapists during their development as *therapeutic artists*. It is titled *The Agony & The Ecstasy*, by Irving Stone, and it is about the life and challenges of one of the world's greatest artists, Michelangelo. There is a section where Michelangelo explains that when he would look at a huge block of marble he was about to sculpt, he would quiet himself and see the shape and beauty within. He would then chip away the extraneous marble, so that the inner beauty could emerge. I see our role with the Myofascial Release Approach as releasing the blockages, the extraneous restrictions, so that the individual's inner beauty and healing power can emerge and express itself, freeing the person to return to a healthy, joyful state. Let your therapeutic artistry spread into all aspects of your being, so that your life will be a *masterpiece!*

I'd like to close with this Native American healer's perspective:

The Path
Whatever you become, my child, may it be rooted in grace.
Whatever your path through life,
May it offer you steepness and rough places
So that you do not become complacent.
Nothing is owed to you, but everything is available to you.
It is up to you to decide.
Your courage will arise if you call it by name,
Just as love will find its way into your heart.
My child, I cannot shoulder your mistakes
In order to keep you free from pain,
But I can open your eyes to beauty,
If you will only take the time.

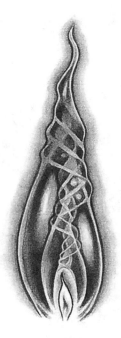

It is with deep love that I encourage you to identify with your essence, stay on your path and enjoy your journey!
Love,
John

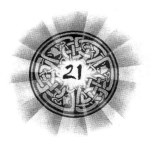

epilogue

An enormous amount of information has emerged since the year 2000 when I wrote my book *Healing Ancient Wounds, The Renegade's Wisdom*. A 'sea change' in awareness has happened since then. I have now trained over 100,000 therapists and physicians in my Myofascial Release Approach®, which has become a very powerful movement. For many years we were bucking the tide, but now the tide has shifted and is propelling us forward at a rapid pace. I am proud of the many therapists offering Myofascial Release. While we will continue to benefit from medicine and surgery, especially in emergency situations, Myofascial Release will become the healthcare of the future.

As you know, the development of my John F. Barnes' Myofascial Release Approach® has been through my own personal experience with pain and trauma and by treating patients from all over the word for over 50 years. I would like to provide a quote that was in my first book, *Myofascial Release, the Search for Excellence* that was published in 1990 which has come to fruition after 25 years. "There is one thing stronger than all of the armies in the world, and that is an idea whose time has come!" Victor Hugo.

Science is verifying the principles of Myofascial Release that I have been teaching for over 40 years. The art of Myofascial Release is to be able to discover the individual's fascial restrictions through feel, which are unique to each human being. This is why protocols do not work. One must engage the restriction with the appropriate amount of pressure and time for each individual. Too much pressure, as used in the older form of Myofascial Release, thrusts the patient into the protection mode. This leads to very limited and temporary results because it attempts to force a system that cannot be forced! Too light a pressure, engages only the muscular and elastic component of the fascial system and not the collagenous component, yielding only superficial and limited short term results.

Information is now emerging that the perineuronal net that was discovered over 130 years ago by scientist Camillo Golgi is now being rediscovered. It is now suggested that it is the fascia's extracellular matrix in our incredible brain that is not only responsible for the health of the neurons, but also may be the storage place of our memories; this explains the phenomena that occurs during Myofascial Structural Release, Myofascial Rebounding and Myofascial Unwinding when memories, sensations, and emotions begin to emerge from the past. These phenomena occur not only in the brain, but also throughout the entire body.

The vital importance to the health of fascia's extracellular matrix and its ground substance has been emphasized in an important new book by one of Germany's leading scientists, Dr. Alfred Pischinger, *The Extracellular Matrix and Ground Regulation; Basis for a Biological Medicine*. Dr. Pischinger's book represents over 30 years of research into the fascial system. Dr. Alfred Pischinger, professor of Histology and Embryology in Vienna, showed that the fascia's extracellular fluids which are called the matrix are the keys to health. His research showed that while cells are certainly important, they are not a separate entity because they cannot exist without being nurtured in the fascial matrix.

Another one of the important points in Dr. Pischinger's book is that there is no nerve or blood vessel that touches any one of the trillions of cells in our body. This completely obliterates the foundational theory called the Neuronal Doctrine which healthcare has been based upon.

I have found over the years just because something is logical doesn't mean it has any basis in reality. All the theories in the world do not have any value if they don't produce consistent, lasting results. The theories of traditional therapy are logical yet terribly flawed and incomplete and unfortunately only produce temporary results for most people.

The fascial system and its ground substance is the main transport medium of our body. Therefore, no matter what food you may ingest, it does not become nutrition until it enters the cell. Hydration does not occur when water goes down our throat, but only when it is capable of entering the cell. If the fascial ground substance has solidified, then all of the nutrition, oxygen, fluid, biochemistry, hormones, information, and energy that are needed by our cells cannot be absorbed. This ultimately means that the cells are in the process of dying.

We were all taught that communication originates in the brain and nerves, which made perfect, logical sense. However, when we start to use our intuition, something feels wrong. How can a nerve that is only capable of conducting one signal at a time at 20 meters per second, stimulate the trillions of cells in our body that must act together in a coordinated fashion instantaneously?

We were taught that our body communicates with words or thoughts, and this is not true. Our body communicates in frequencies of light. The frequencies of light go through the ground substance and the interior of the microtubules of the fascial system at an enormously fast speed. Just for a moment snap your fingers together. Why did I ask you to do this? In the time it took you to snap your fingers, light circled the earth over seven times. The light that flows through the fluidity of the fascial system's ground substance is the primary communication system of our bodies! The brain and nervous system are a slow and secondary communication system working in conjunction with the fascial system. The problem is when the ground substance has solidified from trauma, this blocks the conduction of light and information that the cells need to thrive.

Another fallacy that we were taught is that the brain of the cell was the nucleus. It has been discovered that it is actually the membrane of the cell (fascia) that is its brain. Through the membrane pass minuscule threads called integrins which connect to every one of our body's trillions of cells. This is the mechanism of mechanotransduction. This is how our sustained pressure can reach the entirety of the human mind/body complex.

Furthermore, inside of every cell there is a micro fascial system. If the fascial system, the environment of every cell of the body, has solidified then as cells attempt to excrete, the toxins and waste products cannot be transported into the lymphatic system poisoning the cells.

The pressure from the restricted fascial system interferes with the delicate inner mechanisms of our cells. Recent research shows that debris, waste products, and toxins become trapped in the cells and may be what contributes to the decline that occurs in the ageing process. It seems that excessive pressure and dehydration of the fascia's ground substance forces our molecules to tangle and stiffen with age. Crosslinks form, attaching the molecules together. Crosslinks stiffen our collagen and make our skin look wrinkled. Chemists call this advanced glycation end products. This is why so many people feel younger and also begin to look younger after receiving Myofascial Release.

Going deeper, I believe our mind/body is a hologram and that when we are traumatized; the vibrations of our hologram are altered. The vectors of force go through us and change the flow and frequency of our energy/consciousness that move throughout the body at an incredibly rapid rate. So that change in frequency tends to dehydrate that which is meant to be fluid, the ground substance of the fascia. Over time this ultimately turns into crushing pressure that produces the symptoms of pain, restriction of motion, and malfunction of our physiology.

A voluminous amount of research is now stating that disease begins in the ground substance of the fascia system as a thwarted inflammatory response. What I have said for decades is that it takes 90-120 seconds to even begin to engage the collagenous component, then another 3-5 minutes for a deeper release to produce results that are profound and lasting. My experience and current research has demonstrated that all other forms of therapy have been too quick. They either do not find the barrier or the barrier is not held long enough to produce meaningful change.

Somewhere around 3-5 minutes the phenomenon of piezoelectricity begins to occur. With this in mind, it is a well-known fact that our cells are crystalline in nature. When pressure is applied to a crystal it will create an electrical flow. In our bodies, it is a bioelectrical flow. Piezoelectricity is a Greek word for "pressure electricity", so applying sustained mechanical pressure into a restriction begins to elicit a bioelectrical flow. Then the phenomenon of mechanotransduction creates a biochemical/hormonal effect. At or beyond five minutes of sustained pressure, it has been found that the mind/body begins to produce Interleukin 8, the body's natural anti-inflammatory. Also, Interleukin 3 is produced that stimulates white blood cell formation that can improve the mind/body's natural response to disease as a part of the immune system and Interleukin 1b to enhance vasodilation that is important for tissue recovery, vibrant health and authentic healing.

Next, phase transition occurs. An example of this phenomenon occurs when ice turns into water. Of course, it is not ice in our bodies, but the solidification of the ground substance that has been ignored by everyone which creates crushing pressure on pain sensitive structures. In phase transition there is a chaotic period. Chaos is a bad word in traditional healthcare. As you know healthcare is all about order and control. However, no healing can occur in an orderly controlled environment. Systems Theory states that during this period of chaos there is the potential for change, growth and healing.

You and I were all brought up to believe that there are only three phases of water, namely ice, water and vapor. A new book called The Fourth Phase of Water: Beyond Solid, Liquid and Vapor, by Dr. Gerald H. Pollack, the world's leading expert in fluid dynamics indicates that there is a fourth phase of water that recognizes that fascia is a liquid crystal capable of change as it goes through its chaotic period.

Eventually, as pressure is sustained at the barrier, the person goes into the next phenomenon, resonance or what we call a release. When one human being touches another, the vibratory rates are quite different. As we move into the resonance phase, the vibratory rates match identically and this allows the trapped energy to flow, the tissue to rehydrate and glide to occur releasing the horrendous pressure off of pain sensitive structures.

Look into the research of Paul Standley, PhD who has shown clearly that it is important for the releases to be held 5 minutes or longer to allow for the release of healing messenger cells, cytokines, by way of release of Interleukins after a certain time-frame. I also recommend reading the latest edition of Carol Davis's work *Integrative Therapies in Rehabilitation: Evidence for Efficacy in Therapy, Prevention, and Wellness*. Carol M. Davis, DPT, EdD, MS, FAPTA, Professor Emerita, University of Miami School of Medicine is a wonderful Myofascial Release therapist and an incredible educator. For more information on the scientific rationale and references refer to my chapter in her book titled Myofascial Release, the Missing Link in Traditional Treatment.

A new book has just emerged, by Jean-Claude Guimberteau, MD who has developed endoscopic videos of fascia of living human beings under great magnification. His new book, *Architecture of Human Living Fascia* shows you in vivid detail, the true nature of fascia and its function. Dr. Guimberteau has honored me by asking me to write a section in his book on Myofascial Release.

In Dr. Guimberteau's important book and throughout his videos he states that in decades of research on the fascial system of living human beings, they can find no linearity whatsoever! Yet all of our training as therapists and physicians were based on linear principles. Instead the fascial, neural, vascular systems and every cell of our body is a non-linear system that has a fractal nature. The whole universe has a fractal nature. This is the beauty and importance of Myofascial Release which utilizes totally different principles to engage the fractal nature of the human being and this explains the effectiveness of Myofascial Release.

We spent a lot of time and energy on our education only to find that traditional therapy does not work that well because it is based upon fallacious theories and flawed methodology. There is an old saying that applies to all of us, "No matter how far you have traveled down the wrong road, turn around!"

It has been wonderful to watch the profusion of new books, videos and other inspirational information about Myofascial Release.

As with anything there have been challenges along the way.

I had been in Maui, Hawaii giving a seminar series and while I was away I had some men working on my house. When I returned to Arizona, I was walking barefoot inside and all of a sudden, I felt a horrible pain shoot through me like a lightning bolt. I had stepped on a scorpion! The pain was like an electrical fire. It went up my right leg and then beyond my leg into my etheric field and into my pelvis. It was a pain unlike I had ever felt before. Everything I knew to do for pain did not work. I couldn't sit, walk, or lie down. Breathing exercises didn't help. It lasted for over 30 hours.

I made it through, however, over time, I noticed that I was just not losing weight, but also losing muscle mass. I went for a hike one day noticing that my balance was off and I had mental fogginess. As I was climbing up a rocky ledge, my inner voice said to me, "You are being eaten alive". My linear side discounted this notion. The following day, I went on another hike and my intuition again told me with more urgency that, "You are being eaten alive, do something now!"

I had some blood work done; a sugar level of 100 is considered relatively normal and the scale stops at 500. My sugar was beyond 500 in the category of go to the hospital immediately. I believe my pancreas was damaged by the scorpion. It was a struggle to regain my strength. Life presents all of us with many challenges and the thing that we resist the most is change. We all have to recognize that we cannot change the past. The only constant in life is change, so it is important to embrace change.

Labor Day weekend 2015, I had flown to Cape Cod a few days ahead of time before presenting one of my Myofascial Release seminar series. The resort was very beautiful and tranquil and I was looking forward to some "down time". The afternoon of my arrival, my son Mark called saying that he was concerned about his twin brother Brian. He had been trying to call his brother for some time, but there was no response. Mark communicated that he felt so strange, like a part of him was ripped out energetically. We talked and continued to reach out to Brian. Finally, it was time to call the authorities. Waiting to hear back from the police, I had fallen into a deep sleep. About 2:00 in the morning, I was awakened by a loud banging on the door. The hotel had not set up the phones yet and I was being informed of an emergency. My son Mark called and was very emotional. He told me that Brian had died!

I don't remember anything for days afterwards. I went into shock. I am sure you all can imagine how painful it was for Mark to lose his twin brother at the peak of his life and for me to have lost my incredible son. Brian interacted with many people inspiring them with his loving kindness. The police report stated that they interviewed his neighbors and one of them saw Brian sitting on his deck peacefully petting his dog. He died of ventricular fibrillation where his heart went into chaos. The position of his body indicated that he had run into his bedroom, dove and landed on his bed.

After Brian's death, I went into a very painful, dark place. I struggled to pull myself out. I couldn't, but I had to. The seminar was quickly approaching. I have always had an inner strength and willpower. I realized that I had to go deeper into the pain and into the darkness to access my power. I asked the Myofascial Release therapists to help me and they did. I will never forget that experience. Thank you all again. Through sheer force of will, I pulled myself out of the depths and focused on the seminars. I dedicated the seminars to Brian, disciplined myself, stayed 'centered' and the seminars went well. I am very proud of Mark who showed strength and integrity after the tragedy of losing his twin brother. Brian, we will love you forever!

Over the years there has been a very special connection that has developed between you and I.

Many call it our tribe. This web of life comes from our heart, the Channel 3 experience, your intuitive, instinctive side which is a timeless, spaceless dimension. I may not remember your name, but I know you on a very deep level, energetically, your very essence. I have a photographic memory, not like many people that remember words and numbers, but mine is through pictures and feelings which is the language of the intuitive, instinctive side of our being. This is another benefit of Myofascial Release. When we receive treatment and when we treat someone else, we are at our best when we are in our intuitive, instinctive mode. We grow and we deepen as we help others.

One of the many dysfunctional messages thrust upon us by our society is that we are here to suffer. I do not believe this to be true. We are here to enjoy our life and help others to do the same. Brian would not have wanted me to continue to suffer. A very surprising and shocking experience recently happened. Brian came to me. I was in the back of my house after treating all day, and sat down in a soft padded chair, I was quieting myself, slowing my breathing and allowing my body to soften. I could feel my energy expanding far beyond me and I became aware that something was being cradled in my left arm. I could feel its weight and presence and as I looked down it was Brian as a baby. Brian was looking at me with such love and tenderness and I could see my right index finger touching his lower lip lovingly. I will never forget this moment. It was the most tender, loving moment of my life. Thank you Brian.

Most of you are committed to Myofascial Release and many of you notice that not only does Myofascial Release help you become the ultimate therapist in helping others, but the Myofascial Release principles also permeate into your personal life. When people first learn Myofascial Release some have trouble totally committing initially which is understandable. Be kind to yourself and stick with it. Clarity will come to you and your effectiveness will dramatically increase as your sensitivity increases. Some lose their way trying to perform Myofascial Release from a linear, logical, Channel 5 perspective which is as effective as ramming a square peg into a round hole. It does not work. This is what I call a fence sitter. One foot firmly planted in the tradition paradigm and other foot gingerly dipping into the newer paradigm. This is very weak and distracting. Commit to the Myofascial Release paradigm which will help you have the clarity and accuracy necessary for authentic healing.

You and I as humans are a powerful electromagnetic field of liquid light. Much of this goes back to the incredible insights of Albert Einstein and Nikola Tesla who both stated that everything is energy, different vibrations and frequency of energy. When we go through trauma, a vector of force is thrust into our body. This alters the polarity in the traumatized tissue and the energetic flow while altering the vibrational rate. This then changes what should be fluid, the ground substance of fascia, into a more viscous state and eventually a much more solid state capable of crushing pressure. When we apply sustained pressure at the barrier, for a sufficient amount of time, we are allowing the polarity and vibratory rate to return to its norm and in so doing, the system now rehydrates allowing the tissue to glide which ultimately removes the pressure that creates so many of our symptoms and malfunction of our physiology.

Logic can paralyze your mind if you are not coming from your instincts. A paradigm is a set of shared assumptions. In healthcare, we were taught a set of beliefs as if they were truths because it was logical. We bought the story, including myself, only to find out that the experts did not consider consciousness in the equation or the fascial system, a massive mistake!

It has been said that a paradigm cannot be changed by making some modifications of the existing paradigm. It has to be a totally new paradigm and vision. My vision started over 50 years ago in an instant when my injury ripped away everything I loved, motion and competition. This helped to open my heart to a deeper sense of intuition.

The paradigm of healthcare is based on a false premise. Most scientists don't look at the meta paradigm, that is, the belief that all other theories are based upon. There are two very important questions, does consciousness matter or not matter? The traditional scientific paradigm stated that consciousness does not matter, because there were too many variables.

Science also ignored the fascial system which is the conduit of consciousness and exists as frequencies of light.

Consider discarding the old flawed paradigm of healthcare and replacing it with a more accurate, beautiful picture of yourself and others. The fascial system is actually a powerful liquid crystal lattice. This multi-dimensional web is made up of microtubules of the fascial system. Within these microtubules, even at the tiniest of levels, is a hollow core which is shaped like a vortex. A vortex of liquid light flows at unimaginable speeds carrying nutrition, oxygen, fluids, bio-chemicals, hormones, energy and the information that our trillions of our cells need to thrive.

When the basic fundamental premise is wrong, all of the other theories based on this one premise are also wrong. Logic is a wonderful tool, but not more than that. Go with your gut, go with your instincts and intuition and then apply logic. Einstein said so long ago that all of his incredible ideas never came from his logical, linear mind, but instead came in a flash as pictures and feelings from his intuitive mind. He then applied his logical mind to communicate this knowledge to others.

Too many people spend their life fearfully worrying about what others think of them. This is why, as a Myofascial Release therapist, it is important to be treated regularly by a highly experienced Myofascial Release therapist and live your life in a centered way. It also helps to have an attitude coming from love and not fear. It is not about pleasing others. You don't have to explain yourself and you don't have to defend yourself. You need to be yourself! Myofascial Release helps you identify your true authentic self. Because of our dysfunctional programing, we identify with the intellectual rational side which is basically a survival mechanism. It is a wonderful tool, but it is a tool. We need to learn to move into our intuitive, instinctive and creative side utilizing the incredible wisdom that we all possess.

As you know so much of my knowledge of fascia and consciousness has been through my own personal experiences with pain, trauma and a failed back surgery. As I would treat myself and then others, a lot of the information that I teach came to me through my intuition, like a beautiful mosaic coming together into the Approach that has helped millions of people.

This is the dawn of an important new era and you are a part of it. We are the "point of the spear." Let's all commit to excellence and to live a very joyful, centered life, and teach others to do the same.

Life is precious. I have offered you a very special gift; please use it with love and wisdom.

Enjoy your journey!

ABOUT THE AUTHOR

John F. Barnes, PT, graduated from the University of Pennsylvania as a Physical Therapist in 1960 and he holds physical therapy licenses in Pennsylvania, Arizona, Delaware, Colorado, Hawaii and Minnesota.

He wrote *Myofascial Release: The Search for Excellence* in 1990. He has also been a columnist for the Physical Therapy Forum's *"Therapeutic Insight"* column; he has contributed to *Physical Therapy Today* writing articles for his "Mind & Body" column and has written numerous articles for the *Advance for Physical Therapists* publication, Massage & Bodywork Magazine and Massage Magazine.

John F. Barnes, PT was named one of the most influential persons in the therapeutic profession in the last century, in the national Massage Magazine's featured article "Stars of the Century."

John was so the featured speaker presenting his Myofascial Release Approach® at the American Back Society's symposiums for over twenty-five years whose theme was the most important advances in healthcare this century.

For information on treatment at the Myofascial Release Treatment Centers in Malvern, Pennsylvania or Sedona, Arizona or for information on the international Myofascial Release Seminars call 1-800-FASCIAL.

Myofascial Release Treatment Centers and Seminars
42 Lloyd Avenue
Malvern, PA 19355
Phone 610-644-0136
Fax 610-644-1662
E-Mail: malvern@myofascialrelease.com
Web site address: www.myofascialrelease.com

Therapy on the Rocks
676 North State Route 89 A
Sedona, AZ 86336
Phone 928-282-3002
Fax 928-282-7274
E-Mail: sedona@myofascialrelease.com
Web site addresses: www.myofascialrelease.com
www.therapyontherocks.net